Quantitative Trait Loci

METHODS IN MOLECULAR BIOLOGY™

John M. Walker, SERIES EDITOR

METHODS IN MOLECULAR BIOLOGY™

Quantitative Trait Loci

Methods and Protocols

Edited by

Nicola J. Camp

Genetic Epidemiology, Department of Medical Informatics
University of Utah School of Medicine, Salt Lake City, UT

and

Angela Cox

Institute for Cancer Studies
University of Sheffield Medical School, Sheffield, UK

Humana Press ✳ Totowa, New Jersey

© 2002 Humana Press Inc.
999 Riverview Drive, Suite 208
Totowa, New Jersey 07512

www.humanapress.com

The content and opinions expressed in this book are the sole work of the authors and editors, who have
warranted due diligence in the creation and issuance of their work. The publisher, editors, and authors are not
responsible for errors or omissions or for any consequences arising from the information or opinions presented
in this book and make no warranty, express or implied, with respect to its contents.

This publication is printed on acid-free paper. ∞
ANSI Z39.48-1984 (American Standards Institute)

Permanence of Paper for Printed Library Materials.

Cover design by Patricia F. Cleary.

For additional copies, pricing for bulk purchases, and/or information about other Humana titles, contact Humana
at the above address or at any of the following numbers: Tel.: 973-256-1699; Fax: 973-256-8341; E-mail:
humana@humanapr.com; or visit our Website: www.humanapress.com

Photocopy Authorization Policy:

Printed in the United States of America. 10 9 8 7 6 5 4 3 2 1

Library of Congress Cataloging in Publication Data
Quantitative trait loci: methods and protocols / edited by Nicola J. Camp and Angela Cox.
        p. cm. —(Methods in molecular biology; v. 195)
    Includes bibliographical references and index.
    ISBN 0-89603-927-7 (alk. paper)
    1. Genetics–Statistical methods. 2. Gene mapping. 3. Phenotype. I. Camp, Nicola J.
    II. Cox, Angela, 1961– III. Methods in molecuar biology (Totowa, NJ); v. 195
    QH438.4.S73 Q36 2002
    576.5'07'27–dc21   2001039828

Dedication

For Greggory, Cason, Tim, Alice, and James

Preface

The genetic analysis of quantitative traits in humans began in earnest in the early part of the 20th century, after the rediscovery of Mendel's work, and it was R. A. Fisher's seminal 1918 paper that clarified the main concepts of biometrical genetics. At the start of the 21st century, statistical methods for quantitative trait locus (QTL) analysis are being refined and added to at an astonishing rate. Methods based on the analysis of quantitative traits tend to be more powerful than the equivalent binary trait methods, and, in conjunction with whole-genome screening technologies, are yielding exciting results in agriculture, experimental organisms, and the study of human disease.

Quantitative Trait Loci: Methods and Protocols aims to review the current methodologies available in three main areas: human traits (investigation of QTLs underlying human disease), experimental organisms (as models for human disease), and agriculture (crop and livestock improvement). The aim of each chapter is to provide a practical guide to the topic under discussion, including an overview of the technique in a style that is accessible to the non-mathematician. Thus, investigators will be able to use the book from the study design stage of a project onwards. Each chapter includes a detailed description of how to proceed with a specific analysis, including the use of and where to find appropriate computer software, a guide to the interpretation of the results, and worked examples. The chapters also include citations for the original papers and variations on methods where appropriate. In addition to being a reference for investigators and a text for students starting in the field, this book will prove useful for anyone interested in gaining an overview of the current state-of-the-art in QTL analysis.

Nicola J. Camp
Angela Cox

Contents

Contributors

JENNIFER H. BARRETT • *Genetic Epidemiology Division, Imperial Cancer Research Fund, University of Leeds, UK*

NICOLA J. CAMP • *Genetic Epidemiology, Department of Medical Informatics, University of Utah School of Medicine, Salt Lake City, UT*

WILLIAM COOKSON • *Asthma Genetics, The Wellcome Trust Centre for Human Genetics, University of Oxford, UK*

HEATHER J. CORDELL • *Department of Medical Genetics, University of Cambridge, UK*

ANGELA COX • *Institute for Cancer Studies, University of Sheffield Medical School, Sheffield, UK*

ARIEL DARVASI • *The Life Sciences Institute, The Hebrew University of Jerusalem, Jerusalem, Israel, and IDgene Pharmaceuticals Ltd., Jerusalem, Israel*

ROBERT C. ELSTON • *Department of Epidemiology and Biostatistics, Case Western Reserve University, Cleveland, OH*

CHAD P. GARNER • *Department of Integrative Biology, University of California, Berkeley, CA*

DOMINIQUE GAUGUIER • *The Wellcome Trust Centre for Human Genetics, Oxford, UK*

MARK M. ILES • *Division of Genomic Medicine, University of Sheffield, UK*

ANGELA J. MARLOW • *The Wellcome Trust Centre for Human Genetics, University of Oxford, Oxford, UK*

LYLE J. PALMER • *Channing Laboratory, Brigham and Women's Hospital and Harvard Medical School, Boston, MA, and Department of Epidemiology and Biostatistics, Case Western Reserve University, Cleveland, OH*

DANIEL POMP • *Department of Animal Science, University of Nebraska–Lincoln, Lincoln, NE*

JOAO L. ROCHA • *Department of Animal Science, University of Nebraska–Lincoln, Lincoln, NE*

NILESH SAMANI • *Division of Cardiology, University of Leicester, UK*

AUDREY H. SCHNELL • *Department of Epidemiology and Biostatistics, Case Western Reserve University, Cleveland, OH*

ANNE SHALOM • *The Life Sciences Institute, The Hebrew University of Jerusalem, Jerusalem, Israel*

L. DALE VAN VLECK • *USDA, ARS, USMARC, Lincoln, NE*

ELLEN M. WIJSMAN • *Department of Biostatistics, and Division of Medical Genetics, Department of Medicine, University of Washington, Seattle, WA*

JOHN S. WITTE • *Department of Epidemiology and Biostatistics, Case Western Reserve University, Cleveland, OH*

SHIZHONG XU • *Department of Botany and Plant Sciences, University of California, Riverside, CA*

YOUMING ZHANG • *Asthma Genetics, The Wellcome Trust Centre for Human Genetics, University of Oxford, UK*

I

MAPPING QUANTITATIVE TRAIT LOCI IN HUMANS

1

Association Studies

Jennifer H. Barrett

1. Introduction

A classical case-control study design is frequently used in genetic epidemiology to investigate the association between genotype and the presence or absence of disease. Association studies can also be useful in the investigation of quantitative traits. The aim of such studies is to test for association at the population level between the quantitative trait and genotype at a particular locus. Whether investigating qualitative or quantitative traits, such studies depend on the prior identification of a candidate gene or genes. The genotyped locus could either be a polymorphism within a potentially trait-affecting gene or a marker in linkage disequilibrium with such a gene. Currently, screening of the whole genome is only feasible using linkage analysis, which is discussed elsewhere, because linkage extends over much greater distances than does linkage disequilibrium.

Quantitative trait association studies are based on a sample of unrelated subjects from the population. Various sampling designs are possible, including random sampling and sampling on the basis of an extreme phenotype. The advantages and disadvantages of these alternative designs are discussed.

The basic method of analysis is called analysis of variance (*see* **Subheading 2.1.**) a standard statistical technique for testing for differences in mean between two or more groups, on the basis of the comparison of between- and within-group variances. An alternative if subjects are sampled on the basis of extreme phenotype is to compare *genotypes* between groups with high and low trait values (*see* **Subheading 2.2.**).

From: *Methods in Molecular Biology: vol. 195: Quantitative Trait Loci: Methods and Protocols.*
Edited by: N. J. Camp and A. Cox © Humana Press, Inc., Totowa, NJ

2. Methods

2.1. Analysis of Variance and Linear Regression

The standard approach to the analysis of quantitative trait association studies assumes the following model. The phenotype y_{ij} of individual i with genotype j at the locus of interest is given by

$$y_{ij} = \mu_j + e_i \tag{1}$$

where μ_j is the mean for the jth genotype and e_i represents residual environmental and possibly polygenic effects for individual i, assumed to be Normally distributed with mean 0 and variance σ_e^2. The data required consist of measured phenotypes and genotypes on a sample of unrelated individuals. The parameters μ_j are estimated in the obvious way by the mean values of individuals with genotype j. The F-statistic from analysis of variance (ANOVA), the ratio of between- and within-genotype variances, is used to test for the association between genotype and phenotype, because under the null hypothesis that all genotypes have the same mean and variance, this ratio should be 1. This approach has been called the measured-genotype test (*1*), in contrast to earlier biometrical methods that use information on the distribution of the phenotype only (i.e., with unmeasured genotype) discussed briefly in **Note 1.**

Equivalently, a linear regression analysis of phenotype on genotype can be carried out, possibly including as covariates other factors that may be related to phenotype. Where the genotype is determined by one biallelic polymorphism (with possible genotypes AA, AB, and BB), a test for trend is provided by regressing the phenotype on the number of copies of the A allele.

There are many examples of this type of approach in the literature. For example, O'Donnell et al. (*2*) used multiple linear regression to investigate the relationship between diastolic blood pressure and different genotypes of the angiotensin-converting enzyme (ACE) gene. Hegele et al. (*3*) use analysis of variance to demonstrate association between serum concentrations of creatinine and urea and the gene encoding angiotensinogen (AGT).

2.2 Analysis of Extreme Groups

An alternative approach is to use a sampling scheme that selects individuals on the basis of extreme phenotypes (*4,5*). There is considerable literature on the use of such sampling schemes for sibling pair linkage studies (e.g., **ref. 6**). Extreme sampling is advocated to increase power and efficiency, as extremes are more informative. The approach is particularly useful when the phenotype is relatively easy to measure, so that large numbers of individuals can easily be screened to select extremes for genotyping.

In association studies adopting this method, individuals are randomly selected conditional on their phenotype being below a specified lower threshold or exceeding a specified upper threshold. Alternatively, the upper and lower *n* percentiles of a random sample from the population may be included. A cross-tabulation is then formed by classifying subjects by genotype and by high/low phenotype. The genotype frequencies are then compared between subjects with high and low trait values using a chi-squared test. For example, Hegele et al. (*3*) compared allele and genotype frequencies at the AGT locus in subjects with the lowest and highest quartiles of serum creatinine and urea levels.

3. Interpretation

In common with association studies for qualitative traits, a significant association does not demonstrate an effect of the polymorphism considered, because it may also arise through linkage disequilibrium with another locus. A further similarity is that population admixture can lead to spurious associations. For this reason, family-based approaches, such as the transmission-disequilibrium test for quantitative traits (*7*), have been developed (*see* Chapter 5).

3.1. Heterogeneity

Published results of associations with quantitative as with qualitative traits are not always in agreement. Because for most complex traits the effect of any one locus is likely to be small, individual studies are often not sufficiently powerful to detect association. To address this issue, Juo et al. (*8*) carried out a meta-analysis of studies investigating association between apolipoprotein A-I levels and variants of the apolipoprotein gene, which had produced conflicting results. This is a potentially useful approach, but may be flawed by publication bias, which is likely to be more of an issue in epidemiological studies than in clinical trials. There is also an assumption that patients are genetically and clinically homogeneous, with similar environmental exposures.

3.2. Using Extremes

An important consideration when using extreme sampling strategies (as in outlined in **Subheading 2.2.**) is that extremes may be untypical of the quantitative trait as a whole in that they may be under the influence of other genes. A clear example of this, cited in **ref. *4***, is that studying individuals with achondroplastic dwarfism would be inappropriate if the primary interest were in identifying genes controlling height.

3.3. Power of Association Studies

An attractive feature of association studies is that they may require smaller sample sizes than methods based on linkage (*9*).

Schork et al. (*5*) investigated the power of the extreme sampling method analytically (**Subheading 2.2.**) to detect association between the trait and a single biallelic marker in linkage disequilibrium with a trait-affecting locus. Power depends on many factors, including locus-specific heritability, degree of linkage disequilibrium, allele frequencies, mode of inheritance, and choice of threshold. In some settings, overall sample sizes of less than 500 provided adequate power to detect association with a locus accounting for 10% of the trait variance.

The power of several methods of analysis, variants of those described here, has been compared in a simulation study (*10*). Under the models considered, ANOVA/linear regression (*see* **Subheading 2.1.**) generally performed better than a variant of the extremes method (*see* **Subheading 2.2.**), based on the same number of genotyped individuals, as most of the information on phenotype is lost by categorizing into "high" and "low" values. As with any method based on selective sampling, another drawback is that it is also necessary to phenotype a larger number of subjects to achieve the same sample size for analysis. The same authors suggested a variation on ANOVA/linear regression, the truncated measured genotype (TMG) test, where only extremes are included in the analysis (*see* **Note 4**). This TMG test was found to be more powerful than ANOVA/linear regression for the same sample size of genotyped individuals, although, again, a larger number of subjects must be phenotyped to achieve this. These results are, however, dependent on the underlying genetic model. Allison et al. (*4*) showed that extreme sampling can actually lead to a decrease in power in the presence of another gene influencing the trait.

Page and Amos (*10*) also found that variants of ANOVA/linear regression and of the TMG test, which are based on alleles, were more powerful than the genotype-based methods discussed earlier. In these approaches, the phenotype of each individual contributes to two groups, one for each allele or, in the case of homozygotes, contributes twice to one group. Allele-based methods, which "double the sample size," are generally only valid under the assumption of Hardy–Weinberg equilibrium (*11*). Furthermore, the greater power of this approach is to be expected for the models used in these simulations, all of which assumed an additive effect of the trait allele, and may not apply more generally.

Long and Langley (*12*) investigated the power to detect association using a number of single nucleotide polymorphisms in the region of a quantitative trait locus, but excluding the functional locus itself. Their test statistic was based on ANOVA (*see* ***Subheading 2.1***); the significance of the largest F-statistic obtained from any marker was estimated from its empirical distribution based on 1000 random permutations of the phenotype/marker data. From their simulations, they concluded that, using about 500 individuals, there was generally sufficient power to detect association if 5–10% of the phenotypic variation was attributable to the locus. Furthermore, tests using single markers had greater

Table 1
Summary Data on ACE Levels According to Genotype

ace_geno	Mean	Std. dev.	Freq.
II	74.496732	31.729764	153
ID	90.233871	39.484505	124
DD	103.73913	46.564928	23
Total	83.243333	37.475487	300

power than haplotype-based tests. The latter were based on comparing mean trait values across all distinct haplotypes, and the authors concede that other haplotype-based tests making use of additional information may perform better.

4. Software

The basic methods described in this chapter can be carried out in standard statistical software packages such as Stata (*13*), which is used here, SAS, or SPSS. The data would generally be expected to consist of one record for each subject, recording their measured trait value, their genotype, and any covariates of interest.

5. Worked Example

5.1. Analysis of Variance

An insertion/deletion (I/D) polymorphism of the ACE gene is associated with plasma ACE levels in some populations. Plasma ACE levels were measured and I/D genotype obtained for 300 Pima Indians to investigate the relationship in this population (*14*). The data consist of 300 records, including ACE levels (ranging from 7 to 238 units) and genotype (II, ID, or DD).

In Stata, ANOVA can be carried out by the command

oneway ace_leve ace_geno, tabulate

where *ace_leve* and *ace_geno* are the variables for ACE levels and genotype, respectively. This produces **Tables 1** and **2. Table 1** is produced by specifying the *tabulate* option after the *oneway* command (for one-way analysis of variance) and provides useful summary information. In addition to the mean ACE levels within each genotype group (i.e., estimates of μ_1, μ_2, and μ_3), the standard deviation and the number of subjects with each genotype are displayed. It can be seen that individuals with the DD genotype have much higher levels on average than those with the II genotype, with intermediate levels found in heterozygotes.

Table 2 is the basic ANOVA table. The total variability of the data is measured by the total sum of squares (419,919) (i.e. the sum of squares of the

Table 2
Analysis of Variance Results for the Data in Table 1

Source	SS	df	MS	F	Prob > F
Between groups	27426.3358	2	13713.1679	10.38	0.0000
Within groups	392492.901	297	1321.52492		
Total	419919.237	299	1404.41216		

differences between each of the observations and the overall mean). This figure can be separated into the between-genotype sum of squares (the sum of squares of the difference between the group mean and the overall mean) and the within-genotype sum of squares (the sum of squares of the differences between each observation and the mean for the corresponding genotype). These are used to estimate the corresponding variance, shown in the mean square (MS) column, by dividing by the number of degrees of freedom. [The number of degrees of freedom is one less than the number of groups or observations within groups (i.e., 3−1 for between genotypes and 152+123+22 within genotypes).] The F-statistic (10.38) is the ratio of these estimated variances. Under the null hypothesis of no difference between groups, its expected value is 1 and it should follow an F-distribution with (2, 297) degrees of freedom. In this case, there is overwhelming evidence for a difference in level according to genotype. The differences in the initial table are not the result of random variation.

The analysis of variance table (**Table 2**) can also be obtained by using the Stata command

anova ace_leve ace_geno

This gives the additional information

R-squared = 0.0653

indicating that the I/D genotype explains 6.5% of the variance in plasma ACE levels in this population.

Slightly different output, but exactly the same F-test and estimate of R-squared can alternatively be obtained by carrying out a regression analysis:

xi: regress ace_leve i.ace_geno

The i in front of the ACE genotype variable shows that this is to be treated as a categorical variable in the analysis. If, instead, interest was in testing for a trend in ACE levels with the number of D alleles, then genotype could be

Table 3
Genotype Frequencies in Two Extreme Groups Defined by the Top and Bottom Quintiles of ACE Levels[a]

Five quantiles of ace_leve	ace_geno			
	II	ID	DD	Total
1	39	20	3	62
	62.90	32.26	4.84	100.00
5	17	33	10	122
	28.33	55.00	16.67	100.00
Total	56	53	13	122
	45.90	43.44	10.66	100.00

[a]Pearson chi2(2) = 15.5722, Pr = 0.000.

coded as 0, 1, or 2 to indicate the number of D alleles, and the following regression carried out:

$$regress\ ace\_leve\ ace\_geno$$

This produces an F-statistic of 20.77 on (1, 298) degrees of freedom.

5.2. Analysis of Extremes

Using the same dataset, a new variable is created, recording the appropriate quantile for each subject's ACE level. In this example, quintiles are used, creating 5 groups of approximately 60 subjects. This is easily done in Stata as follows:

$$xtile\ acegp5=ace\_leve,\ nq(5)$$

A chi-squared test is then carried out comparing the top and bottom quintiles:

$$tab\ acegp5\ ace\_geno\ if\ acegp5==1\ |\ acegp5==5,\ chi\ row$$

producing **Table 3**.

The chi-squared statistic of 15.57 on 2 degrees of freedom again indicates very strong evidence of association between ACE levels and genotype, even though only 40% of the original subjects are used in the analysis. Nearly 63% of those with low ACE levels had II genotype compared with only 28% of those with high levels, and the DD genotype was over three times as common in those with high levels compared with those with low levels.

6. Notes

1. Commingling analysis. The model underlying ANOVA (*see* **Subheading 2.1.**) assumes that the data consist of a mixture of Normal distributions, one corresponding

to each genotype, each with the same variance. Even in the absence of genotype data, statistical methods can be used to test for evidence of a mixture of more than one Normal distribution. This "unmeasured genotype" approach is sometimes known as commingling analysis. Evidence for a mixture of two or three distributions is supportive of the hypothesis that a major gene underlies the trait, although, of course, environmental factors could also give rise to distinct distributions. Model fitting allows estimates to be made of parameters of interest such as μ_j and σ_e^2 and the proportion of subjects in each class.

In the presence of genotype data in a candidate gene, the method of commingling analysis can be extended to condition on the measured polymorphism(s). In addition to testing for evidence of a mixture of distributions, this method also provides evidence of whether the measured genotype itself gives rise to the mixture or whether another polymorphism in the gene is a more likely explanation (*15,16*).

2. Distributional assumptions. In view of the underlying model for ANOVA, a Normalizing transformation may be applied to the data. It is important to note that the model assumes a Normal distribution within each genotype rather than overall. (In commingling analysis, Normalizing the data leads to a conservative test for mixture, as this may remove skewness in the overall distribution of the data arising from the mixing of distributions.) The further assumption of a common within-genotype variance can be tested, and homogeneity of variance may sometimes be achieved by transformation. In the worked example in this chapter, there is some evidence for heterogeneity in the variances. One advantage of the extremes method outlined in **Subheading 2.2.** is that it does not rely on these distributional assumptions.

3. Nonparametric alternatives. Another nonparametric alternative to ANOVA is the Kruskal–Wallis test. In this approach, the complete set of N trait values is ranked from 1 to N, and the average rank in each genotype group is calculated. The test statistic is based on comparing the genotype-specific average ranks with the overall average rank of $(N+1)/2$. Under the null hypothesis of no genotype–phenotype association, the test statistic follows a chi-squared distribution with two degrees of freedom (assuming three genotypes), and a significantly higher value indicates that the distributions differ. Applying this method to the example in **Subheading 5.**, the test statistic takes the value 18.2 (p=0.0001). This method is only slightly less powerful than ANOVA when the data are Normally distributed and has the advantage that distributional assumptions are not made. However, the test alone is not very informative, and, in general, the estimates provided by ANOVA are also useful.

4. Analysis of extremes. An alternative suggestion for the analysis of extreme samples, the TMG method mentioned earlier, is to use analysis of variance, ignoring the sampling scheme. The analysis of variance assumption of random sampling from a Normal distribution is violated, but it has been argued that, for large enough sample sizes, the significance level of the test is still correct (*10*). The analogs of this test and of those outlined in **Subheadings 2.1. and 2.2.** based on alleles rather than genotypes, where each individual's phenotype contributes twice to the analysis, violate the further assumption of independence of observations.

Slatkin (*17*) suggested selecting individuals on the basis of unusually high (or low) trait values and testing (1) for a difference in genotype frequency between the selected sample and a random sample and (2) for differences in phenotype distribution according to genotype *within* the selected sample. These two tests are approximately independent and so can be combined into one overall test. This approach is particularly powerful when a rare allele has a substantial effect on phenotype, even though the overall proportion of phenotypic variance attributable to the locus is small.

5. Family-based samples. Although association studies as described in this chapter are applicable to unrelated sets of cases and controls, extensions have been suggested to allow for relatedness between subjects. Tregouet et al. *(18)* suggested using estimating equations, a statistical method for estimating regression parameters based on correlated data. They found that, for nuclear families of equal size, the power of this approach was comparable to maximum likelihood and was similar to the power expected in a sample of the same number of unrelated individuals. However, the type 1 error rate could be substantially inflated in the presence of strong clustering if the number of families is relatively small (<50).

References

1. Boerwinkle, E., Chakraborty, R., and Sing, C. F. (1986) The use of measured genotype information in the analysis of quantitative phenotypes in man. *Ann. Hum. Genet.* **50,** 181–194.

2. O'Donnell, C. J., Lindpainter, K., Larson, M. G., Rao, V. S., Ordovas, J. M., Schaefer, E. J., et al. (1998) Evidence for association and genetic linkage of the angiotensin-converting enzyme locus with hypertension and blood pressure in men but not women in the Framingham Heart Study. *Circulation* **97,** 1766–1772.

3. Hegele, R. A., Harris, S. B., Hanley, A. J. G., and Zinman, B. (1999) Association between AGT codon 235 polymorphism and variation in serum concentrations of creatinine and urea in Canadian Oji-Cree. *Clin. Genet.* **55,** 438–443.

4. Allison, D. B., Heo, M., Schork, N. J., and Elston, R. C. (1998) Extreme selection strategies in gene mapping studies of oligogenic quantitative traits do not always increase power. *Hum. Heredity* **48,** 97–107.

5. Schork, N. J., Nath, S. K., Fallin, D., and Chakravarti, A. (2000) Linkage disequilibrium analysis of biallelic DNA markers, human quantitative trait loci, and threshold-defined case and control subjects *Am. J. Hum. Genet.* **67,** 1208–1218.

6. Risch, N. and Zhang, H. (1995) Extreme discordant sib pairs for mapping quantitative trait loci in humans. *Science* **268,** 1584–1589.

7. Allison, D. B. (1997) Transmission-disequilibrium tests for quantitative traits. *Am. J. Hum. Genet.* **60,** 676–690.

8. Juo, S.-H.H., Wyszynski, D. F., Beaty, T. H., Huang, H.-Y., and Bailey-Wilson, J. E. (1999) Mild association between the A/G polymorphism in the promoter of the apolipoprotein A-I gene and apolipoprotein A-I levels: a meta-analysis. *Am. J. Med. Genet.* **82,** 235–241.

9. Risch, N. J. (2000) Searching for genetic determinants in the new millennium. *Nature* **405,** 847–856.

10. Page, G. P. and Amos, C. I. (1999) Comparison of linkage-disequilibrium methods for localization of genes influencing quantitative traits in humans. *Am. J. Hum. Genet.* **64,** 1194–1205.

11. Saseini, P. (1997) From genotype to genes: doubling the sample size. *Biometrics* **53,** 1253–1261.

12. Long, A. D. and Langley, C. H. (1999) The power of association studies to detect the contribution of candidate gene loci to variation in complex traits. *Genome Res.* **9,** 720–731.

13. StataCorp. 1999. *Stata Statistical Software: Release 6.0.* Stata Corporation, College Station, TX.

14. Foy, C. A., McCormack, L. J., Knowler, W. C., Barrett, J. H., Catto, A., and Grant, P. J. (1996) The angiotensin-I converting enzyme (ACE) gene I/D polymorphism and ACE levels in Pima Indians. *J. Med. Genet.* **33,** 336–337.

15. Cambien, F., Costerousse, O., Tiret, L., Poirier, O., Lecerf, L., Gonzales, M. F., et al (1994) Plasma level and gene polymorphism of angiotensin-converting enzyme in relation to myocardial infarction. *Circulation* **90,** 669–676.

16. Barrett, J. H., Foy, C. A., and Grant, P. J. (1996) Commingling analysis of the distribution of a phenotype conditioned on two marker genotypes: application to plasma angiotensin-converting enzyme levels. *Genet. Epidemiol.* **13,** 615–625.

17. Slatkin, M. (1999) Disequilibrium mapping of a quantitative-trait locus in an expanding population. *Am. J. Hum. Genet.* **64,** 1765–1773.

18. Tregouet, D.-A., Ducimetiere, P., and Tiret, L. (1997) Testing association between candidate-gene markers and phenotype in related individuals, by use of estimating equations. *Am. J. Hum. Genet.* **61,** 189–199.

2

Parametric Linkage Analysis

Lyle J. Palmer, Audrey H. Schnell, John S. Witte, and Robert C. Elston

1. Introduction

"Linkage" describes the situation in which two syntenic loci are inherited together. More specifically, two loci are said to be linked if they are close enough to each other on a chromosome that recombination during meiosis is uncommon enough for their cosegregation to be detectable within families. Thus, linkage is a property of *loci*. All linkage techniques are essentially designed to test for a statistical association between a marker (genetic or biochemical) and a phenotypic trait. Classical model-based (parametric) linkage analysis was developed to investigate the cosegregation of a genetic marker and a binary trait (generally, disease affection status) within pedigrees. Model-based linkage analysis of quantitative traits is also possible and forms the basis of this chapter. Methods based on the exact likelihood calculation are described in this chapter; Markov chain Monte Carlo methods are described in Chapter 6.

Classically, model-based linkage is tested by the calculation of the maximum likelihood log-odds (LOD) score for each marker over a range of recombination fractions (θ). Linkage of a marker to a trait phenotype relies on the detection within families of low levels of recombination between the marker and trait loci. This analysis assumes that a locus having both a major effect on phenotype and a defined Mendelian pattern of inheritance is segregating within families. The detailed model specification required makes model-based LOD score linkage a stringent but nonrobust method for gene discovery. Although linkage analysis can be repeated using many possible models, this constitutes multiple testing; statistical power to detect linkage is reduced once appropriate corrections are made (*1*).

From: *Methods in Molecular Biology: vol. 195: Quantitative Trait Loci: Methods and Protocols.*
Edited by: N. J. Camp and A. Cox © Humana Press, Inc., Totowa, NJ

Model-based linkage analysis may be used for the following: (1) to assess the genetic distance between marker and disease-associated loci by estimating the number of recombination events between them; (2) to order genes in a genetic map if the recombination fractions (θ) are known; and (3) to identify genetic forms of common diseases. The statistical level of significance generally used for evidence of linkage is about 10^{-4}, which corresponds to a LOD score of 3.0, translating to a false-positive rate (i.e., the probability of making an error when inferring the presence of linkage) of around 5% (*2*). Parametric linkage analysis can be performed on nuclear or extended families. Multipoint linkage analysis using more than one marker locus can be performed, which increases statistical power to detect linkage. Similarly, linkage of more than one trait locus is possible (*3*). However, the interpretation of LOD scores is then difficult and somewhat controversial (*4*). It is unclear what level of significance is meaningful for a linkage to a trait determined by multiple genes; there is no clear prior hypothesis to which one may attribute a Bayesian prior probability and genetic studies of complex traits often involve large-scale multiple testing. Lander and Kruglyak (*5*) have suggested that standard linkage analysis of complex traits should use a LOD of 3.3 ($p \approx 0.00005$) as the threshold for statistical significance, in order to give a genomewide false-positive rate of 5%. This assumes linkage analysis with one free parameter (θ), a dense genetic map of markers applied to a large number of informative meioses, and a genome size of 3300 cM.

1.1. Genetic Models

Simple genetic models are derived from Mendelian laws of inheritance. For an individual, the pair of alleles (maternal and paternal) at a locus (the genotype) is homozygous if the two alleles are the same allelic variant and heterozygous if they are different allelic variants. If more than one locus is involved, the patterns of alleles for a single chromosome is called a haplotype; together, the two haplotypes for an individual is called a (multilocus) genotype. Each offspring receives at each locus only one of the two alleles from a given parent; alleles are transmitted randomly (i.e., each with probability 0.5), and offspring genotypes are independent conditional on the parental genotypes. The probability that a parent transmits a particular allele or haplotype to an offspring is called the transmission probability and is the first component of a genetic model.

The second component of a genetic model concerns the relationship between the (unobserved) genotypes and the observed characteristics, or phenotype, of an individual. A phenotype may be discrete or, the focus of this volume, continuous. Penetrance is defined as the probability (in the case of a continuous phenotype, a probability density) of a phenotype given a genotype; a complete genetic model requires specification of the penetrances of all possible genotypes.

The third component of a genetic model is the (distribution of) relative frequencies of the alleles in the population. These allele frequencies are used primarily to determine prior probabilities of genotypes when inferring genotype from phenotype.

These three components, taken together, fully describe the genetic model of a trait. Given a set of phenotypic data on pedigrees, one can estimate the genetic model using statistical techniques collectively known as segregation analysis (*6–8*). Whereas segregation analysis is beyond the scope of this chapter, it is helpful to realize that in a segregation analysis, genotypes are latent variables inferred from trait phenotypes. For simple Mendelian traits, in which only one genetic locus is segregating, estimation of the genetic model is usually straightforward, as only one set of latent variables (genotypes) is involved. For complex quantitative traits, which are the emphasis of many genetic studies today and which are probably the result of the effects of more than one locus, estimation of the genetic model is more difficult, because each locus represents a different set of (possibly interacting) latent variables.

1.2. Single Versus Multipoint Analysis

Assuming that a quantitative trait demonstrates an inheritance pattern consistent with a major gene segregating within families and, further, that the putative major locus can be accurately characterized in terms of its model parameters, then model-based methods of either pairwise linkage analysis (*9*), often referred to as two-point analysis, or multipoint linkage analysis (*10,11*) can be used. In general, multipoint linkage analysis will increase the information available for a linkage analysis and, hence, offers more statistical power to detect linkage.

1.3. Model Specification

In a model-based linkage analysis, it is necessary to completely specify the mode of inheritance of the trait being studied: the number of loci involved, the number of alleles at each locus and their frequencies; and the penetrances of each genotype (which may further depend on age or other covariates). Typically, for computational reasons, we assume that the trait is caused by the segregation of just two alleles at a single locus and that there is no other cause of familial aggregation of the trait. Thus, one allele frequency and three penetrances need to be specified. The marker allele frequencies are also specified, but these have no effect on the evidence for linkage if the marker genotypes of all the pedigree founders (those pedigree members from whom all other pedigree members are descended) are known or can be inferred with certainty. Typically, we assume that the trait and marker genotypes are independently distributed in the pedigree founders.

With this model specification, we can calculate the likelihood for a set of pedigrees, in which we assume that the only unknown parameter is the recombination fraction θ on which the transmission probability depends (we shall assume that θ is scalar [although more generally, it may be a vector if, for example, multiple marker loci are involved] or θ is made sex dependent). Letting L denote likelihood, we base inferences about θ on the likelihood ratio

$$\Lambda = \frac{L(\theta)}{L(\frac{1}{2})} \tag{1}$$

or, equivalently, its logarithm. In human genetics, it is usual to take logarithms to base 10 and we define the LOD score at θ to be

$$Z(\theta) = log_{10}\left(\frac{L(\theta)}{L(\frac{1}{2})}\right) \tag{2}$$

with a maximum $Z(\hat{\theta})$ at the maximum likelihood estimate $\hat{\theta}$. Thus, the LOD as used in genetics is the logarithm of the likelihood for the data if there is linkage divided by the likelihood if there is no linkage. Note that if $L(\frac{1}{2}) > L(\theta)$ for some value of θ, then the corresponding LOD score is negative. Invariably, it is the maximum LOD (sometimes referred to as the maxLOD) that is calculated in linkage analyses, usually with $\hat{\theta}$ bounded at one-half.

When three-generational data are available, more power can be obtained by estimating sex-specific recombination fractions θ_f and θ_m if they are different, using the maximum log likelihood

$$Z(\hat{\theta}_f, \hat{\theta}_m) = log_{10}\left(\frac{L(\hat{\theta}_f, \hat{\theta}_m)}{L(\tilde{\theta}_f, \tilde{\theta}_m)}\right) \tag{3}$$

where $\tilde{\theta}_f$ and $\tilde{\theta}_m$ are maximum likelihood estimates constrained so that $\tilde{\theta}_f + \tilde{\theta}_m = 1$ (*12*).

2. Methods

We will discuss methods of exact likelihood calculations of the LOD score statistics for linkage analysis. Sampling methods will be discussed in Chapter 6.

There are two approaches for model-based linkage analysis of a quantitative trait based on direct maximization of the likelihood that are widely available, have been previously published, and have software available: LODLINK and LINKAGE. In each case, a single gene with two alleles is assumed to contribute to the distribution of the trait.

2.1. The LINKAGE Software Package

In the LINKAGE package version 5.1 (*10*), the quantitative trait is described by the mean for each genotype, the common homozygote variance, and a multiplier for the heterozygote variance (*see* **Note 1**). Commingling analysis is first applied to a quantitative trait using pedigree data in order to estimate mixture parameters—means, standard deviation(s), and admixture proportion(s)—under the assumption of a mixture of two Normal component distributions (*13*). Admixture resulting from two components is often the case of interest in human linkage analysis; the "abnormal" components of the quantitative trait distribution may correspond to one genotype (the recessive case) or to two genotypes (the dominant case). The results of the commingling analysis is used to recode individuals into liability classes, which are then treated as qualitative outcomes in standard LOD-score-based linkage analysis using LINKAGE (*11*) (*see* **Note 2**). The relative frequency of alleles in the two component distributions are also estimated by the commingling analysis and are used to determine genotype probabilities of founder individuals in a pedigree (*14*). The ordinates of the two component Normal distributions for chosen intervals are scaled and are then used as the penetrance probabilities for the respective liability classes.

However, this pseudoquantitative algorithm employed in the LINKAGE package is awkward, has the restriction that it assumes monogenic inheritance of the trait being analyzed (*15*), and, in practice, has proven to result in less statistical power than expected (*16,17*).

2.2. LODLINK Program from the S.A.G.E. Software Package

The S.A.G.E. v3.1 program LODLINK uses genotype/phase elimination algorithms proposed by Lange and Boehnke (*18*) and Lange and Goradia (*19*), together with other enhancements, to perform fast linkage calculations. It checks that markers are consistent with Mendelian inheritance and then performs LOD score calculations for two-point linkage between a main trait and each of a set of markers. The quantitative trait may follow any of the Mendelian regressive models allowed by S.A.G.E. Parameter estimates defining the genetic model from any of the S.A.G.E. REG programs, or some other segregation program, are then required as input (*see* **Subheading 5.**). Additionally, any appropriate penetrance functions can be read in. In our worked example, for simplicity, we will illustrate the option of reading in genotypic means and variances from which the program calculates the penetrances on the assumption of Normality.

3. Interpretation

3.1. Assumptions Implicit in the Genetic Model

Model-based linkage analysis is often used with guessed values of the disease allele frequencies and penetrances, and this will not inflate the significance of a result (i.e., probability statements about the data on the assumption $\theta=\frac{1}{2}$), provided that the quantitative trait being modeled is, in fact, under the control of a major locus in the families being studied and there are no errors in the probability model assumed for the marker [it is not necessary for the marker to be error-free—only that the allele frequencies and marker penetrances are correct (**20,21**)]. Furthermore, given the assumptions underlying the likelihood, we can maximize the LOD score over both θ and the parameters that describe the mode of inheritance of the trait, and, provided the pedigrees are randomly sampled or ascertained on the basis of the trait only, we obtain consistent parameter estimates (**22,23**).

3.2. Statistical Inference

Model-based linkage analysis was originally derived for monogenic diseases and was used exclusively for dichotomous disease affection status. Traditionally, $Z(\hat{\theta})>3$ has been taken as significant evidence for linkage (**24**). From general likelihood theory, under the null hypothesis $\theta=\frac{1}{2}$, the statistic $2[\log_e 10]Z(\hat{\theta})$ is asymptotically distributed as a $\frac{1}{2} : \frac{1}{2}$ mixture of χ_1^2 and a point mass at zero, so that $Z(\hat{\theta})>3$ corresponds asymptotically to a statistic value greater than 13.8, which translates to $p<10^{-4}$ if we allow for the mixture of distributions, which is equivalent to performing a one-sided χ_1^2 test. Use of such an extremely small p-value was chosen in an attempt to limit to 0.05 the probability of making an error when concluding that linkage is present, using the fact that the prior probability of linkage between two random autosomal loci in the human genome is about 0.054. On the assumption that there is no appropriate prior probability of linkage in the case of complex traits, Lander and Kruglyak (**5**) proposed that the appropriate p-value should be based on the multiple testing performed when the whole genome is scanned for linkage, whether or not such a scan has been performed (**25**).

Many linkage programs assume $0\leq\hat{\theta}\leq0.5$. LODLINK obtains the maximum likelihood estimate over the whole interval between 0 and 1 because when most of the data are only two generational, there are usually two maxima, one less than 0.5 and one greater than 0.5. Should the larger maximum occur for $\hat{\theta} > 0.5$, this is evidence *against* linkage. If the maximum occurs for $\hat{\theta} < 0.5$ and the LOD score for $1 - \hat{\theta}$ is smaller, the result is in favor of linkage.

3.3. Power and Efficient Study Design

Linkage studies depend on the availability of families in which at least one parent is a double heterozygote for the two loci being investigated (i.e., the marker and putative disease locus). Families may thus be informative or noninformative with respect to either the genetic marker or trait. Highly polymorphic markers with many, equally frequent alleles are generally most informative for linkage analysis. As is the case with all genetic analysis, model-based linkage analysis is dependent on consistent and accurate phenotypic assessment. Assuming a correctly specified model, model-based linkage analysis is the most powerful test for linkage and provides precise estimates of the putative major gene's location along a genetic map (*26–30*). However, misspecification of the genetic model will lead to loss of statistical power.

Historically, complex genetic disease research has been characterized by failure to replicate linkage findings, particularly those generated using model-based methods. This could be the result, in part, of interpopulation genetic variability or of differences in environmental exposures resulting in expression of a genetic influence in only a proportion of the population studied. However, there are also known statistical difficulties inherent in using LOD-score-based techniques with complex diseases (*31*).

Model-based LOD score statistics critically depend on assumptions about mode of inheritance, gene frequency, and penetrance. One or more of these parameters are likely to be unknown or difficult to define with much certainty in a model-based linkage analysis of a complex phenotype. Such techniques also usually assume a genetic model with one major locus that accounts for all of the genetic variance in the phenotype; if the genetic model is unlikely in a given population, then a previously reported linkage might not be replicated (*4*). There are also limitations inherent in segregation analyses of complex phenotypes. False parameter estimates generated by a segregation analysis of traits under the control of multiple major loci may lead to an incorrect estimate of the recombination fraction in LOD score linkage methods and consequent reduced power to detect linkage (*32*). Both genetic homogeneity and a definable mode of transmission within families are also assumed. Not surprisingly, a clear model for the inheritance of many quantitative traits has not been defined.

4. Software

4.1. The LINKAGE Software Package

The LINKAGE software package is available from ftp://linkage.rockefeller. edu/software/linkage/ and is compiled for the DOS, OS2, Windows, UNIX, and VMS operating systems.

4.2. LODLINK Program from the S.A.G.E. Software Package

LODLINK is available for purchase as part of the S.A.G.E. v3.1 software package (http://darwin.cwru.edu/pub/sage.html) and is compiled for the DOS, Windows, Linux, and UNIX operating systems. S.A.G.E. is a comprehensive software package for statistical analysis in genetic epidemiology currently licensed by the Department of Epidemiology and Biostatistics, Case Western Reserve University, Cleveland, OH. Specific details of the LODLINK package are discussed as part of the worked example (**Subheading 5.**).

5. Worked Example

In this worked example we use dopamine-β-hydroxylase activity as the quantitative trait of interest. Dopamine-β-hydroxylase (DBH) is an enzyme that catalyzes the conversion of dopamine to norephinephrine (*33*). Several studies found evidence that plasma and serum DBH levels are under control of a major locus linked to the ABO blood group locus (*34–36*). In a model-based linkage study of four large Caucasian families (*37*), Wilson and colleagues found strong evidence (LOD=5.88 at θ=0.00) that a gene influencing DBH activity is linked to the ABO blood group locus on chromosome 9q. This analysis of square-root transformed DBH activity (*37*) forms the basis of our worked example.

All of the files used in this example are available on the S.A.G.E. website (http://darwin.cwru.edu/pub/sage.html). Although only a single Caucasian family (HGAR Family 9) is used here because of space constraints, all four families described by Wilson et al. (*37*) are available on our website. The LODLINK program and the Family Structure Program (FSP), both part of the S.A.G.E. v3.1 package of computer programs, will be used to perform the model-based linkage analysis.

5.1. Overview of Programs

The first requirement is a text file for the family data that contains the following information: a study ID (the same for all individuals in the data file), a numeric family ID that is unique to each family, an individual ID, an ID for each of the mother and father, and a code for sex (typically m and f or 1 and 2). In addition, trait and marker information are included. It is the combination of family ID and individual ID that uniquely identifies each individual. Each program also requires a parameter file that is used to select options to configure the program.

In **Fig. 1,** a portion of the data file for this example is listed (*see* **Note 3**). The ruler at the top is given to illustrate the column numbers where the data are located. The study ID is in columns 1–4. The family ID is in column 8. The individual ID is in columns 10–13, the father ID is in columns 15–18, the mother ID is in column 20–23, and the sex code is in column 25. The trait (square root of DBH) is located in columns 31–38 and the marker data are in column 43. Missing values for DBH are coded −1.00000, missing marker data are coded 0, and individuals whose parents are not in the data (founders) have blanks for the parent IDs.

There is a graphic user interface (GUI) that helps to create the parameter files that are used by FSP and LODLINK. This is available from the S.A.G.E.

```
             1            2            3            4
    12345678901234567890123456789012345678901234567



    SVGL    5 0017                1     -1.00000    0

    SVGL    5 0018                2     -1.00000    0

    SVGL    5 0062 0057 0056 2           6.49615    1

    SVGL    5 0063 0054 0055 2           4.94874    6

    SVGL    5 0065 0054 0055 1           5.07937    1

    .

    .

    .

    .

    SVGL    5 0159 0081 0080 2          -1.00000    0

    SVGL    5 0160 0077 0078 2          -1.00000    0

    SVGL    5 0161 0081 0080 2          -1.00000    0
```

Fig. 1. Example DBH data file.

website at http://darwin.cwru.edu/sagegui/main-menu.html. After selecting to create a new parameter file, the first screen asks for the program for which a parameter file is to be constructed (*see* **Fig. 2**). The circle next to the program is clicked to select the program to be used. Then click "continue".

5.2. Family Structure Program

Before executing LODLINK, it is necessary to run the Family Structure Program (FSP) to create the segregation analysis data file (.seg file) required as input for LODLINK (*see* **Note 4**). FSP requires as input the family data file and a parameter file (*see* **Note 5**).

For each screen that can be created with the GUI, the appropriate options are selected using pull-down menus, checking boxes, or typing in a response. After completing each screen, the "next" box is checked to move to the next

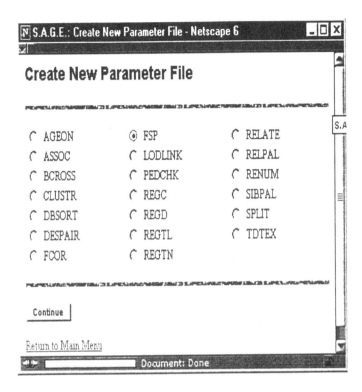

Fig. 2. S.A.G.E. GUI Screen 1.

screen. For FSP screen 1 (**Fig. 3**), the user types in a name for the title of the run. For this example, the box is checked to create the segregation analysis data file. There is one record per individual in the family data file, the symbol for male is 1 and the symbol for female is 2; these numbers are typed into the respective boxes.

For screen 2 (**Fig. 4**), it is necessary to fill in a FORTRAN format statement that tells the program where the data are located and the required format (*see* **Note 6**), The family ID must be numeric. The other parameters are alphanumeric and the maximum length of each (i.e., the maximum number of columns) is listed. **Figure 5** shows the last FSP screen, which outputs the parameter file. When the output parameter file box is clicked, a file download screen appears. The option to save this file to disk should be chosen and the user should note the location where the file is saved. The next step is to run FSP using the parameter file just created and the original family data file to produce the .seg file. How S.A.G.E. is run depends on the computer platform on which S.A.G.E. is installed.

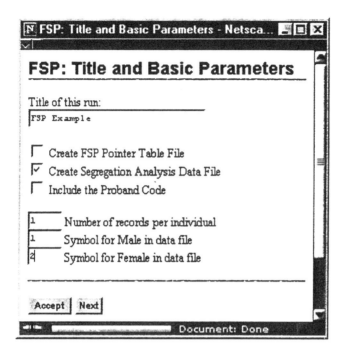

Fig. 3. S.A.G.E. GUI: FSP screen 1.

5.3. Running LODLINK

5.3.1. Input Files for LODLINK v3.1

The following set of records is used to specify the data and analysis to be performed (*see* **Note 3**):

1. ***Parameter File***—used to configure the program execution through parameter records.
2. ***Marker Locus Description File***—contains required information on the various marker loci associated with the data.
3. ***Segregation Analysis Data File (.seg)***—produced by the FSP and containing the pedigree structure information and individual data.

5.3.2. Performing the Linkage Analysis

The locus description file lists the code for missing alleles and other necessary marker information. This includes the marker name, the alleles, and the associated allele frequencies followed by a semicolon (set 1); then the set of all genotypes that give rise to each phenotype, followed by a semicolon. The marker locus description file for the ABO blood group used in this example

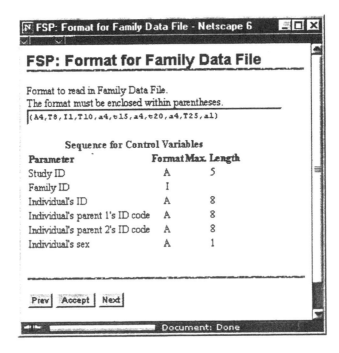

Fig. 4. S.A.G.E. GUI: FSP screen 2.

is shown in **Table 1.** For a completely codominant marker with no errors, only the first set of information is required, followed by the second semicolon (two semicolons total).

Figure 6 shows the first screen used to create the LODLINK parameter file: the title for the run is filled in. For LODLINK screen 2 (**Fig. 7**), Model 7 is selected (*see* **Note 7**). We have chosen to estimate a single recombination fraction for males and females because we know that they are both close to zero. The number 1 is entered for the number of markers and 1 for the number of pedigrees. The number of pairs of recombination fractions at which to compute LODs has been set to the default (i.e., the five values 0.0, 0.01, 0.1, 0.2, 0.3, and 0.4). All other boxes are unselected—no homogeneity tests will be performed and no genotype probabilities will be output.

For screen 3 (**Fig. 8**), the trait name, frequency of allele T1 at the trait locus and the missing value code for the trait are filled in. In screen 4 (**Fig. 9**), no sex effects are chosen (i.e., the boxes are not checked). The estimates of the allele frequency, means, and variances (screens 3, 5, and 6; **Figs. 8, 10,** and **11**) were obtained from prior segregation analysis of these data (*37*). In screen

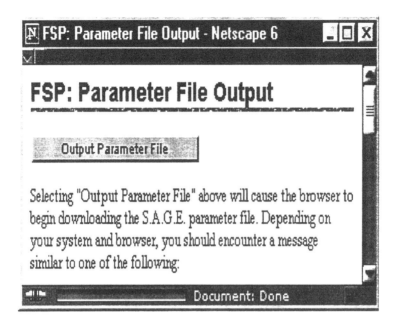

Fig. 5. S.A.G.E. GUI: FSP screen 3.

Table 1
Marker Locus Description File for ABO Blood Group

		Explanation
MISSING=0 ABO	}	ABO is the locus name
A1 = 0.190400 A2 = 0.061200 B = 0.072800 O = 0.675600 ;	}	The alleles and their frequencies
1 = {A1/A1,A1/A2,A1/O}	}	1 is the phenotype code for blood group A_1
2 = {A1/B}		2 is the phenotype code for blood group A_1B
3 = {A2/A2,A2/O}		3 is the phenotype code for blood group A_2
4 = {A2/B}		4 is the phenotype code for blood group A_2B
5 = {B/B,B/O}		5 is the phenotype code for blood group B
6 = {O/O} ;		6 is the phenotype code for blood group O

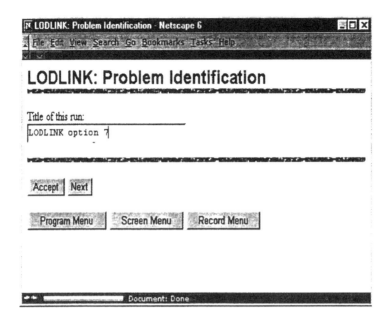

Fig. 6. S.A.G.E. GUI: LODLINK screen 1.

7 (**Fig. 12**), the FORTRAN format statement is filled in. The first five parameters are the family structure information created by FSP. The family ID, trait, and marker phenotype symbols are in exactly the same format (i.e., in the same columns) as the original family data (*see* **Note 8**). **Figure 13** shows the screen to output the LODLINK parameter file again, and the user should save the file and note the location. LODLINK can now be run.

5.3.3. Output from LODLINK

LODLINK produces two output files (*see* **Note 9**). The .out file contains a summary of the options selected, the allele frequencies, and LOD scores family by family for different values of the recombination fraction. The main results are in the .sum file (**Fig. 14**). The first part of the .sum file lists the LOD scores for the values of the recombination fraction selected in the LODLINK parameter file (in this case, the default values were chosen) for each family and the total over all families. (*Note:* There is only one family in this analysis.) The table also lists the number of individuals in each family. The maximum LOD score $[Z(\hat{\theta})]$ occurs at a recombination fraction of 0. The first line of the second part of the output table (**Fig. 14**) gives the equivalent number of fully informative meioses. In this example, the amount of information in the data is equivalent

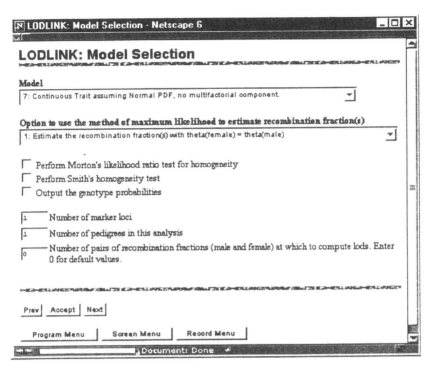

Fig. 7. S.A.G.E. GUI: LODLINK screen 2.

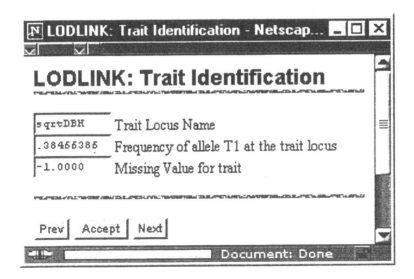

Fig. 8. S.A.G.E. GUI: LODLINK screen 3.

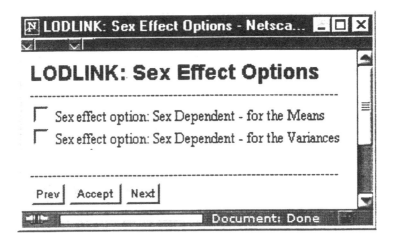

Fig. 9. S.A.G.E. GUI: LODLINK screen 4.

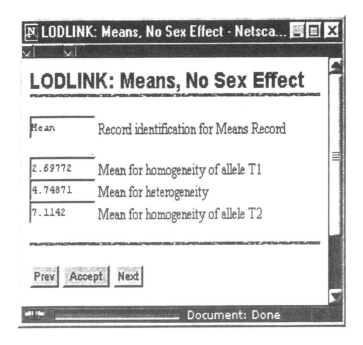

Fig. 10. S.A.G.E. GUI: LODLINK screen 5.

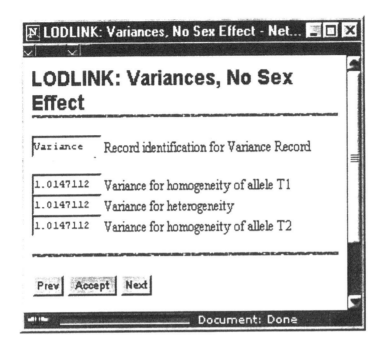

Fig. 11. S.A.G.E. GUI: LODLINK screen 6.

to 7.235 fully informative meioses. The second line of the second part (**Fig. 14**) gives the maximum LOD score for $0 \leq \hat{\theta} \leq 1$. An upper bound for the corresponding *p*-value is given and also the *p*-value that corresponds to the LOD score when the equivalent number of informative meioses is large (e.g., ≥ 50). Provided the estimate $\hat{\theta}$ is neither 0 nor 1, its variance is also calculated. Finally, the LOD score corresponding to $1-\hat{\theta}$ is given.

5.4. Interpretation of Worked Example

The maximum LOD of 2.178 found in our worked example (**Fig. 14**) is suggestive of linkage between ABO blood group genotype and square-root transformed DBH activity in HGAR family 9. For a detailed discussion of this result in HGAR family 9 and in an additional three Caucasian families, see *ref. 37*. In the overall sample of four large Caucasian families (*37*), Wilson and colleagues concluded that there was strong evidence that a gene influencing DBH activity is linked to the ABO blood group locus on chromosome 9q. This was later confirmed by Zabetian et al. (*38*).

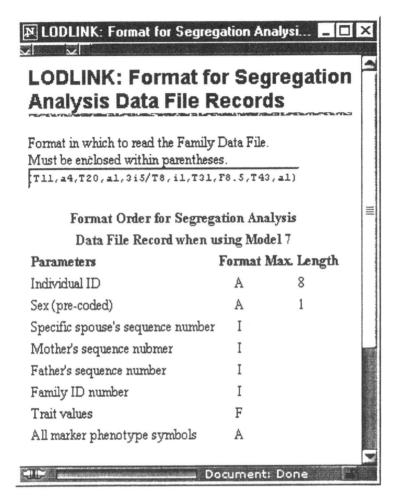

Fig. 12. S.A.G.E. GUI: LODLINK screen 7.

Notes

6.1. Limitations of LODLINK v3.1

This program is limited to the analysis of a single (univariate) main trait, but this may be a linear function that includes covariates. Only pedigree structures that can be generated by FSP are permissible.

At the default settings, LODLINK requires dynamic storage of approximately 2.5 megabytes, which allows for an unlimited number of pedigrees at the default maxima for the modifiable parameters in this program. The dimensions of these

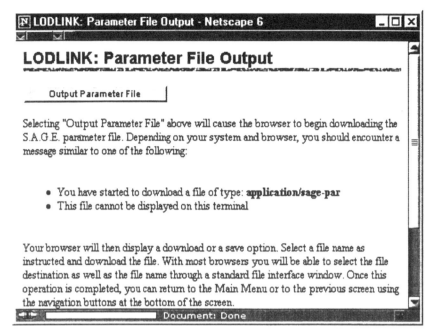

Fig. 13. S.A.G.E. GUI: LODLINK screen 8.

```
LINKAGE ANALYSIS BETWEEN LOCUS sqrtDBH  AND LOCUS ABO
===========================================================
                              --------------------------------------------------
THETA M         !            .0000    .0100    .0500    .1000    .2000    .3000    .4000 !
THETA F         !            .0000    .0100    .0500    .1000    .2000    .3000    .4000 !
----------------------------------------------------------
! PEDIGREE     NUMBER OF  !
!  NUMBER    INDIVIDUALS ! LOD SCORES                                                     !
----------------------------------------------------------
!  00005        88       !  2.1780   2.1362   1.9647   1.7415   1.2685    .7685    .2824 !
----------------------------------------------------------
!               88       !  2.1780   2.1362   1.9647   1.7415   1.2685    .7685    .2824 !
===========================================================================================
                              LOD       CHI    P-VALUE
                            ESTIMATE   SCORE   SQUARE   UPPER BOUND   APPROX. *
                            ========  ======= =======  ===========  ==========
EQUIVALENT NUMBER OF MEIOSES   7.235
THETA IN (0, 1)                 .000    2.178  10.030     .006638     .000770 (ONE-SIDED)
VARIANCE OF THETA             -------
COMPLEMENT (1 - THETA)         1.000   -1.755
* NOTE:  APPROXIMATE P-VALUES ASSUME A LARGE EQUIVALENT NUMBER OF INFORMATIVE MEIOSES.
```

Fig. 14. LODLINK .sum file.

modifiable parameters can be increased to handle larger datasets. The parameters and their default maximum values are shown in **Table 2.**

6.2. *Distributional Assumptions*

The distribution of the quantitative outcome among relatives with the same trait genotype is usually assumed, after transformation if necessary, to be

Table 2
Default Parameter Values for LODLINK

Description	Default value
No. of individuals per pedigree	500
No. of nuclear families in the analysis	100
No. of alleles at the trait locus	6
No. of alleles at any marker locus	10
Maximum number of marker inconsistencies to find	100

multivariate Normal in a segregation or parametric linkage model. If the distributions are skewed and/or kurtotic, this can have a substantial influence on the parameter estimates from a segregation or a linkage model. For instance, the genotype-specific distribution of untransformed DBH activity in the families used in our example is highly skewed, and the transformation used in pedigree analysis has a large effect on the estimate of the gene frequency in our LODLINK analyses (*37*). Overall means and standard errors for the estimated gene frequencies for untransformed DBH activity, square-root transformed DBH activity, and $\log_c$ transformed DBH activity were 0.81±0.11, 0.37±0.07, and 0.22±0.14, respectively (*37*).

7. Notes

1. Although it is the mean of a quantitative trait that is generally assumed to depend on Mendelian genotypes, there are cases in which the means are invariant and the relevant genetic information derives from other aspects of the distribution such as the variance (*39*).
2. GENEHUNTER (*40*) may also be used for this analysis once the quantitative trait has been recoded into liability classes. This has the advantage that multipoint analysis may be performed.
3. All integer-valued data must be right-justified in their fields, with no decimal point. All real-valued data should have a decimal point. The decimal point may be anywhere within the field and will override the given format. Variables read in A format may contain any valid alphanumeric characters. Any numeric fields left blank will be read as zeros.
4. We recommend running PEDCHK (http://darwin.cwru.edu/pub/sage.html) on the Segregation Analysis Data File prior to any analyses in order to detect invalid pedigree structure pointers (see Section 2 of PEDCHK in the TOOLKIT manual).
5. The family data file contains the study ID, individual ID, mother's ID, father's ID, sex code, and other data (e.g., traits, markers). However, FSP only requires the IDs and sex code to be read in. In the next release of S.A.G.E. (S.A.G.E. 4.0), FSP will not be required and parameter files will be constructed differently. At the time of writing, LODLINK is not yet available in S.A.G.E. 4.0.

6. For help with FORTRAN format statements, there is a tutorial on the S.A.G.E. website at http://darwin.cwru.edu/sagegui/help/tutorials.html. FORTRAN. format statements are not required for S.A.G.E. 4.0.

7. In the example used here, the values of the parameters in the model were obtained from a previous segregation analysis (*37*). It is possible to perform segregation analyses within S.A.G.E. 3.1 and use the output from this directly as input into LODLINK. In that case, the allele frequencies, means, and variances would not be specified in the LODLINK parameter file. Thus, the other options are to use direct output from the S.A.G.E. REG segregation programs or to read in the penetrances.

8. In the .seg file, the first record for each individual contains the family structure information. The subsequent record(s) contain(s) the individual data from the original family data file. In other words, FSP creates a record with the family structure information and then appends the data taken from the original family data file. The individual ID, sex, specific spouses sequence number, mothers sequence number, and fathers sequence number are read in with the following FORTRAN format statement: T11, A4, T20, A1, 3I5. A slash is then used to read in data from the next record.

9. When running S.A.G.E. 3.1 under Windows 95 or 98, the program automatically uses the name of the parameter file and adds the appropriate extensions for the output files.

Acknowledgments

This work was supported by grant RR03655 from the National Center for Research Resources and GM28356 from the National Institute of General Medical Sciences.

References

1. Weeks, D., Lehner, T., Squires-Wheeler, E., Kaufmann, A., and Ott J. (1990) Measuring the inflation of the LOD score due to its maximization over model parameter values in human linkage analysis. *Genet. Epidemiol.* **7,** 237–243.

2. Lander, E. and Schork, N. (1994) Genetic dissection of complex traits. *Science* **265,** 2037–2048.

3. Schork, N., Boehnke, M., Terwilliger, J., and Ott, J. (1993) Two trait-locus linkage analysis: a powerful strategy for mapping complex genetic traits. *Am. J. Hum. Genet.* **53,** 1127–1136.

4. Risch, N. (1991) Genetic linkage: interpreting lod scores. *Science* **25,** 803–804.

5. Lander, E. and Kruglyak, L. (1995) Genetic dissection of complex traits: guidelines for interpreting and reporting linkage results. *Nature Genet.* **11,** 241–247.

6. Elston, R. C. (1981) Segregation analysis. *Adv. Hum. Genet.* **11,** 63–120.

7. Khoury, M., Beaty, T., and Cohen, B. (1993) *Fundamentals of Genetic Epidemiology.* Oxford University Press, Oxford.

8. Ginsburg, E. and Livshits, G. (1999) Segregation analysis of quantitative traits. *Ann. Hum. Biol.* **26,** 103–129.

9. Ott, J. (1974) Estimation of the recombination fraction in human pedigrees: efficient computation of the likelihood for human linkage studies. *Am J. Hum. Genet.* **26,** 588–597.

10. Lathrop, G. M., Lalouel, J. M., Julier, C., and Ott J. (1984) Strategies for multilocus linkage analysis in humans. *Proc. Natl. Acad. Sci. USA* **81,** 3443–3446.

11. Lathrop, G. M., Lalouel, J. M., Julier, C., and Ott, J. (1985) Multilocus linkage analysis in humans: detection of linkage and estimation of recombination. *Am. J. Hum. Genet.* **37,** 482–498.

12. Cleves, M. A. and Elston, R. C. (1997) An alternative test for linkage between two loci. *Genet. Epidemiol.* **14,** 117–131.

13. Ott, J. (1999) *Analysis of Human Genetic Linkage,* 3rd ed. The Johns Hopkins University Press, Baltimore, MD.

14. Terwilliger, J. D. and Ott, J. (1994) *Handbook of Human Genetic Linkage.* Johns Hopkins University Press, Baltimore, MD.

15. Goldgar, D. and Oniki, R. (1992) Comparison of a multipoint identity-by-descent method with parametric multipoint linkage analysis for mapping quantitative traits. *Am. J. Hum. Genet.* **50,** 598–606.

16. Curtis, D. and Gurling, H. M. (1991) Using a dummy quantitative variable to deal with multiple affection categories in genetic linkage analysis. *Ann. Hum. Genet.* **55,** 321–327.

17. Devoto M., Shimoya, K., Caminis, J., Ott, J., Tenenhouse, A., Whyte, M. P., et al. (1998) First-stage autosomal genome screen in extended pedigrees suggests genes predisposing to low bone mineral density on chromosomes 1p, 2p, and 4q. *Eur. J. Hum. Genet.* **6,** 151–157.

18. Lange, K. and Boehnke, M. (1983) Extensions to pedigree analysis. IV. Covariance components models for multivariate traits. *Am. J. Med. Genet.* **14,** 513–524.

19. Lange, K. and Goradia, T. M. (1987) An algorithm for automatic genotype elimination. *Am. J. Hum. Genet.* **40,** 250–256.

20. Williamson, J. A. and Amos, C. I. (1995) Guess LOD approach: sufficient conditions for robustness. *Genet. Epidemiol.* **12,** 163–176.

21. Williamson J. A. and Amos, C. I. (1990) On the asymptotic behavior of the estimate of the recombination fraction under the null hypothesis of no linkage when the model is misspecified. *Genet. Epidemiol.* **7,** 309–318.

22. Elston, R. C. (1989) Man bites dog? The validity of maximizing lod scores to determine mode of inheritance [editorial]. *Am. J. Med. Genet.* **34,** 487–488.

23. Hodge, S. E. and Elston, R. C. (1994) Lods, wrods, and mods: the interpretation of lod scores calculated under different models. *Genet. Epidemiol.* **11,** 329–342.

24. Morton, N. E. (1998) Significance levels in complex inheritance. *Am. J. Hum. Genet.* **62,** 690–697.

25. Witte, J. S., Elston, R. C., and Schork, N. J. (1996) Genetic dissection of complex traits. *Nature Genet.* **12,** 355–356; discussion, 357–358.

26. Lange, K., Spence, M. A., and Frank, M. B. (1976) Application of the lod method to the detection of linkage between a quantitative trait and a qualitative marker: a simulation experiment. *Am. J. Hum. Genet.* **28,** 167–173.

27. Boehnke, M. (1990) Sample-size guidelines for linkage analysis of a dominant locus for a quantitative trait by the method of lod scores. *Am. J. Hum. Genet.* **47,** 218–227.

28. Boehnke, M., Omoto, K. H., and Arduino, J. M. (1990) Selecting pedigrees for linkage analysis of a quantitative trait: the expected number of informative meioses. *Am. J. Hum. Genet.* **46,** 581–586.

29. Demenais, F., Lathrop, G. M., and Lalouel, J. M. (1988) Detection of linkage between a quantitative trait and a marker locus by the lod score method: sample size and sampling considerations. *Ann. Hum. Genet.* **52,** 237–246.

30. Demenais, F. and Amos, C. (1989) Power of the sib-pair and lod-score methods for linkage analysis of quantitative traits. *Prog. Clin. Biol. Res.* **329,** 201–206.

31. Morton, N. E. (1992) Major loci for atopy? *Clin. Exp. Allergy* **22,** 1041–1043.

32. Dizier, M.-H., Bonaiti-Pellie, C., and Clerget-Darpoux, F. (1993) Conclusions of segregation analysis for family data generated under two-locus models. *Am. J. Hum. Genet.* **53,** 1338–1346.

33. Kaufman, S. and Friedman, S. (1965) Dopamine-beta-hydroxylase. *Pharmacol. Rev.* **17,** 71–100.

34. Elston, R. C., Namboodiri, K. K., and Hames, C. G. (1979) Segregation and linkage analyses of dopamine-beta-hydroxylase activity. *Hum. Heredity* **29,** 284–292.

35. Goldin, L. R., Gershon, E. S., Lake, C. R., Murphy, D. L., McGinniss, M., and Sparkes, R. S. (1982) Segregation and linkage studies of plasma dopamine-beta-hydroxylase (DBH), erythrocyte catechol-*O*-methyltransferase (COMT), and platelet monoamine oxidase (MAO): possible linkage between the ABO locus and a gene controlling DBH activity. *Am. J. Hum. Genet.* **34,** 250–262.

36. Asamoah, A., Wilson, A. F., Elston, R. C., Dalferes, E., Jr., and Berenson, G. S. (1987) Segregation and linkage analyses of dopamine-beta-hydroxylase activity in a six-generation pedigree. *Am. J. Med. Genet.* **27,** 613–621.

37. Wilson, A. F., Elston, R. C., Siervogel, R. M., and Tran, L. D. (1988) Linkage of a gene regulating dopamine-beta-hydroxylase activity and the ABO blood group locus. *Am. J. Hum. Genet.* **42,** 160–166.

38. Zabetian, C. P., Anderson, G. M., Buxbaum, S. G., Elston, R. C., Ichinose, H., Nagatsu, T., ed al. (2001) A quantitative-trait analysis of human plasma-dopamine beta-hydroxylase activity: evidence for a major functional polymorphism at the DBH locus. *Am. J. Hum. Genet.* **68,** 515–522.

39. Murphy, E. A. and Trojak, J. L. (1986) The genetics of quantifiable homeostasis: I. The general issues. *Am. J. Med. Genet.* **24,** 159–169.

40. Kruglyak, L., Daly, M., Reeve-Daly, M., and Lander, E. (1996) Parametric and nonparametric linkage analysis: A unified multipoint approach. *Am. J. Hum. Genet.* **58,** 1347–1363.

3

Nonparametric Linkage Analysis

I. Haseman–Elston

Chad P. Garner

1. Introduction

The original nonparametric (or model-free) method of linkage analysis that was described by Haseman and Elston in 1972 (*1*) was designed for analysis of quantitative traits using the sib-pair study design. In the following subheading, a brief introduction to linear regression precedes a description of the traditional and new Haseman–Elston theory. The Methods, Interpretation, and Worked Example sections of the chapter are all based on the programs GENIBD and SIBPAL2 from the S.A.G.E. Version 4.0 *Beta 5* software package. SIBPAL2 is currently the only software publicly available for carrying out the new Haseman–Elston method.

1.1. Linear Regression

Regression is used to explore the dependence of one or more variables on another. The term *linear* implies that the relationship between the variables is linear and the adjectives *simple* and *multiple* describe a regression model with one or more than one predictor variable, respectively. In simple linear regression, the relationship is of the form

$$Y = \alpha + \beta x + e \tag{1}$$

where Y (referred to as the response or dependent variable) and x (referred to as the predictor or independent variable) are observable random variables. The quantities α and β, are the y-intercept and slope (also referred to as the regression coefficient or parameter) of the regression line, respectively, and e is the residual error. β and α are fixed and unknown parameters and e is a random variable

From: *Methods in Molecular Biology: vol. 195: Quantitative Trait Loci: Methods and Protocols.*
Edited by: N. J. Camp and A. Cox © Humana Press, Inc., Totowa, NJ

with expectation $e = 0$ and assumed to follow a Normal distribution. The objective of linear regression is to estimate the values of α and β that gives the best fit for the joint distribution of the dependent and independent variables. The population parameters, α and β, are approximated by the parameters a and b that are estimated from the sample. Finding the values of a and b that best fit the data requires a mathematical method for minimizing the error in the model; one method that is commonly used for simple linear regression models is called least squares.

Least squares regression makes no statistical assumptions about the observations x and y. For any line $y = a + bx$, the residual sum of squares (RSS) is defined to be

$$RSS = \sum_{i=1}^{n} (y_i - (a + bx_i))^2 \tag{2}$$

The least squares estimates of α and β are defined as those values of a and b such that the line $a + bx$ minimizes the RSS. By writing

$$\sum_{i=1}^{n} (y_i - (a + bx))^2 = \sum_{i=1}^{n} ((y_i - bx_i) - a)^2 \tag{3}$$

the value of a that gives the minimum RSS can be found for any fixed value of b. The minimized value of a is

$$a = \frac{1}{n} \sum_{i=1}^{n} (y_i - bx_i) = \bar{y} - b\bar{x} \tag{4}$$

where $\bar{y}$ and $\bar{x}$ are the sample means of y and x, respectively. For any given value of b, the minimum value of the RSS is

$$\sum_{i=1}^{n} ((y_i - bx_i) - (\bar{y} - b\bar{x}))^2 = \sum_{i=1}^{n} ((y_i - \bar{y}) - b(x_i - \bar{x}))^2 \tag{5}$$

$$= Var(y) - 2b\,Cov(x, y) + b^2\,Var(x)$$

The value of b that gives the minimal value of RSS is obtained by setting the derivative of the quadratic function of b equal to zero and solving. The least squares estimators of a and b are thus

$$a = \bar{y} - b\bar{x} \tag{6}$$
$$b = \frac{Cov(x, y)}{Var(x)}$$

The least squares estimators of the *y*-intercept and slope of a simple linear regression are functions of the observed means, variances, and covariance.

The multiple regression model is of the form

$$Y = \alpha + \beta_1 x_1 + \beta_2 x_2 + ... + \beta_n x_n + e \tag{7}$$

where Y is a function of n predictor variables and the terms $\beta_1,..., \beta_n$ are the partial regression coefficients. Like simple linear regression, the task in multiple regression is to find the values for the parameters (a and the b_i) that give the best fit of the conditional expectation of Y given $x_1,..., x_n$ using the least squares approach. The partial regression coefficients are functions of the observed variances and covariance; however, unlike simple linear regression, each partial regression coefficient is a function of the variances and covariances of all the measured variables in the model. Multiple regression models are most often expressed as matrices and vectors.

For statistical simplicity, it is desirable to work with Normally distributed data. Tests for Normality include the small-sample *W*-test of Shapiro and Wilk and the large-sample *D*-test of D'Agostino. In situations where the raw data do not fit the Normal distribution, the data may be transformed by changing scale. Commonly used transformations include the log transformation and the Box–Cox transformation.

1.2. The Traditional Haseman–Elston Method

The Haseman–Elston method for linkage analysis is based on the hypothesis that sib pairs having similar trait values will also have greater than average genetic similarity in a region that is linked to a locus that is affecting the observed trait values. It is assumed that the trait is influenced by a locus (quantitative trait loci [QTL]) that has two alleles, B and b, having frequencies p and q. Each genotype has a genotypic value that represents the effect on the trait that can be attributed to the genotype, in the absence of any additional sources of variation. For a biallelic locus with alleles B and b, convention defines the genetic values for BB, Bb and bb be a, d, and $-a$, respectively. Letting x_{1j} and x_{2j} be the trait values of the first and second sibs, respectively, of the jth sib pair,

$$x_{1j} = \mu + g_{1j} + e_{1j} \tag{8}$$
$$x_{2j} = \mu + g_{2j} + e_{2j}$$

where μ is the overall mean of the trait and g_{1j} and e_{1j} are the genetic and environmental effects, respectively. Assuming that only one locus determines g_{1j} and that there is random mating, the genetic effects are the genotypic values described above. Letting $e_j = e_{1j} - e_{2j}$ and $E(e_j^2) = \sigma_e^2$, σ_e^2 is a function of environmental variance, the environmental covariance between sibs and any

Table 1
Conditional Probabilities of Y$_j$ and π_j

Sib 1	Sib 2	Y$_j$	$\pi_j = 0$	$\pi_j = 0.5$	$\pi_j = 1$
BB	BB	e_j^2	p^4	p^3	p^2
bb	bb	e_j^2	q^4	q^3	q^2
Bb	Bb	e_j^2	$4p^2q^2$	pq	$2pq$
BB	Bb	$(a - d + e_j)^2$	$2p^3q$	p^2q	0
Bb	BB	$(-a + d + e_j)^2$	$2p^3q$	p^2q	0
Bb	bb	$(a + d + e_j)^2$	$2pq^3$	pq^2	0
bb	Bb	$(-a - d + e_j)^2$	$2pq^3$	pq^2	0
BB	bb	$(2a + e_j)^2$	p^2q^2	0	0
bb	BB	$(-2a + e_j)^2$	p^2q^2	0	0

order effect. The similarity in trait values for sib pair j is measured by their squared mean-corrected trait difference, expressed as

$$Y_j = [(x_{1j} - \mu) - (x_{2j} - \mu)]^2 = (x_{1j} - x_{2j})^2 \tag{9}$$

which is equivalent to the squared trait difference.

The mean number of alleles shared identical by descent (IBD) by a sib pair is more commonly expressed in terms of the proportion of alleles shared IBD, π; the expected value of π for sib pairs is 0.50. Haseman and Elston (**1**) proposed a Bayesian estimator for π given by

$$\hat{\pi}_j = f_{j2} + \tfrac{1}{2}f_{j1} \tag{10}$$

where f_{j2} and f_{j1} are the probabilities that the jth sib pair share two and one alleles IBD, respectively. More recently, multipoint methods have been proposed that use information from linked markers to estimate the IBD at any point on a chromosome.

Assuming a fixed e_j, the conditional distribution of Y_j and the conditional probabilities of $\pi_j = 0$, 0.5, and 1 are given for the nine possible sib-pair genotype configurations in **Table 1.** The table can be used to calculate the expected value of Y_j conditional on π_j. Omitting much algebra that can be found in **ref. 1,**

$$E\,(Y_j|\pi_j = 1) = E\{e_j^2\,[p^2 + q^2 + 2pq]\} = E(e_j^2) = \sigma_e^2$$
$$E(Y_j|\pi_j = (\tfrac{1}{2})= E\{e_j^2[p^3 + q^3 + pq] + [(a - d + e_j)^2 + (-a + d + e_j)^2]p^2q$$
$$+\, [(a + d + e_j)^2 + (-a - d + e_j)^2]pq2\}$$
$$= \sigma_e^2 + \sigma_a^2 + 2\sigma_d^2$$

$$E(Y_j|\pi_j = 0) = E(\{e_j^2[p^4 + q^4 + 4p^2q^2] + [(a - d + e_j)^2 + (-a + d + e_j)]\ 2p^3q$$
$$+ [(a + d + e_j)^2 + (-a - d + e_j)^2]\ (2pq^3) \tag{11}$$
$$+ [(2a + e_j)^2 + (-2a + e_j)^2]\ p^2q^2\}$$
$$= \sigma_e^2 + 2\sigma_a^2 + 2\sigma_d^2$$

where σ_e^2, σ_a^2, and σ_d^2 are the environmental, additive genetic, and dominance genetic variances, respectively. From these equations, one can see that the expected value of Y_j increases as π_j decreases; the degree to which the sibs differ in trait value is expected to increase as the IBD sharing at the QTL decreases. If there is no dominance variance, the expected value of Y_j can be written in the general form

$$E(Y_j|\pi_j) = (\sigma_e^2 + 2\sigma_g^2) - 2\sigma_g^2\pi_j, \quad \pi_j = 0,\ \tfrac{1}{2},\ 1 \tag{12}$$

This can be written in the form of a simple regression model

$$E(Y_j|\pi_j) = \alpha + \beta\pi_j \tag{13}$$

where $\alpha = \sigma_e^2 + 2\sigma_g^2$, $\beta = -2\sigma_g^2$, and σ_g^2 is the total genetic variance, $\sigma_g^2 = \sigma_a^2 + \sigma_d^2$. The least squares estimate $-\beta/2$ is an unbiased estimator of σ_g^2. The null hypothesis represents a slope $\beta = 0$, and a statistically significant negative slope is evidence for linkage. The theory presented so far has related π_j to Y_j. Haseman and Elston (*1*) derived the expectation of $\hat{\beta}$ when $\hat{\pi}_j$ is estimated from a single linked marker and found that $\hat{\beta}$ is a function of the genetic variance and the recombination fraction between the QTL and the marker. With multipoint methods, the IBD status at the QTL can be estimated so that the regression is no longer a function of the genetic distance. For families with three or more siblings, each of the sib pairs in the sibship are not independent and treating them as such increases the type I error rate of the linkage test. Single and Finch (*2*) proposed a generalized least squares approach that accounted for the correlation between multiple relationships in a family without the type I error rate exceeding the nominal value.

1.3. The New Haseman–Elston Method

Drigalenko (*3*) proposed an extension of the Haseman–Elston method that uses the squared mean-corrected sib-pair sum as well as the difference and he showed that this value is linearly related to the proportion of alleles shared IBD. He also showed that the model gives equivalent information to the sib-pair covariance modeled by the variance component methods (*see* Chapter 4).

The squared mean-corrected sum is expressed in an analogous way to the difference shown earlier, such that

$$Y_j[(x_{1j} - \mu) + (x_{2j} - \mu)]^2 \tag{14}$$

Drigalenko (**3**) and Elston et al. (**4**) showed that the combined information from the sums and differences can be expressed as the mean-corrected cross product, giving

$$Y_j = (x_{1j} - \mu)(x_{2j} - \mu). \tag{15}$$

The expectation of the cross-product is the sib covariance and the regression coefficient is half as large in magnitude than and opposite sign to the model where Y_j is the traditional squared-trait difference. The model for the new Haseman–Elston was defined by Elston et al. (**4**) to be the multiple regression

$$E(Y_j|\hat{\pi}_{j1}, \hat{f}_{2j}) = \alpha + \beta_1\hat{\pi}_j + \beta_2\hat{f}_{2j} + e \tag{16}$$

where $\hat{\pi}_j$ is the proportion of alleles shared IBD and $\hat{f}_{2j}$ is the probability that a relative pair shares two alleles IBD. Elston et al. (**4**) showed that β_1 and β_2 in Eq. (16) are estimates of σ_a^2 and σ_d^2, respectively, where $\sigma_a^2 = \sigma_g^2 - \sigma_d^2$ is the additive genetic variance. Additional regression terms can be added to the model to include covariate effects.

2. Methods

This section describes the steps for carrying out a linkage analysis with the new Haseman–Elston method using S.A.G.E. Ver. 4.0 *Beta 5* software package. Three programs will be used in the analysis: PEDINFO generates a summary of the pedigree data, GENIBD computes the IBD allele-sharing probabilities, and SIBPAL2 does the regression-based linkage analysis. Instructions for downloading and setting up the programs for the UNIX and Linux operating systems is given in **Subheading 4.** It is recommended that one reads **Subheading 4.** if unfamiliar with the S.A.G.E. software package.

2.1. Preparing the Raw Data for Linkage Analysis

The trait data should be looked at before linkage analysis is performed. The distribution of the raw trait values can be plotted as a histogram using most general statistical analysis software packages. A plot of the data will identify two potentially confounding factors: (1) a large deviation from the Normal distribution and (2) the existence of extreme outliers. Specific tests are available within most statistical software packages to assess the fit of the data to the Normal distribution (*see* **Subheading 1.1.**). The data should be rescaled (or transformed) when significant deviations from the Normal distribution are observed (*see* **Subheading 1.1.** for suggested transformations of scale). The effects of covariates on the data can be estimated and accounted for in this initial stage of the analysis. Extreme outliers (data points that are much more than three standard deviations from the mean) often occur in the raw data either because of a transcription error or for a real biological reason. Extreme data points can have a large effect on the results of the analysis and it is recommended that they are changed to missing values if it cannot be determined that they are transcription problems and can be corrected. The extreme cases may be biologically significant, but their existence will only make the statistical interpretation of the results more difficult.

Prior to a linkage analysis, the marker data should be analyzed for misspecified relationships and genotyping errors. Publicly available programs are described in **Subheading 6.** that can be used to carry out both of these types of analysis.

In the absence of fully informative marker data, the IBD sharing estimates will be dependent on the marker allele frequencies; therefore, it is very important that the allele frequencies used in the analysis be as accurate as possible.

2.2. Preparing the Input Files

Detailed descriptions of the input files needed for PEDINFO, GENIBD, and SIBPAL2 are given in **Subheading 4.** Briefly, the programs require the parameter file, the pedigree data file, the marker locus description file, and the genome map file (if one is estimating multipoint IBD sharing probabilities). The input files do not have to be given specific names, but it is recommended that the user call them something relating to the analysis that is being performed. The parameter file describes the format and contents of the pedigree file and the types of analysis that are to be performed. The pedigree file includes all of the family, trait, and marker data. The locus and map files define the marker allele frequencies and the genetic map, respectively. All three programs can use the same set of input files. GENIBD will generate an output file that will then be used to run SIBPAL2. Individuals may wish to use other programs to estimate the IBD sharing probabilities and convert the output from these programs into the IBD files required by SIBPAL2. A description of the IBD files is given in **Subheading 4.** and other methods and programs for estimating the IBD sharing are discussed in **Subheading 6.**

2.3. Running PEDINFO

The PEDINFO program reports the numbers of each relationship type in the data and calculates some simple summary statistics describing the input data. If the report given by the program is not consistent with what the investigator knows about the data, then this is an indication that there may be problems with the pedigree data file.

To run the program, type the program name followed by the names of the parameter and pedigree files at the command line:

% pedinfo *parameter_file pedigree_file*

The program will print "Analysis complete!" to the screen when the program is finished. The output of the program will be in a file called *pedinfo.out.*

2.4. Estimating the IBD Sharing with GENIBD

GENIBD can do single-point and multipoint IBD estimation. Multipoint IBD methods capture more information than single-point methods; however, one must be certain of the map order and have good estimates of the genetic distances between the markers in order to get reliable IBD sharing estimates. GENIBD can calculate single-point or multipoint IBD probability estimates using an exact-likelihood-based algorithm for small pedigrees or a Markov chain Monte Carlo (MCMC)-based algorithm of larger pedigrees. The exact approach is recommended for nuclear family data. The type of IBD analysis to be carried out is specified in the analysis definition section of the parameter file (*see* **Subheading 4.1.3.** for a description of the file format). It is possible to specify both single-point and multipoint analyses in the parameter file and the program will execute both. GENIBD requires a parameter, pedigree, marker locus description, and genome map file (if one is carrying out a multipoint analysis). Descriptions of these files and some of the program options are described in **Subheading 4.**

To run the program, type the program name followed by the names of the parameter, pedigree, locus and map files at the command line:

% genibd *parameter_file pedigree_file locus_file map_file*(optional)

The program will print an error message to the screen if it is unable to run. The error message will give a general idea of the problem that the program has encountered. A description of common problems is given in **Subheading 6.** Program execution information is written to a file called *genibd.inf.* Errors that cause the program to terminate are described in this file. The program also writes a file called *genome.inf,* which has marker genotype and map information.

As the program is running, it will print its progress to the screen. The results of the IBD analysis are in a file with the naming scheme *output.region*.ibd. The *output* is specified in the parameter file. The *region* is the name of the region defined by the user in the genome map and parameter files. It is helpful to use the chromosome name as the region name if one is carrying out a genomewide multipoint analysis. The format of the IBD file is described in **Subheading 4.** No modification to this file is necessary prior to linkage analysis.

2.5. Testing for Linkage with SIBPAL2

Once the IBD file is generated, running SIBPAL2 is straightforward. If GENIBD ran successfully, the only reason why SIBPAL2 would be terminate as a result of an error would be if the analysis were not specified correctly in the analysis definition section of the parameter file or if an IBD file that was not created by GENIBD were being used and it had not been formatted correctly.

To run the program, type the program name followed by the names of the parameter, pedigree, and IBD files at the command line:

$$\% \text{ sibpal2 } \textit{parameter\_file pedigree\_file ibd\_file}$$

The program will print its progress to the screen and announce a successful completion. A log file called *sibpal2.inf* will be generated with each run of the program. The results of the linkage analysis are written to a file called *traits.out*. An interpretation of the results is given in **Subheading 3.** and a description of the output file is given in **Subheading 4.**

3. Interpretation

When evaluating the results of a Haseman–Elston linkage analysis, there are two important considerations. The first is the statistical significance, or *p*-value, of the estimated regression coefficients; this is equivalent to the amount of evidence for linkage. The *p*-value associated with the estimate is derived from a Student's *t*-distribution and represents the probability of the null hypothesis, $\beta = 0$. The threshold one wishes to use for declaring their results significant will depend on the number of markers tested as multiple testing should be accounted for in the interpretation of the results. Guidelines for interpreting and reporting linkage results have been given by Lander and Kruglyak (**5**) and by Sawcer et al. (**6**). The second consideration is the size of the estimated regression coefficient. The regression coefficients indicate the extent to which a linked QTL is affecting the trait; the simple regression parameter is a function of the genetic variance and the multiple-regression parameters are functions of the additive and dominance variances. With a large sample, it is possible to get a small regression coefficient with a significant *p*-value. This would be evidence for linkage to a QTL of small effect. Alternatively, with small sample sizes, it is possible to have a nominally significant *p*-value associated with a large regression coefficient. The standard error of the parameter estimate is an indication of the quality of the parameter estimate. The standard errors of the estimates should always be considered, especially if one has a small sample. In statistical inference, it is important to consider the value of the estimated parameter and its significance.

The outcome of a linkage analysis will be dependent on power. The amount of power a study has depends on the genetics of the trait and the sample being used to search for QTL affecting the trait. Sample size (including both the size and number of families) and the number of genotyping errors, relationship specification errors, phenotyping errors, and the accuracy of the marker allele frequency estimates are characteristics of the sample that will affect power. The number of QTLs affecting the trait, the size of their effects, interactions both between QTLs and between QTLs and the environment, and genetic and allelic heterogeneity are characteristics of the genetics of the trait that will affect power.

4. Software

4.1. Getting the S.A.G.E. Software

The S.A.G.E. Ver. 4.0 *Beta 5* programs are currently available free of charge and can be downloaded from the following URL: http://darwin.cwru.edu/beta. Versions of the programs are available for Digital UNIX, Sun Solaris, and Linux operating systems. The files are downloaded in a tarred and compressed form. To create the files, type the following at the command line:

% uncompress *filename*.tar.Z

where *filename*.tar.Z is the name of compressed S.A.G.E. file. Then, type

% tar xvf *filename*.tar

and a directory will be created that has the same name as the filename. Inside this directory is a subdirectory called bin/ that will contain the program files. The documentation for the programs are in a PDF file that is called *beta5.pdf.*

4.2. The Input File Formats

4.2.1. The Pedigree File

The pedigree file will be described first, as it is usually the first file created before a linkage analysis is performed. The programs are very flexible as to the format of the pedigree file as long as it correctly described in the parameter file. The programs can either read character delimited files or column delimited files. The difference between the two files types is simple; character-delimited files have a character (examples include a space, comma, or tab) separating fields, and in a column-specified file, the fields are in specific columns described by a formatting statement. It is recommended that the character-delimited file in which the fields are delimited by spaces is used because this type of file is easily created with Microsoft Excel and because similar formats are used by the more popular genetic analysis programs like LINKAGE (*7*) and GENE-HUNTER (*8*). Also, the formatting statement required by the column-delimited file could be difficult for individuals who are not familiar with the FORTRAN

programming language. Character-delimited files have the following requirements: Each record must be exactly one line (a record being an individual);
there must be at least one delimited character between fields; and there can be
no empty fields.

The file includes three types of information: the pedigree data, the trait data,
and the marker data. The pedigree information includes a unique pedigree
identification number, an individual's identification code that is unique within
the pedigree, the individual's parents' identification codes, and a code for the
individual's sex. For each relative pair included in the pedigree file, there must
be records for the relatives that connect them. An individual that does not have
a genetic relative in the family (excluding parent–offspring relationships) is
called a founder and everyone else is a nonfounder. Nonfounders need to have
their parents specified in the pedigree file and founders do not. An example
of the pedigree data section of a space-delimited pedigree file for a pair of
sisters follows:

```
PID ID P1 P2 SEX
  1  1  0  0  1
  1  2  0  0  2
  1  3  1  2  2
  1  4  1  2  2
```

The first line of the pedigree file defines what is in each field. The order of
the fields is given in the following order: the unique pedigree number (PID),
the individual's identification number (ID), the father's identification number
(P1), the mother's identification number (P2), and the sex code (SEX). The
pedigree number is 1. The sex code is 1 for male and 2 for female, so that
individual 1 is the father of the two sisters (individuals 3 and 4), and individual
2 is the mother. The sex code is defined in the parameter file. The mother and
father are founders; therefore, they do not have parent records and have zeros
in the mother and father columns to represent missing values. The missing
value code is defined in the parameter file. The sisters each have their father's
identification number followed by their mother's in fields 3 and 4.

The trait and marker data follow the pedigree data as shown:

```
PID ID P1 P2 SEX TRAIT1 MARKER1 MARKER2
  1  1  0  0  1   5.324   1/3     1/2
  1  2  0  0  2  -3.876   4/5     3/4
  1  3  1  2  2  -0.287   3/4     1/4
  1  4  1  2  2   4.678   1/4     2/3
```

The trait (TRAIT1) and markers (MARKER1 and MARKER2) follow the sex
field. Multiple traits and markers can be included in one pedigree file. The

order of the traits and markers is given in the parameter file. Each marker has two alleles that are separated by an allele delimiter (a forward slash in the example). The field and allele delimiters cannot be the same. The allele delimiter is defined in the parameter file. The above format is only a recommendation; examples and explanations of other formats are given in the program documentation.

4.2.2. The Parameter File

The parameter file tells the program what the data are and what analyses to perform. The file has two main sections: the configuration information and the analysis definition. The configuration information tells the programs what the format and content of the pedigree file is and defines parameters.

The general syntax for the parameter file is

```
parameter[=value][,attribute[=value]]
[{
        [statement]
}]
```

where syntax enclosed in brackets represents optional information.

An example of the configuration information section of a parameter file that corresponds to the above pedigree file example is given by

```
pedigree, character
{
        individual_missing_value="0"
        sex_code, male="1", female="2"
        delimiters=" "
        delimiter_mode=multiple

        pedigree_id=PID
        individual_id=ID
        parent_id=P1
        parent_id=P2
        sex_field=SEX
        trait=TRAIT1,missing="-99"
        marker=MARKER1,missing="0"
        marker=MARKER2,missing="0"
}
```

The first line of the example specifies the *pedigree* parameter with an attribute defined as *character* to indicate that the pedigree file is character delimited. This is followed by several statements; the first four are setting options that describe how the pedigree file should be read. The *individual_missing_value* statement defines the code for missing individuals; missing individuals would be the parents of founders in the pedigree file. Statements or attributes that sets a value to be read from the pedigree file should indicate the value in quotation marks. In the next line, *sex_code* is defined to be 1 for males and 2 for females. The third statement defines the delimiter to be a space. The value of the *delimiter_mode* parameter can either be single or multiple. This parameter tells the program how many consecutive delimiters it can read. Setting the value to multiple allows one to leave multiple spaces between fields.

The next eight statements define the contents of the pedigree file. The parameters correspond to the different data types and these are set equal to the names that they have been assigned in the first line of the pedigree file. The parameters *pedigree_id, individual_id, parent_id*, and *sex_field* are associated with the pedigree data part of the pedigree file. The parameters *trait* and *marker* indicate fields as such. Missing values for the traits and markers are defined as attributes of the trait and marker parameters as shown in the example.

The analysis definition section of the parameter file appears after the configuration information. The following is an example of a parameter file with the parameters for running GENIBD and SIBPAL2:

```
scantype=interval
Distance=2
ibd_analysis
{
        mode=multipoint
        title="multipoint analysis of chr5"
        output="MP"
        region=chr5
}
trait_regression,simple
```

The *scantype* parameter instructs the program to compute IBD probabilities at intervals and not just at the marker, and Distance defines the size of the intervals in cM. The *ibd_analysis* parameter gives directions to the GENIBD program. The parameter *mode* tells the program if *multipoint* or *singlepoint* analysis is to be conducted. The *title* and *output* will appear in the output file and in the name of the output file, respectively. The *region* parameter corresponds to a parameter in the genome map indicating to which chromosome or chromosome region the analysis corresponds. The last line of the file instructs SIBPAL2 to carry out a simple-regression analysis. Recall from the **Subheading 1.** that the simple-regression analysis estimates the total genetic variance as a result of the locus and the multiple-regression estimates the additive and dominance variance separately. Replacing the word "multiple" by "simple" in the above command would result in a multiple-regression analysis being conducted. However, it is strongly recommended that multiple regression not be carried out with multipoint IBD estimates. This is because a problem may occur that is the result of the fact that linked markers can be extremely linearly correlated, resulting in a singular design matrix during the regression. Many other options are available that have not been included in the sample parameter file given earlier. One should refer to the program documentation if they are interested in experimenting with the full range of options offered by the program. The parameter file given earlier will carry out the type of linkage analysis described in **Subheading 1.3.** It is possible to put comments in the parameter file that the program will not read. Comments are helpful reminders of what the file is instructing the program to do. Each line that the user does not want the program to read should begin with the # symbol.

4.2.3. The Locus File

The locus file includes the marker allele frequency data. Each marker to be analyzed must be represented in the locus file in order for the program to run. The locus file has a very specific format; the following is an example for two markers.

```
MARKER1
1 = 0.17
2 = 0.31
3 = 0.22
4 = 0.05
5 = 0.25 ;
;
MARKER2
1 = 0.61
2 = 0.23
3 = 0.08
4 = 0.08 ;
;
```

The marker names are given first followed by the frequency data. The marker names must be the same as the names defined in the pedigree and parameter files, and the allele names must be the same as they are in the pedigree file. Two semicolons must come after each marker in the file. All of the alleles that appear in the pedigree file must be specified in the marker locus file and the sum of the frequencies for each marker should be 1. The alleles can be numbers or characters as long as they correspond to what is in the pedigree file.

4.2.4. The Genome Map File

The genome map file is required for multipoint IBD analysis. The file defines the order of the markers and the genetic distances between them. The syntax of the genome file is very similar to the parameter file. An example of a genome map file for two markers separated by 10 cM is as follows:

```
genome
        {
        region=chr5
                {
                marker="MARKER1"
                distance=10.0
                marker="MARKER2"
                }
        }
```

In the example, the *region* parameter corresponds to the *region* parameter defined in the parameter file. The *region* parameter tells the program what group of markers to use in the multipoint analysis. The map of markers is then given by each marker followed by the distance to the next marker and so on for the region. The order of the markers in the pedigree file does not have to correspond to the map order, only the names. One could also define the map in terms of recombination fraction by substituting the *distance* for *theta*. The program is told to use a *Kosambi* or *Haldane* mapping function by adding an attribute to the *region* parameter. It is very important that the marker order be correct and the best estimates of the distances between markers be used for a multipoint analysis. An example of a genome map file that is specified in terms of recombination fraction is as follows:

```
genome
        {
        region=chr5,map=Haldane
                {
                marker="MARKER1"
                theta=0.10
                marker="MARKER2"
                }
        }
```

4.3. The Output Files

4.3.1. The Output File from GENIBD

The following file was generated by GENIBD. This file does not correspond to the earlier example files and is for a single-point analysis; this is because the GENIBD output file from a multipoint analysis is too large to show.

```
BD File 1.0: This File is automatically generated. Do NOT edit!
#=================================================================
#
MARKERS
#------
MARKER1
MARKER2
#========================================
# Pedigree  Ind 1 Ind 2   MARKER1 f0,   MARKER 1 f2,   MARKER 2 f0,   MARKER 2
f2.
#--------- ------ -----   -----------   ------------   ------------   ------------
        1,     3,    4,   0.000000000   0.000000000   1.000000000   0.000000000
```

A list of the locations where the IBD was estimated is given in the header of
the file. The results for the one pedigree analyzed appear on the last line. The
probabilities of the pair sharing 0 or 2 alleles IBD (f0 and f2) are shown at
each location where the IBD is estimated, with each line representing the
sharing between a pair of relatives in a family.

4.3.2. The Output File from SIBPAL2

A file generated by SIBPAL2 for a multipoint analysis follows. The data
used in the analysis that generated the results shown below were from 100
families similar to the one in the example pedigree file shown in **Subheading
4.3.1.** The parameter file used is the same as the one shown in **Subheading 4.3.1.**

```
S.A.G.E. RELEASE 4.0 Beta 5 -- Sibpal2 JUNE 2000
COPYRIGHT (C) 1999 CASE WESTERN RESERVE UNIVERSITY.

ANALYSIS OF FULL SIB COVARIANCE: Single regression
Using all markers since none were specified.
Using all traits since none were specified.
Regression for continuous trait 'Trait'.
----------------------------------------
Traits Phenotypes: Trait
Dependent variable: Mean-corrected trait cross-product
```

Marker, Covariate or Interaction	Pairs	Genetic Variance	Estimate	Std Error	P-value	
MARKER1	100	Total	2.2355	0.7662	0.00218250430	**
chr1 2.0	100	Total	2.2375	0.8224	0.00384826069	**
chr1 4.0	100	Total	2.1125	0.8639	0.00811925136	**
chr1 6.0	100	Total	1.8525	0.8824	0.01916059378	**
chr1 8.0	100	Total	1.4937	0.8736	0.04521613161	**
MARKER2	100	Total	1.1022	0.8397	0.09616221260	

The header of the file provides information about the analysis that was carried out, followed by the table of results. Two markers were used in the analysis, MARKER1 and MARKER2, and the IBD sharing was estimated at the markers and every 2 cM across the interval between the markers. The table shows the number of pairs used in the analysis and indicates that the "Total" genetic variance is being estimated in the analysis. The column under the heading "Estimate" is the estimate of the b parameter in the regression with the standard error of the estimate given in the next column. The "P-value" is the probability of the t-statistic and describes the significance of the regression parameter.

5. Worked Example

5.1. The Data

Data were simulated for the following example. The data consisted of 200 nuclear families having a single sibling pair. Three markers, each having four equally frequent alleles, were simulated at 20-cM intervals. A QTL was simulated to lie between two of the markers. Instructions for the preparation of real data are given in **Subheading 2.1.**

5.2. The Input Files

The pedigree, parameter, locus and, genome map files were called *chr1.ped, chr1.par, chr1.loc,* and *chr1.gen,* respectively. Only the first two pedigrees in the pedigree file are shown in the following followed by the full parameter, locus, and map files.

chr1.ped

```
PID  ID  P1  P2  SEX  TRAIT   MARKER1  MARKER2  MARKER3
  1   1   0   0   1     0.146    1/4      4/1      4/1
  1   2   0   0   2     1.466    1/2      2/4      4/2
  1   3   1   2   1     2.447    1/2      4/4      1/2
  1   4   1   2   2    -1.636    1/4      2/1      4/1
  2   1   0   0   1     0.861    2/4      2/3      1/3
  2   2   0   0   2    -0.323    2/2      1/2      3/4
  2   3   1   2   1    -1.475    2/2      1/2      4/1
  2   4   1   2   2    -1.541    2/2      2/2      3/3
```

chr1.par

```
pedigree,character

    individual_missing_value="0"
    sex_code, male="1", female="2"
    delimiters=" "
```

```
      delimiter_mode=multiple
      pedigree_id=PID
      individual_id=ID
      parent_id=P1
      parent_id=P2
      sex_field=SEX
      trait=Trait,missing="-99"
      marker=MARKER1,missing="0"
      marker=MARKER2,missing="0"
      marker=MARKER3,missing="0"
}
scan_type=interval
Distance=2
ibd_analysis
{
      Title="Multi-point"
      output = "MP"
      mode = multipoint
      region = chr1
}
trait_regression,simple
```

chr1.loc

```
MARKER1
1 = 0.25
2 = 0.25
3 = 0.25
4 = 0.25 ;
;

MARKER2
1 = 0.25
2 = 0.25
3 = 0.25
4 = 0.25 ;
;

MARKER3
1 = 0.25
2 = 0.25
3 = 0.25
4 = 0.25 ;
;
```

chr1.gen

```
genome
{
   region=chr1
      {
         marker  =  "MARKER1"
         distance = 20.0
         marker  =  "MARKER2"
         distance = 20.0
         marker  =  "MARKER3"
      }
}
```

5.3. Checking the Pedigree Data with PEDINFO

The following command was typed to start the PEDINFO program:

% pedinfo chr1.par chr1.ped

The program wrote a message to the screen saying that the program run was successful and it created the files *pedinfo.inf* and *pedinfo.out*. The *pedinfo.inf* file shows what the program read for the first 10 individuals, which confirmed that it had read the data correctly. The *pedinfo.out* file provides a table of counts and simple statistics that were calculated from the pedigree data. Running PEDINFO is not required for the analysis and is only recommended as a means of checking the data.

5.4. Estimating the IBD Allele Sharing

The parameter file has instructed the program to compute multipoint IBD estimates at 2-cM intervals across the 60-cM region defined in the map file. The program GENIBD requires all of the input files and was run by typing

% genibd chr1.par chr1.ped chr1.loc chr1.gen

For each unique pedigree in the pedigree file, the program printed the following message to the screen:

```
Multi-point: Pedigree 1
        Generating Marker Likelihoods       ...................Done.
        Generating Multipoint Information  ...................Done.
        Generating Multipoint Combined Info...................Done.
        Generating Multipoint IBDs         ...................Done.
```

The program created the files *genibd.inf* and *genome inf*. The *genibd.inf* file is similar to the *pedinfo.inf* file. The *genome.inf* file reports the frequencies of each genotype it has found in the sample. The *genome.inf* file is as follows:

```
S.A.G.E. RELEASE 4.0 Beta 5—GENIBD JUNE 2000
COPYRIGHT (C) 1999 CASE WESTERN RESERVE UNIVERSITY.

LOCUS DESCRIPTION:
--------------
Locus MARKER1
1 = 0.25, 2 = 0.25, 3 = 0.25, 4 = 0.25
 No. Genotype Genotypic Frequency
  0         1/1 0.062500
  1         1/2 0.125000
  2         1/3 0.125000
  3         1/4 0.125000
  4         2/2 0.062500
  5         2/3 0.125000
  6         2/4 0.125000
  7         3/3 0.062500
  8         3/4 0.125000
  9         4/4 0.062500

Locus MARKER2
1 = 0.25, 2 = 0.25, 3 = 0.25, 4 = 0.25
 No. Genotype Genotypic Frequency
  0         1/1 0.062500
  1         1/2 0.125000
  2         1/3 0.125000
  3         1/4 0.125000
  4         2/2 0.062500
  5         2/3 0.125000
  6         2/4 0.125000
  7         3/3 0.062500
  8         3/4 0.125000
  9         4/4 0.062500

Locus MARKER3
1 = 0.25, 2 = 0.25, 3 = 0.25, 4 = 0.25
 No. Genotype Genotypic Frequency
  0         1/1 0.062500
  1         1/2 0.125000
  2         1/3 0.125000
  3         1/4 0.125000
  4         2/2 0.062500
  5         2/3 0.125000
  6         2/4 0.125000
  7         3/3 0.062500
  8         3/4 0.125000
  9         4/4 0.062500
```

The IBD sharing information is contained in a file called MP.CHR1.ibd; the naming scheme is described in **Subheading 2.4.** All of the estimates for a sibling pair are reported on a single line of the IBD sharing file; therefore, the file is too large to show, but it is of similar format to the file shown in **Subheading 4.1.3.** The IBD file was used as input for SIBPAL2 program.

5.5. The Linkage Analysis

In the parameter file, the SIBPAL2 program was instructed to run the simple-regression linkage analysis. Recall that it is not recommended that multiple-regression analysis be carried out with multipoint IBD estimates. The program used the IBD file created by GENIBD along with the parameter and pedigree files. Typing the following command ran the program:

% sibpal2 chr1.par chr1.ped MP.CHR1.ibd

The program printed its progress to the screen and announced its completion. The program created a file called *sibpal2.inf* that is identical to the *pedinfo.inf* file created by the PEDINFO file. The results of the linkage analysis were written to a file called *traits.out* as follows:

```
S.A.G.E. RELEASE 4.0 Beta 5 -- Sibpal2 JUNE 2000
COPYRIGHT (C) 1999 CASE WESTERN RESERVE UNIVERSITY.

ANALYSIS OF FULL SIB COVARIANCE: Single regression

Using all markers since none were specified.
Using all traits since none were specified.
Regression for continuous trait 'Trait'.
----------------------------------------------------
Traits Phenotypes: Trait
Dependant variable: Mean-corrected trait cross-product
```

Marker, Covariate or Interaction	Pairs	Genetic Variance	Estimate	Std Error	P-value	
MARKER1	200	Total	1.6929	0.6028	0.00273672906	**
chr1 2.0	200	Total	1.8651	0.6482	0.00222480331	**
chr1 4.0	200	Total	2.0240	0.6906	0.00188787881	**
chr1 6.0	200	Total	2.1483	0.7263	0.00173532931	**
chr1 8.0	200	Total	2.2145	0.7513	0.00179236653	**
chr1 10.0	200	Total	2.2042	0.7622	0.00212629696	**
chr1 12.0	200	Total	2.1139	0.7573	0.00288087929	**
chr1 14.0	200	Total	1.9566	0.7375	0.00430805247	**
chr1 16.0	200	Total	1.7577	0.7054	0.00676637575	**
chr1 18.0	200	Total	1.5439	0.6652	0.01064846876	*

Marker, Covariate or Interaction	Pairs	Genetic Variance	Estimate	Std Error	P-value
MARKER2	200	Total	1.3362	0.6205	0.01624267046 *
chr1 22.0	200	Total	1.3758	0.6702	0.02070150866 *
chr1 24.0	200	Total	1.3729	0.7164	0.02837257574 *
chr1 26.0	200	Total	1.3124	0.7545	0.04176330209 *
chr1 28.0	200	Total	1.1861	0.7796	0.06486583045
chr1 30.0	200	Total	1.0004	0.7875	0.10272396376
chr1 32.0	200	Total	0.7773	0.7770	0.15914608937
chr1 34.0	200	Total	0.5470	0.7497	0.23322994088
chr1 36.0	200	Total	0.3363	0.7101	0.31813616303
chr1 38.0	200	Total	0.1611	0.6632	0.40417365652
MARKER3	200	Total	0.0257	0.6133	0.48329721794

The most significant evidence for linkage to the QTL ($p=0.0017$) is at the position 6 cM from marker 1; the locus was simulated to be at 10 cM from this marker. The asterisks next to the p-value symbolize the degree of significance of the results; one for p-values <0.05 and two for p-values <0.01. For the simple-regression model used in this analysis, the estimate of the regression coefficient is an estimate of the genetic variance resulting from the QTL. The total phenotypic variance of the simulated trait was approximately 3.0; therefore, with a regression parameter estimate of 2.1483, this QTL would account for 72% of the total variance in the trait. This would be considered a QTL of large effect. Given the standard error of 0.7263 on the estimate of the regression parameter, the QTL could account for as much as 96% or as little as 47% of the total phenotypic variance in the trait (mean estimate ± standard error).

6. Notes

1. Premature termination of S.A.G.E. S.A.G.E. generally gives a good indication of why it terminated early in the error messages printed in the *.inf* files. Should one of the programs fail to run, the first step should be to read these error messages. The most common reason for the failure of any analysis program to run is errors in the format or syntax of the input files. A description of the input files was given in **Subheading 4.2.** and it is important that the directions be followed closely. It is also recommended that the documentation for the program always be referenced when generating the input files, as formats may change. When data files have been manually typed into a computer, there may be typographical errors in the files; for example, a character in a field that requires numbers would cause most programs to terminate. When declaring the markers and traits in the parameter file, ensure that the definition that is given for the missing values are not a variable that might occur as a true value in the data. If you define 0 to be the missing value for the trait and there are individuals that have a trait value equal to 0, then these individuals

will be treated as having missing trait values and you will lose power. If files are created in a word processing or spreadsheet program like MS Word and Excel, the files must be saved as text in order to be read by the analysis programs. It is very common to have problems in trying to run a program the first time, so do not get discouraged if it happens to you.

2. Error reduction.   It is very important that the data be as free from errors as possible before one undertakes a linkage analysis.

   a. Pedigree structure errors.   Programs exist for checking that the relationships that one has designated in the pedigrees are consistent with the genotype data. The most common relationship problems associated with sib-pair analysis are half-sibs and monozygotic twins being defined as siblings. The program RELCHECK (**9**) is recommended for relationship checking.

   b. Genotyping errors.   The power of linkage analysis is greatly affected by geno-type errors. The first analysis of the genotype data should always be a search for genotype errors. Genotype errors become easier to detect as more pedigree members are typed, with single-marker genotypes in a single sib pair without parents giving no error detection information. The program PEDCHECK (**10**) is recommended for genotype error analysis.

3. Other software.   This chapter has used the GENIBD and SIBPAL2 programs for the linkage analysis. There are alternative ways of carrying out the new Haseman–Elston method. Other programs exist for conducting the IBD analysis, the most popular being the GENEHUNTER program (**8**). GENEHUNTER can print a file with the IBD sharing probabilities and this file would then have to be formatted for SIBPAL2. This would not be recommended for individuals who are not familiar with the file formats. If one is dedicated to using an alternative program for computing the IBD probabilities, they should run GENIBD as well and compare the results of the two programs and to get an example of the file format needed by SIBPAL2. SIBPAL2 is currently the only program that will do the new Haseman–Elston linkage analysis; however, individuals with good computer and statistical skills may wish to carry out the regression analysis using a statistical software package or write their own program to do the analysis. It is recommended that one check the results of their program to the results given by SIBPAL2 if they wish to use their own program.

Acknowledgment

   This work was supported by National Institutes of Health (NIH) grant GM-40282.

7. References

1. Haseman, J. K. and Elston, R. C. (1972) The investigation of linkage between a quantitative trait and a marker locus. *Behav. Genet.* **2**, 3–19.

2. Single, R. M. and Finch, S. J. (1995) Gain in efficiency from using generalized least squares in the Haseman–Elston test. *Genet. Epidemiol.* **12**, 889–894.

3. Drigalenko, E. (1998) How sib-pairs reveal linkage. *Am. J. Hum. Genet.* **63,** 1243–1245.

4. Elston, R. C., Buxbaum, S., Jacobs, K. B., and Olson, J. M. (2000) Haseman and Elston revisited. *Genet. Epidemiol.* **19,** 1–17.

5. Lander, E. and Kruglyak, L. (1995) Genetic dissection of complex traits: guidelines for interpreting and reporting linkage results. *Nature Genet.* **11,** 241–247.

6. Sawcer, S., et al. Empirical genomewide significance levels established by whole genome simulations. *Genet. Epidemiol.* **14,** 223–229.

7. Lathrop, G. and Lalouel, J. (1984) Easy calculations of lod scores and genetic risks on small computers. *Am. J. Hum. Genet.* **36,** 460–465.

8. Kruglyak, L., Daly, M. J., Reeve-Daly, M. P., and Lander, E. S. (1996) Parametric and nonparametric linkage analysis: a unified multipoint approach. *Am. J. Hum. Genet.* **58,** 1347–1363.

9. Boehnke, M. and Cox, N. J. (1997) Accurate inference of relationships in sib-pair linkage studies. *Am. J. Hum. Genet.* **61,** 423–429.

10. O'Connell, J. R. and Weeks, D. E. (1998) PedCheck: a program for identification of genotype incompatibilities in linkage analysis. *Am. J. Hum. Genet.* **63,** 259–266.

4

Nonparametric Linkage Analysis

II. Variance Components

Angela J. Marlow

1. Introduction

1.1. Background

R. A. Fisher combined Galtonian biometrics with Mendelian inheritance to establish what is known today as biometrical genetics. In his article "The Correlation Between Relatives on the Supposition of Mendelian Inheritance" (*1*), Fisher demonstrated that the normal distribution observed for many biological and behavioral traits could result from the inheritance of many individual loci. This formed the polygenic biometrical model, however, it should be noted that none of the biometrical expectations depend on the number of genes involved.

In general, the Fisher model specifies that any continuous phenotype, P, can be considered as a function of the effects of genes, G, and the environment, E:

$$P = G + E \tag{1}$$

Fisher extended this simple trait model into the context of analysis of variance, which provides a mechanism to partition observed variance into component parts. In the biometrical framework, this variance partitioning involves

$$V_P = V_G + V_E \tag{2}$$

where V_P represents the total phenotypic variance, V_G the genetic variance, and V_E the environmental variance.

With the appropriate data types (i.e., families), it is possible to estimate the genetic variance, V_G, and environmental variance, V_E, even though the pheno-

From: *Methods in Molecular Biology: vol. 195: Quantitative Trait Loci: Methods and Protocols.*
Edited by: N. J. Camp and A. Cox © Humana Press, Inc., Totowa, NJ

typic variance is the only observed quantity. This unobserved estimation is the essence of "variance components analysis" (VC) and is the main focus of this chapter. In order to appreciate the VC method and applications, however, it is useful to briefly review the principles of the biometric model that underlie variance components modeling.

1.2. The Biometrical Model

The biometrical model defines a quantitative trait in terms of the allele frequencies and genotypic values of a causative locus or loci. The simplest form of the model is one with a single locus and two alleles (A_1 and A_2). Two parameters define the measurable effects of the three possible genotypes, a and d. The parameter a, known as the "additive genetic value," is half the measured difference between the homozygotes' trait values, with the midpoint between $-a$ and $+a$ being the mean effect of the homozygous genotypes. The parameter d, the dominance deviation, represents the deviation of the heterozygous genotype from the midpoint. The allele frequencies of A_1 and A_2 are given by q and p, respectively. Loci that result from such effects are often referred to as quantitative trait loci (QTL).

The relationship between genotypes, effect parameters a and d, and their allele frequencies are shown in **Fig. 1** and **Table 1**.

The mean effect of the locus (here represented by g) is given by

$$\mu_g = \sum_{i=0}^{2} f_i x_i = a(p - q) + 2dpq \tag{3}$$

The variance of the genetic effects is given by

$$\begin{aligned}
\sigma_g^2 &= \sum f_i(x_i - \mu_g)^2 \\
&= \sum f_i x_i^2 - \mu_g^2 \\
\sigma_g^2 &= 2pq[a+(q - p)d]^2 + 4p^2q^2d^2 \\
\sigma_g^2 &= V_{ga} + V_{gd}
\end{aligned} \tag{4}$$

The genotypic variance at a locus can be partitioned further into additive and dominance components, as shown in Eq. (4), where $2pq[a+(q - p)d]^2$ and

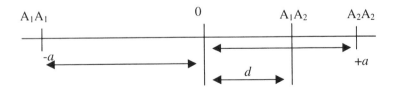

Fig. 1. Assignment of genotypic values

Table 1
Parameters of the Biometrical Model

No. of A_2 alleles (i)	0	1	2
Genotypes	A_1A_1	A_1A_2	A_2A_2
Frequency (f_i)	q^2	$2pq$	p^2
Genotypic effect (x_i)	$-a$	d	$+a$

$4p^2q^2d^2$ are termed the additive and dominance variance components, respectively. Under the assumption that many such loci contribute to a trait, the genetic variance in Eq. (2) can be partitioned into the cumulative additive genetic and dominance variance at many loci:

$$V_G = V_A + V_D \tag{5}$$

Similarly, the environmental variance, V_E, can be partitioned into unique, individual specific, environmental variance, V_S, and environmental variance that derives from common family effects, V_C:

$$V_E = V_S + V_C \tag{6}$$

When Eqs. (5) and (6) are inserted into Eq. (2), the full biometrical model (excluding interactions) becomes:

$$V_P = V_A + V_D + V_C + V_S \tag{7}$$

1.2.1. Covariance for Sib Pairs

The covariance between any pair of relatives can also be expressed in terms of the biometrical model. For example, the expected genetic covariance between sibling pairs can be expressed in terms of the values and frequencies of the nine possible sibling pair genotype combinations (2). The expected frequencies for the genotypes of the sibling pair (f_{ij}) are calculated taking into consideration the fact that sibs may share zero, one, or two alleles identical by descent (IBD) with probability 0.25, 0.5, and 0.25, respectively (*see* **Table 2**).

Given a locus with two alleles, the covariance for sibs reduces to

$$\text{Cov(sibs)} = \sum_{i=0}^{2} \sum_{j=0}^{2} f_{ij} \, (x_{1i} - \mu_g)(x_{2j} - \mu_g) \tag{8}$$
$$= pq[a+(q-p)d]^2 + p^2q^2d^2$$

When the sum of many such loci are considered, this covariance becomes

$$\text{Cov(sibs)} = \tfrac{1}{2}V_A + \tfrac{1}{4}V_D \tag{9}$$

Table 2
Expected Genetic Covariance for Sibling Pairs

				P(observing sibs' genotypes $\mid k$ alleles IBD)			
Sib 1	Sib2	x_{1i}	x_{2j}	$k=0$	$k=1$	$k=2$	f_{ij}
A_1A_1	A_1A_1	$-a$	$-a$	q^4	q^3	q^2	$V_4 q^2(q+1)^2$
A_1A_1	A_1A_2	$-a$	d	$2pq^3$	pq^2	0	$V_2 pq^2(q+1)$
A_1A_1	A_2A_2	$-a$	a	p^2q^2	0	0	$V_4 p^2q^2$
A_1A_2	A_1A_1	d	$-a$	$2pq^3$	pq^2	0	$V_2 pq^2(q+1)$
A_1A_2	A_1A_2	d	d	$4p^2q^2$	pq	$2pq$	$V_4 pq(pq+2)$
A_1A_2	A_2A_2	d	a	$2p^3q$	p^2q	0	$V_2 p^2q(p+1)$
A_2A_2	A_1A_1	a	$-a$	p^2q^2	0	0	$V_4 p^2q^2$
A_2A_2	A_1A_2	a	d	$2p^3q$	p^2q	0	$V_2 p^2q(p+1)$
A_2A_2	A_2A_2	a	a	p^4	p^3	p^2	$V_4 p^2(p+1)^2$

1.3. Heritability

Heritability is simply the proportion of observed variance attributed to genetic variance. In the "broad sense," it is $\dfrac{(V_A + V_D)}{V_P}$. In the more commonly used "narrow sense," it is simply $\dfrac{V_A}{V_P}$. The VC method can be used to estimate the heritability of a quantitative trait and this can and should be carried out before any marker data are obtained. Prior evidence for heritable effects is valuable, as it can be costly to initiate a large collection of pedigrees for linkage analysis only to discover that the trait of interest does not reveal any familial resemblance. Heritability is strictly relative and population-specific.

1.4. Linkage Analysis

The biometrical model underlies the analyses using the VC approach. Consider a phenotypic trait with a continuous distribution and known mean and variance in a population. Following the basic Fisher model, it is supposed that a number of loci are involved in the determination of an individual's trait value, along with a number of environmental factors. In order to estimate the variance parameters, family data are required. It is the known genetic structure of family data that provides the experimental design required to tease genetic and environmental effects apart.

The VC method can be extended in order to search for evidence of linkage to a particular locus. In this case, the estimate for overall heritability can be partitioned into a linked major gene effect and an unlinked remaining genetic effect. The latter may be the result of many genes (polygenic effect). At this point, the number of alleles shared at the locus by a pair of relatives determines the extent to which their trait value covaries. If the loci under investigation affects the trait, then it is expected that as the number of alleles shared increases, the covariance of the trait increases.

The linkage model is simply the full biometric model shown in Eq. (7), but incorporating direct observed effects from a putative QTL g as in Eq. (4):

$$V_P = V_A + V_D + V_C + V_S + V_{ga} + V_{gd} \tag{10}$$

or as parameters to be estimated:

$$\sigma_p^2 = \sigma_A^2 + \sigma_D^2 + \sigma_C^2 + \sigma_S^2 + \sigma_{ga}^2 + \sigma_{gd}^2 \tag{11}$$

Often, the environmental and polygenic effects are not partitioned, so the model becomes

$$
\begin{aligned}
\mathrm{Cov}(x_i, x_j) &= \sigma_{ga}^2 + \sigma_{gd}^2 + \sigma_G^2 + \sigma_E^2 \quad \text{if } i{=}j \\
\mathrm{Cov}(x_i, x_j) &= \pi_{ij}\sigma_{ga}^2 + \Delta_{ij}\sigma_{gd}^2 + \Phi_{ij}\sigma_G^2 \quad \text{if } i{\neq}j
\end{aligned}
\tag{12}
$$

where $x_{i\,or\,j}$ is the trait value for pedigree members i or j, σ_{ga}^2 is the major gene additive effect, $2pq[a-d(p-q)]^2$, σ_{gd}^2 is the major gene dominance effect, $4p^2q^2d^2$, σ_G^2 is the polygenic component, σ_E^2 is the residual environmental component, π_{ij} is the the proportion of genes shared IBD, Δ_{ij} is the probability that the pair shares both alleles IBD, and Φ_{ij} is the coefficient of relationship between the pairs of individuals, the mean probability that they share alleles IBD based on their relationship.

Simultaneously, the model can include the estimation of the trait mean and covariate effects, which are referred to as "fixed effects" in mixed-model terminology. The variance estimates are the "random effects" of the model; they are assumed to have zero correlation.

Assuming multivariate normality, the likelihood for the variances and covariances can be written. Using numerical methods, maximum likelihood estimates can be obtained for the major gene (σ_g^2) for each locus under investigation, as well as the polygenic (σ_G^2) and environmental (σ_E^2) variance components. The variance components are all constrained to have values greater than or equal to 0 to avoid meaningless estimates (**3**). Two likelihoods are compared: (1) allowing free estimation of the major gene effect and (2) assessing that there is no major gene effect (i.e., when σ_g^2 is constrained to be 0). When only the additive genetic component is estimated, minus twice the $\log_e$ likelihood ratio has an asymptotic distribution that is a 50:50 mixture of a χ^2 variable, with one degree of freedom and a point mass at 0 (**4**).

As well as identifying the location of any QTL, the relative size of the estimated variance component provides a measure of the magnitude of the effect of a detected locus. Generally these estimates show a small downward bias (5–7). This appears to be the result of the incorrect attribution of some variance to polygenic factors.

1.5. Advantages and Disadvantages of the Variance Components Method.

One of the advantages of the VC method is that it treats each family as a unit, explicitly allowing for statistical non-independence among sibs, and is less liable to type 1 error than are statistics based on pairs of relatives (*8*).

However, the assumption of multivariate normality can be a major constraint. Several factors can lead to markedly non-normal phenotypic distributions, including the presence of a major gene, some gene–environment interactions, and methods of selective sampling. It has been shown that the likelihood ratio test of the VC method is relatively robust to some types of non-normality but not to others (*9*). For example, the presence of a major gene induces platykurtosis, but simulations have shown that the VC method is robust to moderate platykurtosis. However, non-normality resulting from leptokurtosis does increase the type 1 error rates in excess of the nominal levels; the degree of inflation appears to be directly related to the residual sibling correlation (*9*). Also, in the presence of sibling correlation, marked kurtosis or skewness leads to a significant increase in the type 1 error rate. Therefore, when VC analysis is used, care should be taken that the distribution of the trait will not adversely affect the method. Transformation of the trait data to a normal distribution before the VC analysis can be performed. Otherwise, procedures that do not rely on specific distribution assumptions can be used such as quasi-likelihood methods (*5*) or simulation (*9*). When ascertainment has induced non-normality this can sometimes be corrected for if the ascertainment criteria are known (*10*). However, a failure to correct for ascertainment tends to lead to a loss of power rather than to inflation of the rate of type 1 error (**ref.** *11*; C. Amos, personal communication).

1.6. Type of Data

Family data are required for VC analysis. The smallest family unit could be nuclear families with either twin or sib-pair data. Genotypic and phenotypic information is required for the offspring; the parents are coded in the file to link the children. The presence of genotypic information for the parents is not essential but can help with both the accuracy and speed of the analysis; phenotypic information for the parents is also not essential.

The method generalizes to pedigrees of any size, however, the limiting factor is computing power. Estimating the identity by descent (IBD) probabilities and handling matrices for the variance components can prove computationally intensive. When extended families are used, both phenotypic and genotypic data are required for as many individuals in the family as possible; some individuals with missing data may need to be included in the pedigree to maintain the structure.

2. Methods

2.1. Explore Trait Data

Before beginning the analysis, it is very important to understand the trait under investigation. For the method to be unbiased, the trait must be a continuous variable and normally distributed.

It is important to carry out some exploratory statistics on the trait data. The simplest thing to do is to plot a histogram of the data and assess whether it appears to be normally distributed. Other diagnostic plots are available, such as the boxplot, the density plot, and the normal qq-plot, these provide an indication of the distribution and possible outliers. Higher order of moments such as skewness and kurtosis also help with assessing the distribution, as well as formal tests of normality, such as the Kolmogrov–Smirnov test. An example of the exploration of trait data is given in **Subheading 5.1**.

Summary statistics, such as the mean and variance, are also important, knowing these allows verification that the parameters estimated in the variance component model are reasonable.

Transformation of the trait data may be necessary in order to make its distribution normal, useful transformations include the log and square root. Statistical procedures are also available to determine the most appropriate transformation (e.g., Box–Cox).

2.2. Covariates

As mentioned, an individual's trait value may be influenced by a number of covariates. Typically, these include age, sex, smoking, and so forth. Scatter plots of the trait value against the covariate value for each individual allows visual inspection of any relationship between them. Regression analysis can determine the exact relationship and whether it is significant. It is often useful to adjust the trait for any known covariates, which can either be carried out by performing a regression analysis and then using the residuals in the VC analysis, or by including the covariates in the main analysis.

Alternatively, one may standardize the sample trait using a standard population (e.g., with family data for developmental dyslexia, one may adjust the reading ability by age using the relationship between reading ability and age in a matched normative population). This can be done if the relationship between reading ability and age is known in an equivalent standard population (regression equation) (*11*). In this case, the residuals for each family member can then be calculated and used in the VC analysis.

2.3. Ascertainment

The distribution of a number of traits is normal in human populations if the sample is randomly ascertained from the population. However, in many of the QTL mapping experiments of today, the ascertainment criteria are seldom random.

Either because of a desire to increase power or because we are interested in the genes that cause disease where, over some threshold value, a continuous trait indicates a clinical disorder, alternative experimental designs are often implemented, such as the extreme discordant design (*12*). Alternatively, single ascertainment may be used (i.e., based on families containing at least one individual with a trait value at or above a threshold with their relatives showing variation in their trait value).

Ascertainment often results in the departure of the trait data from normality. Adjustment for ascertainment where the criteria are known can be made and this can circumvent this problem. For example, if families are ascertained on the trait value of a single individual exceeding some threshold, then this can be adjusted for in the maximum likelihood estimation of the model. However, different schemes of ascertainment are often difficult to deal with in practice. By correcting for ascertainment, the parameters estimated in the sample (e.g., heritability) can be applied to the general population from which the sample was drawn. If no correction can be made, then the parameters estimated are appropriate only to the sample. In fact, some derived quantitative measures may have little meaning outside of a clinical sample (e.g., diagnostic question-naires of some behavioral traits).

Non-normal trait data can also be dealt with using a simulation procedure to determine the significance of the test statistic empirically (*9*). This procedure can be automated, but it may prove computationally infeasible. Alternatively, quasi-likelihood methods that relax the assumptions of multivariate normality can be used (*5*). This approach should provide more efficient estimates of the parameters, but it does depend on large samples for correct hypothesis testing.

2.4. Overview of Standard Variance Components Analysis

2.4.1. Estimating Identity-by-Descent Probabilities

Before the models are constructed, the probabilities that relatives share alleles identical by descent (IBD) are calculated from the marker data. This information as well as the trait values are used to estimate the required variance components.

2.4.2. Estimating the Variance Components and Assessing Linkage Evidence

The basic analyses involves the fitting of two models (as described in **Subheading 1.4.**). The first is the null model, where the major gene effect is constrained to be 0. The polygenic additive effect and an environmental effect are included in this model. Second, the alternative model is fitted, in which the size of the major gene effect is estimated. This model includes a QTL additive genetic effect (major gene effect), a residual polygenic additive effect (unlinked genetic effect), and an environmental effect. These two models are fitted at regular intervals along a chromosome, and minus twice the $\log_e$ likelihood ratio between the two models is calculated at each point. The degree of significance of the corresponding χ^2 value (or, equivalently, the log odds [LOD] score) can be used to determine the most likely position of the QTL affecting the trait.

2.4.3. Estimating Heritability

With regard to heritability, the most interesting values are the overall heritability of the trait and the heritability of a trait that can be attributed to the major gene at the location of interest. The first of these, the overall heritability of the trait, is estimated by the polygenic additive variance as calculated under the null hypothesis. The heritability attributable to a specific locus is estimated by the additive major gene effect variance (also called the additive QTL effect) under the alternative hypothesis, with the additive polygenic effect under the alternative hypothesis estimating the heritability not accounted for by the QTL.

These estimates are important because they indicate the effect size of the QTL located by the analysis (i.e., the proportion of the genetic variance [or total variance] that is accounted for by the identified locus).

2.4.4. Notes on the Variance Components Software Programs

The standard genetic VC analyses can be carried out using three widely available software packages: GENEHUNTER (*7, 13*), SOLAR (*14*) and ACT (*5*). **Subheadings 2.5., 2.6.,** and **2.7.** will demonstrate the use of these three software packages. The ease of use of these three programs relates to the complexity of the analysis that each can perform. However, when familiarizing oneself with the method and the program, it can become frustrating if all that is required is a basic analysis.

Although better documentation and the use of a standard format for input files and clearer output can be a criticism, it should be noted that these programs, along with most other genetic analysis packages, are freely available from research groups whose sole interest is not the development of software.

2.5. GENEHUNTER

2.5.1. Introduction to GENEHUNTER

GENEHUNTER (GH) is probably the simplest of the three programs to use in terms of the file format, the steps involved in the analysis, and the output.

The file format is of a standard form that has long been used in linkage programs (*15*). As the extent of the options for the VC analysis is limited, this helps with the ease of getting to grips with the basic analysis. The documentation is clear with regard to the commands available and there is on-line help available, but there is limited description of the output files.

The IBD sharing estimates use an exact multipoint approach to extract the full probability distribution of allele sharing at every point (*16*); however, because of this exact calculation the size of the families is limited. No single-point option (two-point analysis; one marker locus, one trait locus) is available for the quantitative analysis in GH 2.0 (beta) as it is for the qualitative analysis.

Covariates can be included in the analysis, although there is no option to incorporate ascertainment correction. Estimates of the mean can be switched between a single mean for both sexes or sex specific means. Estimates of the variance components for both the polygenic and major gene can include the effect of dominance variance. This can be important when estimating the effect of a putative QTL, as a trait with dominance variance analyzed under a model lacking this component can result in an inflated estimate of the additive effect. This is the result of the dominance variance being incorrectly specified. There is an option to input start values for the VC analysis, but the default is to use a constant fraction of the total phenotypic variance.

2.5.2. File Formats

Two files are required to run GH: the locus (datain) file and a pedigree file.

2.5.2.1. THE LOCUS FILE

The locus file describes the marker data, the affection locus, the traits, and the covariates. The affection locus needs to be present, although it is not used in the QTL analysis. The order and layout of the locus or datain file is important, as is the corresponding order of the loci between the locus file and the pedigree file.

The following is an example of the file format that was used to analyze the simulated Q4 trait data (see **Subheading 5.** for details on the trait Q4). The format is standard linkage (*15*) except that the third line contains only listings for the disease locus (numbered 1) and the 50 genotypic markers (numbered

2 to 51). The traits and covariates are not included in this list. Briefly, the first number on line 1 contains the total number of disease loci, marker loci, traits, and covariates. In the example, this is 52: 1 disease locus, 50 genotypic markers, and 1 trait (Q4). The third line, as noted earlier, numbers only the disease and marker loci. The disease locus lines start with "1 2" and below the allele, frequencies are given, followed by the number of liability classes and the penetrances. These are ignored for the VC analysis. Each marker locus lines starts with a number 3, followed by the number of alleles for that marker, the frequencies of the alleles follow on the line below. Each phenotype trait requires a line starting with "0 2 #" followed by five lines containing either the standard linkage information for a trait or five empty lines, as GH does not use this information. In the example locus file in **Fig. 2**, the five lines beneath "0 2 #" are consistent for the linkage file format. The penultimate line contains the intermarker distances. In **Fig. 2**, these are given in Haldane cM.

2.5.1.2. THE PEDIGREE FILE

The pedigree data file is a standard linkage premakeped format. It contains the necessary information to construct each pedigree. Parents must be defined in order to structure the pedigree even if no information is known about them. A single row is required for each individual in a family containing the following information: Pedigree, IndividualID, FatherID, MotherID, Sex, Affection, Alleles of Marker1,..., Alleles of Marker$n$, Trait1,..., Trait$k$,, Covariate1,..., Covariate$m$. The order of the fields is important, as the pedigree structure is established first, then the gender (1 male, 2 female), then the affection status (2 affected, 1 unaffected, 0 is unknown). The affection status will not be used in a quantitative analysis, so a dummy value can be used, but it must be included. The marker information follows and, finally, the traits and covariates. As already mentioned, it is essential that the order of the loci correspond to the order in the locus file. The code for missing variables is 0, except for the quantitative variables (traits, covariates) when the code is a dash (-).

The following is an example of a pedigree file with two nuclear families, five markers, one trait, and no covariates:

```
1 1 0 0 1 2 2 3 4 5 1 3 3 4 1 2   -
1 2 0 0 2 2 2 4 2 6 1 3 4 4 3 5   -
1 3 1 2 2 2 2 3 2 5 1 1 3 4 1 3 11.047
1 4 1 2 1 2 2 4 4 6 3 3 4 4 1 5 12.1438
2 1 0 0 1 2 2 3 3 5 2 3 3 7 3 3 10.28
2 2 0 0 2 2 2 5 4 6 2 4 4 5 1 3 10.7452
2 3 1 2 2 2 2 5 4 5 2 2 3 5 3 3 11.0479
2 4 1 2 2 2 2 2 5 6 2 2 3 5 1 3 10.6258
```

```
                    Total number of markers, traits, covariates and affection status.

52 0 0 5

0 0.000 0.000 0

1 2 3 4 5 6 7 8 9 10 11 12 13 14 15 16 17 18 19 20 21 22 23 24 25 26 27 28 29 30 31

32 33 34 35 36 37 38 39 40 41 42 43 44 45 46 47 48 49 50 51

1 2 # Aff

0.500000 0.500000              "these numbers should not include the traits or covariates"

1

1.0000 1.0000 1.0000

3 5 # D8G1

0.093800 0.406200 0.250000 0.156200 0.093800

~

~

3 6 # D8G50

0.233300 0.300000 0.300000 0.133300 0.033300 0.000100

0 2 # Q4                              Only this line is required to define a trait

0.500000 0.500000                    the following five lines may be left blank

1

0.250000 0.500000 0.250000 << GENOTYPE MEANS

0.500000

1.000000

0 -1

0.50000 0.02200 0.03200 0.00901 0.02199 0.02300 0.03000 0.02499 0.01001 0.00800

0.01300 0.02200 0.01500 0.01800 0.02400 0.01800 0.02200 0.02500 0.01199 0.01300

0.02500 0.02400 0.02199 0.02300 0.01800 0.02801 0.01500 0.01300 0.02200 0.02100

0.02100 0.01700 0.01200 0.01100 0.02299 0.02801 0.02500 0.02199 0.02300 0.01300

0.01700 0.02200 0.02200 0.02499 0.02101 0.02199 0.03300 0.03200 0.00801 0.01800

0.50000 Haldane

1 0.10000 0.45000
```

Fig. 2. Locus file format for GH

2.5.3. Running GENEHUNTER.

This section illustrates how to run an analysis using GENEHUNTER. The program may be run interactively, and the following example illustrates such an interactive run. The trait data that are being analyzed is trait Q4 from the GAW10 data analysis workshop (*17*). See **Subheading 5.** for more details.

```
***********************************************************************
*                                                                     *
*         GENEHUNTER - Complete Linkage Analysis                      *
*              (version 2.0 beta (r2))                                *
*                                                                     *
***********************************************************************
Type 'help' or '?' for help.

npl:1> load gh_dat.08
Parsing Linkage marker data file...
50 markers read (last one = D8G50)

npl:2> use
Current map (50 markers):
D8G1 2.2 D8G2 3.3 D8G3 0.9 D8G4 2.2 D8G5 2.4 D8G6 3.1 D8G7 2.6 D8G8 1.0 D8G9
0.8 D8G10 1.3 D8G11 2.2 D8G12 1.5 D8G13 1.8 D8G14 2.5 D8G15 1.8 D8G16 2.2
D8G17 2.6 D8G18 1.2 D8G19 1.3 D8G20 2.6 D8G21 2.5 D8G22 2.2 D8G23 2.4 D8G24
1.8 D8G25 2.9 D8G26 1.5 D8G27 1.3 D8G28 2.2 D8G29 2.1 D8G30 2.1 D8G31 1.7
D8G32 1.2 D8G33 1.1 D8G34 2.4 D8G35 2.9 D8G36 2.6 D8G37 2.2 D8G38 2.4 D8G39
1.3 D8G40 1.7 D8G41 2.2 D8G42 2.2 D8G43 2.6 D8G44 2.1 D8G45 2.2 D8G46 3.4
D8G47 3.3 D8G48 0.8 D8G49 1.8 D8G50

npl:3> incre dist 1.0
Scanning will now be done in constant increments of 1.0 cM

npl:4> disp off
Screen display of NPL scores, LOD scores, and haplotypes is now 'off'

npl:5> scan gh_ped.08
analyzing pedigree 1...
using non-originals: 3 4
~
~
~
~
analyzing pedigree 239...
using non-originals: 3 4

npl:6> means by sex

Genehunter currently estimates male and female means separately.

1. Estimate a single mean
2. Estimate male and female means separately
Enter the index of the option you want to use [2]: 1

npl:7> variance components

include polygenic dominance variance component? y/n [y]: n
include QTL dominance variance component? y/n [y]: n

file to store variance components [vc.out]:vc.out
file to store parameter correlations [corr.out]:corr.out
Manually enter starting values for means and variances? y/n [y]: n
```

```
Analysis complete
text output file successfully written

npl:8> quit

    ...goodbye...
```

2.5.4. *GENEHUNTER Output*

GENEHUNTER outputs a file with the default name vc.out unless the user specifies an alternative name. Chromosomal position is indicated in the first column. The second column indicates the LOD-score evidence for a QTL gene at each specific chromosomal position. The third and fourth columns indicate the trait mean (and standard deviation), followed by the fifth and sixth columns, which indicate the additive polygenic variance estimate (and standard deviation) under the alternative hypothesis. The seventh and eighth columns show the environmental variance estimate, with its standard deviation, and the ninth and tenth column indicates the additive QTL variance estimate (and standard deviation) under the alternative hypothesis. The final column indicates whether the run converged or not.

Beneath the estimates under the alternative hypothesis (free model), the estimates for mean trait value, additive polygenic variance, and environmental variance are given under the null hypothesis (additive QTL variance constrained to zero).

```
vc.out

pos LOD     Mean            Additive (P)    Environmental    Additive (QTL)   C

0 0.16617 11.54885(0.04132) 0.44351(0.10502) 0.40871(0.04990) 0.07321(0.07865) Y

1 0.19447 11.54891(0.04133) 0.43835(0.10545) 0.40818(0.04988) 0.07906(0.07934) Y

2 0.21962 11.54893(0.04134) 0.43527(0.10482) 0.40765(0.04986) 0.08281(0.07861) Y

~

52 1.0899 11.54703(0.04123) 0.31476(0.11142) 0.41046(0.04995) 0.20022(0.08718) Y

53 1.2705 11.54668(0.04122) 0.29573(0.11099) 0.41113(0.04999) 0.21896(0.08655) Y

54 1.3906 11.54687(0.04121) 0.28047(0.11224) 0.41258(0.05008) 0.23270(0.08788) Y

55 1.3893 11.54736(0.04123) 0.27731(0.11351) 0.41181(0.05005) 0.23688(0.08953) Y

56 1.2579 11.54797(0.04125) 0.29364(0.11305) 0.41035(0.04998) 0.22202(0.08907) Y

~

100   0   11.54796(0.04129) 0.51452(0.10638) 0.41019(0.04993) 0.00000(0.07979) Y

101   0   11.54796(0.04129) 0.51452(0.10668) 0.41019(0.04993) 0.00000(0.08024) Y

Parameter estimates under null hypothesis:

 Mean trait value = 11.547963 (0.041291)

  Polygenic additive variance = 0.514516 (0.069893)

  Environmental variance = 0.410193 (0.049926)
```

2.6. Solar

2.6.1. Introduction to SOLAR

Like GH, the user can run SOLAR interactively. The file format is not standard linkage format, but it is easily formatted and is described in the documentation and on-line help. There are extensive options available in SOLAR, although some require considerable understanding of the program and are not well documented. However, the documentation that is available includes clear descriptions of the basic commands, together with example runs. GAW10 test data are also provided.

Standard options available include the ability to estimate the heritability before doing any linkage analysis and the inclusion and significance testing of covariates. SOLAR automatically corrects for any significant covariates in the analysis, unless specified otherwise. The trait values in SOLAR appear to be adjusted by covariates using regression outside of the VC analysis, unlike GH and ACT. This procedure has implications when there are extensive missing data. Ascertainment correction for single selection is available. Two-point and multipoint analyses are available. For two-point analyses, the IBD estimate at the marker loci uses the method of Curtis and Sham (*18*) as the default or a Monte Carlo procedure (*19*), depending on the pedigree structure. For multipoint analyses, SOLAR uses an approximation to a multipoint method to estimate the IBD sharing at positions along the chromosome by means of regression on the IBD values at marker loci (*20*).

Estimating the dominance variance at the QTL or polygenes is possible from the extension of the model, however, this is not a straightforward option. Other options available include the estimation of any household effects, bivariate trait analysis, and a Bayesian approach to oligogenic modeling.

2.6.2. File Formats

SOLAR requires at least four files and an optional fifth file if you provide the allele frequencies rather than allowing the program to estimate them from the data. The five files are the pedigree file, phenotype file, marker file, map file, and the frequencies file. It is very important that the pedigree structure remains consistent across files. Marker names and order must also be consistent between files, although they do not have to be in map order, as this is taken from the map file.

2.6.2.1. PEDIGREE FILE

This file contains the pedigree structure defined by pedigreeID, individualID, fatherID, motherID, and gender. Founders of pedigrees have their parents coded as 0, the fields are comma delimited, and the header is required.

```
FAMID,ID,FA,MO,SEX
1,1,0,0,M
1,2,0,0,F
1,3,1,2,F
1,4,1,2,M
2,1,0,0,M
2,2,0,0,F
2,3,1,2,F
2,4,1,2,F
```

2.6.2.2. PHENOTYPE FILE

This file contains the pedigreeID and individualID, which must match those of the pedigree file, followed by any trait values. It also contains any covariates and proband status if required; the file is comma delimited with missing values as blanks and the header is required.

```
FAMID,ID,Q4
1,1,
1,2,
1,3, 11.04700
1,4, 12.14380
2,1, 10.28000
2,2, 10.74520
2,3, 11.04790
2,4, 10.62580
```

2.6.2.3. MARKER FILE

This file contains the marker information for each individual, and again, the IDs must correspond to the pedigree file. The missing code is 0 and the fields are comma delimited, alleles are separated by a back slash, and the header is required.

```
FAMID,ID,D8G1,D8G2,D8G3,  . . . . . . . . . . .  D8G49,D8G50
1,1,2/ 3,4/ 5,1/ 3,  . . . . . . . . . .  2/ 4,1/ 2
1,2,2/ 4,2/ 6,1/ 3,  . . . . . . . . .  6/ 6,3/ 5
1,3,2/ 3,2/ 5,1/ 1,  . . . . . . . . .  2/ 6,1/ 3
1,4,2/ 4,4/ 6,3/ 3,  . . . . . . . . .  2/ 6,1/ 5
2,1,2/ 3,3/ 5,2/ 3,  . . . . . . . . .  5/ 5,3/ 3
2,2,2/ 5,4/ 6,2/ 4,  . . . . . . . . .  6/ 7,1/ 3
2,3,2/ 5,4/ 5,2/ 2,  . . . . . . . . .  5/ 6,3/ 3
2,4,2/ 2,5/ 6,2/ 2,  . . . . . . . . .  5/ 7,1/ 3
```

2.6.2.4. MAP FILE

The file contains the chromosome number (e.g., chromosome 8) and then the markers are listed in map order, followed by their cumulative position in Kosambi cM. The names must correspond to the names given in the marker file.

```
8
   D8G1 0.000000
   D8G2 2.201548
   D8G3 5.405937
   ~
   ~
   D8G50 98.969506
```

2.6.2.5. FREQUENCY FILE

This file contains the name of each of the markers, followed by the name of each allele and its frequencies. The order of the markers must match the order of the markers in the marker file. The fields are spaced delimited and no header is required.

```
D8G1 1 0.093800 2 0.406200 3 0.250000 4 0.156200 5 0.093800
D8G2 1 0.035700 2 0.107100 3 0.107100 4 0.107100 5 0.464300 6 0.178600 7
0.000100
D8G3 1 0.250000 2 0.250000 3 0.343800 4 0.093800 5 0.062500
~
~
D8G50 1 0.233300 2 0.300000 3 0.300000 4 0.133300 5 0.033300 6 0.000100
```

2.6.3. Running SOLAR

This section illustrates how to run an analysis using SOLAR. The program may be run interactively, and the following example illustrates such an interactive run. The trait data that are analyzed here are for trait Q4 from the GAW10 data analysis workshop, as earlier (*17*). See **Subheading 5.** for more details.

```
SOLAR version 1.5.7, compiled on Mar 8 2000 at 15:21:46.
Copyright (c) 1995-2000 Southwest Foundation for Biomedical Research
Enter help for help, exit to exit.
solar> load ped solar_ped.08
solar> load freq solar_freq.08
solar> load marker solar_marker.08
solar> load map solar_map.08
solar> load phen solar_phen.08
solar_phen.08: FAMID ID Q4
solar> automodel solar_phen.08 Q4
solar> polygenic -s
*******************************************************************
* (Screening) Get starting beta values using sporadic type model *
* with diagonal covariance matrices (default for sporadic)       *
*******************************************************************

*******************************************************************
* (Screening) Maximize polygenic model with all covariates       *
*******************************************************************
```

```
**********************************************************************
* (Screening) Maximize polygenic models                             *
* one with each covariate deactivated                               *
**********************************************************************
  *** Testing covariate sex by suspending it ***

  *** Loglikelihood w/o covar sex is -410.041622
  *** chi = 0.8640, deg = 1
  *** p = 0.3526089 (Not Significant)

**********************************************************************
* Covariate screening completed                                     *
* Now using models with only significant or fixed covariates        *
* Maximize sporadic model                                           *
**********************************************************************

  *** Loglikelihood of sporadic model is -460.857697

*******************************************************************
* Maximize polygenic model                                        *
*******************************************************************

  *** Loglikelihood of polygenic model is -410.041622
  *** H2r in polygenic model is 0.5564083

  *** Determining significance of H2r
  *** Comparing polygenic and sporadic models
  *** chi = 101.6321, deg = 1, p < 0.0000001

*******************************************************************
*            Summary of Results                                   *
*******************************************************************
    Pedigree:   solar_ped.08
    Phenotypes: solar_phen.08
    Trait:   Q4              Individuals: 1000

            H2r is 0.5564083 p < 0.0000001 (Significant)
       H2r Std. Error: 0.0586150

                    sex p = 0.3526089 (Not Significant)

    The following covariates were removed from final models:

sex
    No covariates were included in the final model
    Output files and models are in directory Q4/
    Summary results are in Q4/polygenic.out
    Best model is named Q4/poly or null0 (currently loaded)
    Final models are named poly, spor
    Constrained covariate models are named no<covariate name>
```

```
solar> mkdir ibds
solar> ibddir ibds
solar> ibd
Computing IBDs for D8G1 ... pedigree 239
Computing IBDs for D8G2 ... pedigree 239
Computing IBDs for D8G49 ... pedigree 239
Computing IBDs for D8G50 ... pedigree 239
solar> twopoint
        Model          LOD         Loglike       H2r       H2q1
  --------------    ---------   -----------   --------   --------
        D8G1          0.0041     -410.032  0.541479  0.014943
        D8G2          0.0084     -410.022  0.537041  0.020323
  ~

  ~

        D8G49         0.0020     -410.037  0.547319  0.008985
        D8G50         0.0000     -410.042  0.556408  0.000000
                 Highest New Result
        D8G27         2.0828     -405.246  0.211719  0.344942
    *** Results have been written to Q4/twopoint.out
solar> mkdir mibd
solar> mibddir mibd
solar> mibd 1
Creating relative-class file ...

Merging marker IBDs ...
Computing mean IBD by relative-class ...
Computing multi-point IBDs:
solar> chromosome 8
solar> interval 1
solar> multipoint 3
         Model          LOD         Loglike       H2r       H2q1
  --------------    ---------   -----------   --------   --------
         polygenic               -410.042  0.556408  0.000000
         Model          LOD         Loglike       H2r       H2q1
  --------------    ---------   -----------   --------   --------
chrom 8 loc    0      0.0239     -409.987  0.522277  0.034762
chrom 8 loc    1      0.0326     -409.967  0.517250  0.040094
  ~

  ~

chrom 8 loc   98      0.0000     -410.042  0.556408  0.000000
chrom 8 loc   99      0.0000     -410.042  0.556408  0.000000
    *** Highest LOD in pass 1 was 1.4988 at Chrom 8 Loc 52
    *** Additional information is in files named Q4/multipoint*.out
solar> quit
```

2.6.4. SOLAR Output

Numerous files are output from SOLAR and it also creates a number of directories for each marker and trait analyzed. The files required are in the directory under the trait name (Q4). The polygenic.out and poly.mod file, contain the results for the analysis before fitting marker data, including parameter estimates and their standard errors. The files twopoint.out, multipoint.out, and the last model.out contain the results when fitting a QTL. The file null1.out has the parameters estimates and standard errors under the alternative hypothesis containing one QTL (the file null0.out contains the results for no linkage components, null2.out would be for two QTLs and so forth).

2.6.4.1. POLYGENIC.OUT

```
Pedigree: solar_ped.08
Phenotypes: solar_phen.08
Trait:   Q4 Individuals: 1000

        H2r is 0.5564083 p < 0.0000001 (Significant)
    H2r Std. Error: 0.0586150

                  sex p = 0.3526089 (Not Significant)

The following covariates were removed from final models:

sex
No covariates were included in the final model
Loglikelihoods and chi values are in Q4/polygenic.logs.out
Final models are named poly, spor
Initial sporadic and polygenic models are s0 and p0
Constrained covariate models are named no<covariate name>
```

2.6.4.2. POLY.MOD.

```
solarmodel 1.5.7
trait Q4
parameter   mean = 11.54796336  Lower 8.4764   Upper 14.4849
parameter   mean         se 0.04129878331  score -7.73110338e-08
parameter   sd  = 0.9616178908 Lower 0      Upper 4.808069294
parameter   sd           se 0.02371642557  score -5.671905994e-07
parameter   e2  = 0.4435916656 Lower 0.01    Upper 1
parameter   e2           se 0.05861500703  score -3.720608479e-07
parameter   h2r = 0.5564083344 Lower 0      Upper 1
parameter   h2r          se 0.05861500703  score -1.935039784e-07
parameter  h2q1  = 0             Lower -0.01   Upper 1
constraint h2q1  = 0
constraint e2 + h2r = 1
omega = pvar*(phi2*h2r + I*e2)
# Mu is determined by covariates only
loglike set -410.041622
```

2.6.4.3. TWOPOINT.OUT.

Model	LOD	Loglike	H2r	H2q1
D8G1	0.0041	-410.032	0.541479	0.014943
D8G2	0.0084	-410.022	0.537041	0.020323
~				
D8G26	1.0788	-407.558	0.310498	0.244510
D8G27	**2.0828**	**-405.246**	**0.211719**	**0.344942**
~				
D8G49	0.0020	-410.037	0.547319	0.008985
D8G50	0.0000	-410.042	0.556408	0.000000

2.6.4.4. MULTIPOINT1.OUT.

Model		LOD	Loglike	H2r	H2q1
chrom 8 loc	0	0.0239	-409.987	0.522277	0.034762
chrom 8 loc	1	0.0326	-409.967	0.517250	0.040094
chrom 8 loc	2	0.0440	-409.940	0.511962	0.045720
~					
chrom 8 loc	46	0.9279	-407.905	0.340474	0.215403
chrom 8 loc	47	1.0722	-407.573	0.323335	0.232023
chrom 8 loc	48	1.2131	-407.248	0.308344	0.246829
chrom 8 loc	49	1.3365	-406.964	0.297270	0.258105
chrom 8 loc	50	1.4181	-406.776	0.290665	0.264718
chrom 8 loc	51	1.4790	-406.636	0.283202	0.272212
chrom 8 loc	**52**	**1.4988**	**-406.590**	**0.275729**	**0.279684**
chrom 8 loc	53	1 .3353	-406.967	0.284180	0.270827
chrom 8 loc	54	1.2004	-407.278	0.296141	0.259599
chrom 8 loc	55	1.0350	-407.658	0.316016	0.240630
chrom 8 loc	56	0.9520	-407.849	0.327536	0.229269
~					
~					
chrom 8 loc	98	0.0000	-410.042	0.556408	0.000000
chrom 8 loc	99	0.0000	-410.042	0.556408	0.000000

*** Highest LOD in pass 1 was 1.4988 at Chrom 8 Loc 52

2.6.4.5. LAST.MOD

This file contains the final model estimated in SOLAR.

```
solarmodel 1.5.7

trait Q4
parameter mean = 11.54739378  Lower 8.4764        Upper 14.4849
parameter   sd = 0.9620326041 Lower 0             Upper 4.808069294
parameter   e2 = 0.444586964  Lower 0.3445862523 Upper 0.5407575693
parameter  h2r = 0.275728541  Lower 0             Upper 0.6120491678
parameter h2q1 = 0.279684495  Lower 0             Upper 0.3722121489
constraint e2 + h2q1 + h2r = 1
omega = pvar*(phi2*h2r + I*e2 + mibd1*h2q1)
# Mu is determined by covariates only
```

2.6.4.6. NULL1.MOD

This file contains the parameters for the alternative hypothesis assuming one QTL. It contains the upper and lower value of these estimates and their standard errors.

```
solarmodel 1.5.7
matrix load /tmp/angela/mibd/mibd.8.52.gz mibd1
trait Q4
parameter  mean = 11.54739378  Lower 8.4764        Upper 14.4849
parameter  mean            se 0.04120648496    score -7.496902402e-05
parameter    sd = 0.96203261  Lower 0            Upper 4.808069294
parameter    sd            se 0.02385084992    score -0.01785785247
parameter    e2 = 0.4445869498 Lower 0.3445862523 Upper 0.5407575693
parameter    e2            se 0.05879505211    score -0.008254964227
parameter   h2r = 0.2757285431 Lower 0           Upper 0.6120491678
parameter   h2r            se 0.1302041715    score -0.008312984156
parameter  h2q1 = 0.2796845071 Lower 0           Upper 0.3722121489
parameter  h2q1            se 0.1081721848    score -0.009394667769
constraint e2 + h2q1 + h2r = 1
omega = pvar*(phi2*h2r + I*e2 + mibd1*h2q1)
# Mu is determined by covariates only
loglike set -406.590401
```

2.7. ACT

2.7.1. Introduction to ACT

The ACT package comes as a series of programs. The function and how they interact with each other need to be established before any analysis can be embarked upon. The sheer amount of files can be daunting, and although documentation is provided in each directory for that specific program, a document giving the overall structure of the package would be useful. The documentation for the Multic program comes closest to this. Example data are also provided with the ACT package.

Multic is the program that carries out the VC analysis. It does this one position at a time so it needs to be put in a script to loop through the analysis if analyzing more than one marker or multipoint analysis; this means that two-point analysis can be performed.

The file format depends on the program used, for the following example, the input data to calculate the IBD probabilities are in a GH format. The files for Multic have default names fort.12 (pedigree information) and multic.par (the control file). The format for these files is not standard, but the availability of utility programs makes the process easier.

Covariates can be included in the analysis, as can proband status for ascertainment correction. Additional features offered by the ACT package include quasi-likelihood, double ascertainment, bivariate/multivariate trait analysis, and longitudinal data analysis.

2.7.2. File Formats

In our example, the IBD sharing estimates have been generated by a modified GH program supplied in the ACT distribution, these are then fed to Multic to perform the VC analysis. To do this, the following files are required: a pedigree file and locus file as used for GH (*see* **Subheading 2.5.2.**), a specific Multic file called fort.12, an analysis parameter file called multic.par, and an instruction file multic.in. As GH is only being used to calculate the IBD sharing estimates, information about the trait or covariates is not required in the pedigree and locus GH files, however, if these are present, they can be left. The purpose of the fort.12 file is to check that the pedigree ordering is consistent in the modified GH run, and for the Multic runs, it provides the phenotypic data.

2.7.2.1. FORT.12

The format of the fort.12 file is pedigreeID, personID, fatherID, motherID, sex, affection status, dummy marker information, and trait values. The GH pedigree file can be used as the fort.12 file, provided it contains the trait. Here, we have reformatted the file to contain a single dummy marker, rather then the 50 markers typed, for ease of reading. The pedigree structures must be consistent between the GH pedigree file and the fort.12 file. In our example, the important information contained in fort.12 is the trait value, although it may also contain covariate and proband information if this is pertinent. The user specifies the missing code, and in this example, it is −999.

```
fort.12
1 1 0 0 1 2 3 5 -999
1 2 0 0 2 2 2 3 -999
1 3 1 2 2 2 2 5 11.047
1 4 1 2 1 2 3 3 12.1438
2 1 0 0 1 2 2 2 10.28
2 2 0 0 2 2 3 6 10.7452
2 3 1 2 2 2 2 6 11.0479
2 4 1 2 2 2 2 3 10.6258
```

2.7.2.2. MULTIC.PAR AND MULTIC.IN

A control file for Multic is also required and this can be built using the interactive program Premultic provided with the ACT package. Premultic queries the user with a series of questions and the responses build the multic.par file. The first record in multic.par is the title of the run. The second record has the analysis choices; in this example, these are n = no ascertainment, 3 = run both the null and alternative hypothesis using the starting values in the file, 1 = break value for convergence (10E-5), y = program fixes the boundary, 2 =

multic. The third record contains the number of traits, markers, covariates, and repeat measurements. In this example, there is one trait and only one dummy marker, because the IBD estimates are obtained separately. The fourth line has the trait description; this is repeated for each trait with the name, then the missing value code. Record 5 is the same as the above but for the markers. Record 6 would be used for any covariates if used, again using the same format. Record 7 is the fixed format statement for the family data file, t(number) tells you what column the values begin in, then the F(number) gives the length of any real number (e.g., for traits and covariates), whereas a4 refers to a genotype of length 4. Records 8–11 give the initial values for the parameters to be estimated (E), the others are fixed (F). The final value is the number of iterations. This file needs to be renamed multic_par when using the shell script, which subsequently renames it multic.par. Multic.par is the control file fed to the program Multic for each position of IBD estimates.

```
(9-8-0) ← Name of the file, the date is used otherwise.
n31y2
   1   1   0   1
Q4        -999.000000
dummy           0
(t39,F9,t50,a4)

x_mu(E)   = 8
x_poly(E) = 2
x_mg1(E)  = 2
x_mg2(F)  = 0
x_env(E)  = 2
x_sib(F)  = 0
x_pp (F)  = 0
x_po (F)  = 0
N1 = 500
```

The file multic.in is also provided, it is an instruction file for Multic replacing the interactive response of a user. It contains just the value "1," indicating multivariate data.

2.7.3. Running ACT

In the previous sections, the analyses for GH and SOLAR were run using interactive commands. For ACT, the analysis does not involve interactive commands and, instead, the procedure to perform the analysis is explained.

To run the ACT analysis, the shell script go.csh provided in the directory ~/Act/Gh/Demo1/ of the package can be used. Before running the shell script, it is important to check that all of the programs called from within the script are in the correct path. Check that all of the required input files are present within the directory from which the script will be run and that the script is executable. Typing go.csh at the prompt runs the script.

The first thing the script does is run the modified version of GH. The file called gh_in is used to instruct GH in performing the IBD calculations. The commands are the same as if running GH interactively and can be edited, as in this example, to provide IBD estimates at 1 cM intervals.

```
GH instruction file gh_in:

load gh_dat.08
use
incre dist 1.0
scan gh_ped.08
dump ibd

y
quit
```

This produces the three required files; share.out, mloci.out and npoints.out shown next. The first column of share.out provides the degree of relatedness between the pair of relatives:

```
0.000 0 1 0
0.500 0 0 1
0.500 0 0 1
0.500 0 0 1
0.500 0 0 1
0.500 1 0 0
```

The file, mloci.out, contains the IBD sharing probabilities based on the marker data for all the relative pairs within a pedigree for each of the positions scanned. The number of positions scanned is stored in the file npoints.out.

When the shell script continues, it calls a program cutloci, which cuts mloci.out into a file the same length as share.out, called loci.out. The order in these files corresponds to one another, so that for each relative pair, we have the coefficient of relationship and the IBDs. The following is the layout of the file mloci.out / loci.out containing the probability of sharing 0, 1, and 2 alleles identical by descent:

```
0.000 0.000 0.000
1.000 0.000 0.500
1.000 0.000 0.500
1.000 0.000 0.500
1.000 0.000 0.500
1.000 0.000 0.500
```

The file fort.12 is modified by a program called getheader, which adds a header to the file that includes the total number of pedigrees followed by the number of individuals in each family.

The files share.out, loci.out, and fort.12 file are finally fed to Multic along with the Multic control and instruction file, multic_par and multic_in, respectively, one scan position at a time. This is repeated depending on the number of positions scanned.

2.7.4. ACT Output

Numerous files are output from Multic and some contain the value of only one parameter at each position; unfortunately, the position is not given in these files. However, the majority of the output is contained within the file multic.log. The following is the output for the position giving the maximum likelihood:

```
Multic.log

      Fri Sep 15 10:55:43 2000

   Analyze Multivariate Traits with Covariance Program (MULTIC)
   ACT: Analysis for Complex Traits Package
   Revision 5.0 (30-12-99)
   Copyright(C) 1997
   Department of Epidemiology
   UT M.D. Anderson Cancer Center
   All rights reserved.

   The program used cpu time: 4.780000 seconds
      =====================
      | SUMMARY OF ANALYSIS |
      =====================
      ( multivariate data )
   ----------------
   INPUT FILES
   ----------------
   (1). Parameter file: 'multic.par'
      ------------------
      (9-8-100)
      n31y2
       1 1 0 1
      ...
      ------------------
   (2). Family data file: 'fort.12'
      (Total number of families : 239
       Total number of individuals: 1164)
```

```
------------------
PARAMETERS FOR THE ANALYSIS
------------------
(1). 1 Trait(s): q4.
(2). 1 Marker(s): dummy.
(3). 0 Covariate(s): .
(4). Ascertainment: NO.
------------------
RESULTS FOR THE ANALYSIS (H_0)
------------------
(1). Covariate coefficients:
                        Estimate      S.E.
Trait 1 (q4):
    mean(0)1     =      11.547963   0.041291
(2). Variance components:
                        Estimate      S.E.
    Polygenic:
    s(0)11       =      0.514516    0.069893

    First Major gene:
    m1(0)11      =      0.000000 (FIXED EXTERNALLY)

    Second Major gene:
    m2(0)11      =      0.000000 (FIXED EXTERNALLY)

    Environment:
    t(0)11       =      0.410193    0.049926

(3). Shared common environmental variance components:
                        Estimate      S.E.
    Shared Sibship:
    sib(0)11     =      0.000000 (FIXED EXTERNALLY)

    Shared Spouse:
    p(0)11       =      0.000000 (FIXED EXTERNALLY)

    Shared Parent-Offspring:
     q(0)11      =      0.000000 (FIXED EXTERNALLY)

(3). Log Likelihood after convergence:
    L(0)         =      -410.041622

    --------------------------------
    RESULTS FOR THE ANALYSIS (H_A)
    --------------------------------
    (1). Covariate coefficients:
                        Estimate      S.E.
    Trait 1 (q4):
        mean(A)1   =    11.546876 0.041209
```

```
(2). Variance components:
                              Estimate      S.E.
        Polygenic:
        s(A)11          =     0.280370   0.112238

        First Major gene:
        m1(A)11         =     0.232794   0.087869

        Second Major gene:
        m2(A)11         =     0.000000   (FIXED EXTERNALLY)

        Environment:
        t(A)11          =     0.412577   0.050078
(3). Shared common environmental variance components:

                              Estimate      S.E.
        Shared Sibship:
        sib(A)11        =     0.000000   (FIXED EXTERNALLY)

        Shared Spouse:
        p(A)11          =     0.000000   (FIXED EXTERNALLY)

        Shared Parent-Offspring:
        q(A)11          =     0.000000   (FIXED EXTERNALLY)

(3). Log Likelihood under the hypothesis of
     with major gene component(s):
     L(A)               =      -406.836219

     LRT = -2*(L(0)-L(A)) = 6.410807
```

3. Interpretation

3.1. GENEHUNTER

The output file vc.out (*see* **Subheading 2.5.4.**) shows, for each scan position, the LOD score, estimates of the means, variance components, and covariate regression coefficients for any covariates, if included in the analysis. Standard errors are also given for each of the parameter estimates. The final column of the file indicates if the program converged or not. The corresponding estimates for the null model are also shown at the end of this file.

From this output, it can be seen that the maximum LOD score of 1.3906 occurs at scan position 54 (54 cM Haldane, close to marker D8G27). At this position, the maximum likelihood estimates give an overall trait mean (11.547 ± 0.041), an additive polygenic effect (0.280 ± 0.112), an environmental effect (0.413 ± 0.050), and an additive QTL effect (0.233 ± 0.088). The parameters of the null model give a similar estimate of the mean (11.548 ± 0.041), as expected, and this is almost identical to the mean trait value in the summary statistics, so this is a good indication that the VC analysis was carried out correctly. The successful convergence at each scan position is also reassuring. The polygenic additive variance component (0.515 ± 0.070) under the null gives an estimate of the trait's heritabilty and the environmental variance (0.410 ± 0.050).

3.2. SOLAR

The file polygenic.out (*see* **Subheading 2.6.4.1.**) contains the estimate of the overall additive heritability, H2r (0.556 ± 0.059). SOLAR is the only program of the three that tests the significance of this heritability estimate. In this example, the heritability is significant. The program also tests the significance of any covariates; sex is the only covariate in this file and it is not significant. The file poly.mod (*see* **Subheading 2.6.4.2.**) contains the parameter values and standard errors under the polygenic model (null hypothesis model with the QTL variance constrained to zero). The parameters estimates for the overall mean for Q4 (11.548 ± 0.04), the heritability (additive) h2r (0.556 ± 0.059), and the environmental component e2 (0.444 ± 0.059) are given. The results for the alternative hypothesis for two-point analyses and multipoint analyses are found in twopoint.out (*see* **Subheading 2.6.4.3.**) and multipoint1.out (*see* **Subheading 2.6.4.4.**), respectively. For the multipoint analyses, IBD estimates are used at regular intervening intervals across the chromosome. For the two-point analysis, the maximum LOD score of 2.0828 occurs at the marker D8G27. The estimated linked QTL effect H2q1 (0.345) with a residual genetic effect H2r (0.212). The multipoint results localizes the QTL to 52 cM (Kosambi cM) close to D8G27, with a maximum LOD score (1.4988). The file null1.out give the estimates for the maximum LOD score, with their standard errors, H2q1 (0.280 ± 0.108) and H2r (0.276 ± 0.130) and e2 (0.445 ± 0.059), respectively.

3.3. ACT

The file multic.log produces output at each scan position. The largest maximum likelihood ratio indicates the most likely position of the putative QTL 54cM (Haldane cM) near D8G27. For each position, the output echoes the options specified in the multic.par file; it also gives the number of families and individuals in the file. Then, the results for the null hypothesis are output, the mean (11.548 ± 0.0413), the polygenic effect (0.515 ± 0.070), the environmental effect (0.410 ± 0.0499), and the log likelihood. The output for the alternative hypothesis follows: the major-gene (QTL) effect (0.280 ± 0.112), the unlinked polygenic effect (0.233 ± 0.088), and the environmental effect (0.413 ± 0.050), with the log likelihood for this model. Finally, the likelihood ratio test (LRT) is given, which compares the two models, this is χ^2 distributed. It can be converted to a LOD score [$\chi^2/2(\log_e 10) \sim$ LOD] to compare with the results from the other programs (e.g., 6.410807/4.6=1.3937). If a p-value is required, the χ^2 value with one degree of freedom gives the p-value for a two-sided test. This is divided by 2 because the test is one-sided (variance components must be greater than 0).

3.4. Summary of Results

All three programs correctly localized the position (close to D8G27, approx 52 cM Kosambi, approx 54 cM Haldane) of the QTL (MG4) affecting the trait Q4. The LOD scores obtained were modest (1.3906–1.3937) and would not be significant at a genomewide level. The analysis also provided estimates of effect size. These can be biased and their standard error needs to be considered when assessing their significance. For the true generating model, the total heritability accounted for 55% of the variance of Q4, and the QTL on chromosome 8 accounted for 28% of that variance, therefore, the unlinked polygenes accounted for the remaining 27%.

The estimates from GH, SOLAR, and ACT for the total heritability (additive) were 51.5%, 55.6%, and 51.5% respectively. Estimates for the linked QTL (additive effect) were 23.3%, 34.5%, 28.0%, and 23.3% for GH, SOLAR (two-point), SOLAR (multipoint), and ACT, respectively. For the unlinked polygenes, the respective estimates were 28.0%, 21.2%, 27.6%, and 28.0%, respectively. SOLAR's multipoint estimates were the most accurate, although all of the estimates were close.

The difference in the results between the three programs should only be the result of the IBD estimates. For both GH and ACT, these are identical because they are both using the same exact-multipoint algorithm from GH; therefore, the VC analysis should be very similar, indeed, the estimates are identical (**Table 3**). SOLAR uses an approximate multipoint IBD estimating method, which has been shown to compare favorably to the exact method (*21*) and has the advantage of not being limited by pedigree size. The complete marker information present in this stimulated dataset would also prove favorable to SOLAR. However a dataset with missing information should benefit from exact IBD estimates.

The LOD scores for the length of chromosome for the three programs are shown in **Fig. 3**. For GH and ACT, the LOD scores are almost identical (as expected) and cannot be distinguished from one another in the figure. The maximum LOD score for SOLAR is slightly higher than the other two, but not significantly so.

All three programs localized the Q4 trait to the correct position, the slight difference is the result of the different mapping functions used between GH and SOLAR when estimating the IBD probabilities. Table 4 lists the corresponding Kosambi and Haldane map positions for the region where the MG4 is located.

Table 3
Comparison of Results from GENEHUNTER, SOLAR (Multipoint), and ACT

			Alternative hypothesis			Null hypothesis	
	LOD	Mean	Additive QTL	Additive polygenic	Environmental	Additive polygenic	Environmental
GH	1.3906	11.547±0.041	0.233±0.088	0.280±0.112	0.413±0.050	0.515±0.070	0.410±0.050
SOLAR (multipoint)	1.4988	11.547±0.962	0.280±0.108	0.276±0.130	0.445±0.059	0.556±0.059	0.444±0.059
ACT	1.3937[a]	11.547±0.041	0.233±0.088	0.280±0.112	0.413±0.050	0.515±0.070	0.410±0.050

[a] Converted to a LOD score from the likelihood ratio statistic (6.411).

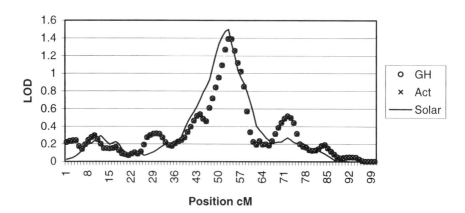

Fig. 3. LOD scores from GH, Solar, and Act_multic.

Table 4
Map Positions for Corresponding Mapping Functions

Theta	Kosambi cM	Haldane cM
0.028	50.335	51.450
0.015	51.836	52.973
0.013	53.136	54.290
0.022	55.337	56.540
0.021	57.439	58.686
0.021	59.539	60.831

The Kosambi mapping function incorporates the effect of interference, which is why the map is shorter compared to the Haldane map.

4. Software

The software used in this chapter included GH, SOLAR, and ACT. These can all be downloaded via Jurg Ott's linkage software site at Rockefeller: http://linkage.rockefeller.edu/soft/list.html. Much of the software listed there can also be downloaded from the "Linkage and Mapping Software Repository of the EBI" whose web address is ftp://ftp.ebi.ac.uk/pub/software/linkage_and_mapping/

The summaries from the linkage sites of the three programs as presented next.

4.1. GENEHUNTER

Full name: Genehunter
Version: 2.0 beta (Nov. 1998)

Descriptions: multipoint analysis of pedigree data, including nonparametric linkage analysis, LOD-score computation, information-content mapping, haplotype reconstruction

Authors: Leonid Kruglyak (leonid@genome.wi.mit.edu), Mark Daly (mjdaly@ genome.wi.mit.edu), Mary Pat Reeve-Daly (mpreeve@genome.wi.mit.edu), and Eric Lander (lander@genome.wi.mit.edu) (Whitehead Institute)

Web: ftp: http://waldo.wi.mit.edu/ftp/distribution/software/genehunter/gh2/; see also, Falling Rain Genomics, Inc.

Source code language: C

Operating systems: UNIX

Executables: gh

On-line documentation (2.0 beta)

Documentation (in PDF) (2.0 beta).

On-line instruction (1.1, from Falling Rain Genomics, Inc.)

4.2. SOLAR

Full name: Sequential Oligogenic Linkage Analysis Routines

Version: 1.4.0 (June 1999)

Descriptions: SOLAR is a flexible and extensive software package for genetic variance components analysis, including linkage, analysis, quantitative genetic analysis, and covariate screening. Operations are included for calculation of marker-specific or multipoint identity-by-descent (IBD) matrices in pedigrees of arbitrary size and complexity, and for linkage analysis of quantitative traits which may involve multiple loci (oligogenic analysis), dominance effects, and epistasis

Authors: John Blangero (john@darwin.sfbr.org), Kenneth Lange, Laura Almasy (almasy@darwin.sfbr.org), Tom Dyer (tdyer@darwin.sfbr.org), and Charles Peterson (charlesp@darwin.sfbr.org).

Web: http://www.sfbr.org/sfbr/public/software/solar/index.html

Source code language: FORTRAN, C, C++, TCL

Operating systems: UNIX (Solaris)

Executables: solar, ibdprep, ibdmat, relate, multipnt

4.3. ACT

Full name: Analysis of Complex Traits

Version: 1.1 (Mar 17, 2000)

Descriptions: It contains the following modules: ibd, calculates the proportion of gene shared identical by decent for a nuclear family; ibdn (modified program of ERPA), which implements a method for assessing increased allele sharing between all pairs of affected relatives within a pedigree; multic, multivariate analysis for complex traits; ml, estimation of variance components using maximum likelihood; ql, estimation of variance components using quasi likelihood; relcov, generates first-degree relationship coefficients for extended families, sim2s, the simulation program that was used to test ACT; cage, Cohort Analysis for Genetic Epidemiology; gh: GeneHunter, heavily modified to assist multipoint calculation using Multic

TDT: TDT programs written in SAS

Authors: Christopher I. Amos (camos@request.mdacc.tmc.edu), Mariza de Andrade (mandrade@request.mdacc.tmc.edu), and Jianfang Chen (cjf@ request.mdacc.tmc.edu)

Web: http://www.epigenetic.org/Linkage/act.html; http download: http:// www.epigenetic.org/Linkage/act.tar.gz. gcc and f77 compilers are necessary. Executable programs are included for compatible operating system (i.e., Solaris2.6).

Source code language: Fortran77, C++

Operating systems: UNIX (Solaris 2.4/..)

Executables: ibd, ml, ql, he, ibdn, multic

4.4. Additional Comments

The complete source code is provided for both GENEHUNTER and ACT; no code is provided with SOLAR, just an executable version.

The approximate run time for the three programs to perform the VC analysis using the Q4 example run on a Dual Sun SPARC Workstation II, CPU (400Mhz) with 2GB RAM was of the order of GH, 10 min; ACT, 15 min; SOLAR, 1 h, 45 min (reflects the time taken to obtain the IBDs).

5. Worked Example

The pedigree data analyzed in the previous sections was taken from a simulated dataset (problem 2A) produced for the Tenth Genetic Analysis Workshop (GAW10). A limited description of the model is given here, for those interested in the complete model, they are referred to the original article (*17*).

A common disease was simulated using an underlying model thought to reflect the situation underlying many of the complex disorders attempting to be mapped today. Affection status was assigned using a threshold model based on an individuals value for the quantitative trait Q1 exceeding a value $T = 40$. Four other intervening quantitative traits were involved in the model (Q2, Q3, Q4, Q5); some of these traits were influenced by age, sex, and an environmental factor (EF). Pedigrees were randomly ascertained, subject to the constraint that there were at least two living offspring, with individuals younger than 16 years old excluded from the study. Phenotypic data were provided for all living individuals; of these, 7% were affected.

Genotypic data were also simulated for all individuals (both dead and alive) for 367 highly polymorphic markers (average heterozygosity of 0.77), averagely spaced (2.03 cM) across 10 chromosomes, totaling 726 cM in length. Two hundred replicates were simulated and each of these replicates comprised 239 nuclear families, with 1164 individuals (1000 living). One of the intervening traits, Q4, genetically uncorrelated with the other intervening traits (Q2–Q5), but environmentally correlated (0.4) with Q5, it was influenced by three major genes (MG4, MG5, and MG6). Fifty-five percent of the variance was attributed to these genes (MG4 28%, MG5 16% and MG6 11%); the remaining variance (45%) was the result of random variation. MG4 thus accounted for the largest genetic variance of the trait Q4 and it was not affected by any covariates or by the EF. It is located on chromosome 8, 0.9 cM from D8G26 and 0.6 cM from D8G27.

To demonstrate the variance components method, the phenotypic data of trait Q4 and the genotypic data from chromosome 8 of the first replicate were analyzed. Each of the three VC methods correctly localized MG4 to the correct position on chromosome 8, as well as providing good estimates of the genetic effect and remaining variance components.

5.1. Exploring Trait Data

All analyses in this chapter were demonstrated with a trait called Q4, which is part of a simulated dataset from GAW10 (*17*). The distribution, summary statistics, and normality test are shown for Q4 in the following.

5.1.1. A Histogram for Trait Q4

A histogram and density plot of Q4 is presented in **Fig. 4**.

5.1.2. Summary Statistics for Q4

```
              Q4
      Min:  8.47640000
  1st Qu.:  10.85060000
     Mean:  11.55671120
   Median:  11.57270000
  3rd Qu.:  12.18237500
      Max:  14.48490000
  Total N:  1000.00000000
     NA's:  0.00000000
 Variance:  0.92562684
 Std Dev.:  0.96209503
 Skewness:  0.06055284
 Kurtosis:  -0.11824515
```

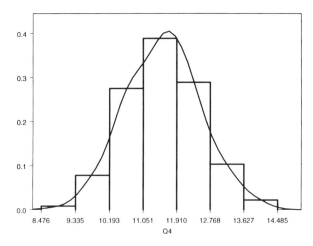

Fig. 4. A histogram and density plot of Q4.

5.1.3. The Kolmogorov–Smirnov Test for normality

```
One sample Kolmogorov-Smirnov Test of Composite normality

data: Q4
ks = 0.0213, p-value = 0.5
alternative hypothesis:
 True cdf is not the normal distn. with estimated parameters
sample estimates:
 mean of x standard deviation of x
  11.55671            0.962095
```

The Kolmogorov–Smirnov test is not significant for Q4. We, therefore, accept the null hypothesis that the distribution is normal.

6. Notes

1. File format. Mega2 is a data-handling program for facilitating genetic linkage and association analyses written by N. Mukhopadhyay, L. Almasy, M. Schroeder, W.P. Mulvihill, and D.E. Weeks (University of Pittsburgh). It is available via the web at http://watson.hgen.pitt.edu/register/soft_doc.html; ftp: registration page at http://watson.hgen.pitt.edu/register [Reference: *Am. J. Hum. Genet.* **65(Suppl.)** (1999) (abstract).]

   Mega2 can presently provide the correct formatted files for 19 different analysis programs, including GH and SOLAR. It is a menu-driven program that requires a minimum of three files. Two of these files are standard linkage format: a pedigree file (pedin.dat) that has been run through makeped and a locus file (datain.dat). The third file, the map file, is mega2-specific and is of the following format:

```
Map file
chr pos     name
08  0       D8G1
08  2.25    D8G2
08  5.557   D8G3
~
~
08  98.52   D8G48
08  99.327  D8G49
08  101.16  D8G50
```

The cumulative positions of the markers are given in cM (Haldane) and the name of the markers must correspond exactly to the name used in the locus file.

If the three files are given, the default names pedin.xx, datain.xx, and map.xx, where the xx refers to the chromosome number (e.g., pedin.08, etc). The first menu of mega2 option 1 allows the user to enter the chromosome number (in this case, "8"), mega2 then automatically finds these default named files. The rest of the menus are fairly self-explanatory.

Makeped is a utility program that is part of the linkage package; it takes a standard linkage pedigree file and adds three pointer fields and a proband field to each individual; these fields are used for reconstructing pedigrees.

2. Hints on the Programs

a. GENEHUNTER. GENEHUNTER uses an exact multipoint algorithm to calculate the full probability distribution of allele sharing at every point. The time and memory required to do this means that the size of the families that can be used is limited. The requirements are directly proportional to the number of meioses being examined. This number is $2N - F$, where F is the number of founders in the pedigree and N is the number of nonfounders. GH can rapidly analyze general pedigrees of moderate size (i.e., up to 16 nonfounding members, on current workstations).

The default mapping function in GH is Haldane. The Kosambi mapping function is still available; however, this has been shown to give errors (*22*).

Covariates are coded in the same way as trait data in the pedigree file, within the locus description file covariates are coded up with just a single line with no proceeding blank lines, e.g. 4 0 # AGE

Covariates should be listed immediately after the phenotypes. The maximum number of traits and covariates that can be included are given by the constants max_phenotypes and max_covariates in the file npl.h; the default is 10.

If convergence is a problem for which different starting values should be tried; also, it is possible to increase the number of iterations (MAXITS in the file varcom.c). Different start values can also be tried to confirm that the true maximum likelihood estimates were found.

b. SOLAR. The limit on the size of pedigree depends on whether or not the class of relative required by the data has been coded up. For this dataset of nuclear families, the IBD estimates were relatively slow compared to GH. However, as the data were simulated and no data were missing, the analysis could have been sped up by not loading the allele frequency files and by using the Monte Carlo method.

The map function for SOLAR should be specified in Kosambi cM.

Covariates are coded up in the solar_phen file in the same way as trait values. When carrying out an analysis, all of the variables in the phen file will be used as covariates, if you use the automodel and polygenic –s option. Therefore, you need to make sure you define the trait and only include the covariates you want, the exclude command can be used to remove those not required.

```
solar > load phen solar_phen.08
solar tells you what was loaded.
ped, per, sex, var1, var2, var3, var4 etc
solar > exclude var2 var3 etc
solar > automodel solar_phen.08 var1
solar > polygenic -s                    (-s option means screen).
solar > model
```

The command "model" will show you what the current model is.

Ascertainment correction can be carried out for single ascertainment if the proband status is known. It is coded up in the phen file under the header "proband, probnd, or prband" in uppercase or lowercase. In this proband field, a blank or 0 signifies non-proband and anything else indicates a proband. If SOLAR detects such a field, then it will use this in the analysis, unless the following command is issued or the field is renamed:

solar> field probnd –none

Probands must have all of the required quantitative variables; probands missing any quantitative variables are not included in the proband count and, except for defining the pedigree structure, do not enter into the calculations.

c. ACT. The limit on pedigree size depends on the method used to obtain the IBD sharing estimates. Multic also has a limit of 20 family members for extended families. Programs available to obtain IBD sharing estimates include a modified ERPA (*18*) and modified GH. The maximum number of traits at present is five for multivariate data and one for longitudinal data. If any trait value is missing, this current version of Multic eliminates that individual's data record.

Covariates can be included in the analysis, as can the proband status for ascertainment correction. Covariates are coded up in the same way as the trait phenotypes are in the fort.12 file; the user assigns the missing code and this should be something obvious like –999. In the multic.par control file, the number of covariates and the column position is specified. The maximum number of covariates is 10.

For ascertainment correction, the proband must have trait information; if this is missing, the program will exit with an error message. Individual proband status is coded up in the last eight columns of each family record in the file fort.12 file, 1 = proband and 0 = non-proband. For ascertainment to be used, the second record of the multic.par file needs to be coded "y".

Acknowledgments

The author would like to thank Dr. Lon Cardon for his helpful comments on this chapter.

Angela J. Marlow is funded by the Wellcome Trust. The simulated data came from the GAW10 work supported by the GAW grant, NIH grant GM31575.

References

1. Fisher, R. A. (1918) The correlation between relatives on the supposition of Mendelian inheritance. *Transl. R. Soc.* Edinburgh **52**, 399–433.
2. Neale, M. C. and Cardon, L. R. (1992) *Methodology for Genetic Studies of Twins and Families.* NATO ASI Series. Kluwer Academic, Dordrecht, pp. 55–70.
3. Searle, S. R., Casella, G., and McCulloch, C. E. V (1991) *Variance Components.* Wiley, New York.
4. Self, S. G. and Liang, K. Y. (1987) Asymptottic properties of maximum likelihood estimators and likelihood ratio tests under non-standard conditions. *J. Am. Stat. Assoc.* **82**, 605–610.
5. Amos, C. I. (1994) Robust variance-components approach for assessing genetic linkage in pedigrees. *Am. J. Hum. Genet.* **54**, 535–543.
6. Amos, C. I., Zhu, D. K., and Boerwinkle, E. (1996) Assessing genetic linkage and association with robust components of variance approaches. *Ann. Hum. Genet.* **60**, 143–160.
7. Pratt, S. C., Daly, M. J., and Kruglyak, L. (2000) Exact multipoint quantitative-trait linkage analysis in pedigrees by variance components. *Am. J. Hum. Genet.* **66**, 1153–1157.
8. Wijsman, E. M. and Amos, C. I. (1997) Genetic analysis of simulated oligogenic traits in nuclear and extended pedigrees: summary of GAW10 contributions. *Genet. Epidemiol.* **14**, 719–735.
9. Allison, D. B., Neale, M. C., Zannolli, R., Schork, N. J., Amos, C. I., and Blangero, J. (1999) Testing the robustness of the likelihood-ratio test in a variance-component quantitative-trait loci-mapping procedure. *Am. J. Hum. Genet.* **65**, 531–544.
10. de Andrade, M., Thiel, T. J., Yu, L. P., and Amos, C. I. (1997) Assessing linkage on chromosome 5 using components of variance approach: univariate versus multivariate. *Genet. Epidemiol.* **14**, 773–778.
11. Fisher, S. E., Marlow, A. J., Lamb, J., Maestrini, E., Williams, D. F., Richardson, A. J., et al. (1999) A quantitative-trait locus on chromosome 6p influences different aspects of developmental dyslexia. *Am. J. Hum. Genet.* **64**, 146–156.
12. Risch, N. and Zhang, H. (1995) Extreme discordant sib pairs for mapping quantitative trait loci in humans. *Science* **268**, 1584–1589.
13. Kruglyak, L. and Lander, E. S. (1995) Complete multipoint sib-pair analysis of qualitative and quantitative traits. *Am. J. Hum. Genet.* **57**, 439–454.
14. Almasy, L. and Blangero, J. (1998) Multipoint quantitative-trait linkage analysis in general pedigrees. *Am. J. Hum. Genet.* **62**, 119–1211.

15. Terwilliger, J. D. and Ott, J. (1994) *Handbook of Human Genetic Linkage.* The John Hopkins University Press, Baltimore, MD.

16. Kruglyak, L., Daly, M. J., Reeve-Daly, M. P., and Lander, E. S. (1996) Parametric and nonparametric linkage analysis: A unified multipoint approach. *Am. J. Hum. Genet.* **58**, 1347–1363.

17. MacCluer, J. W., Blangero, J., Dyer, T. D., and Speer, M. C. (1997) GAW10: simulated family data for a common oligogenic disease with quantitative risk factors. *Genet. Epidemiol.* **14**, 737–742.

18. Curtis, D. and Sham, P. C. (1994) Using risk calculation to implement an extended relative pair analysis. *Ann. Hum. Genet.* **58**, 151–162.

19. Davis, S., Schroeder, M., Goldin, L. R., and Weeks, D. E. (1996) Non-parametric simulation-based statistics for detecting linkage in general pedigrees. *Am. J. Hum. Genet.* **58**, 867–880.

20. Fulker, D. W., Cherny, S. S., and Cardon, L. R. (1995) Multipoint interval mapping of quantitative trait loci, using sib pairs. *Am. J. Hum. Genet.* **56**, 1224–1233.

21. Fulker, D. W. and Cherny, S. S. (1996) An improved multipoint sib-pair analysis of quantitative traits. *Behav. Genet.* **26**, 527–532.

22. Ott, J. (1996) *Linkage Newsletter.* Rockefeller University, Volume 10, No 6.

5

Linkage and Association

The Transmission/Disequilibrium Test for QTLs

Mark M. Iles

1. Introduction

1.1. Genetic Association

Usually, the probability of observing a particular allele at one locus is independent of the alleles observed at another locus. However, this is not the case when two alleles are 'associated.' For instance, let the frequency of allele 1 at locus 1 by p_1 and the frequency of allele 2 at locus 2 be p_2. If the two alleles are not associated, then the frequency with which they appear together is $p_1 p_2$. If their joint frequency is greater than $p_1 p_2$ the two alleles are said to be positively associated. If their joint frequency is less than $p_1 p_2$, the two alleles are said to be negatively associated. Association is the nonindependence of allele frequencies at different loci.

Association between two alleles can arise by a number of mechanisms. However, in a randomly mating population, association between noninteracting alleles will only persist if they are linked. This type of association is termed *linkage disequilibrium.* Association between linked loci will dissipate at a rate determined by the characteristics of the population. In a randomly mating, outbred population linkage disequilibrium may only span a few thousand bp, whereas in a population isolate, it may exist at distances up to 5 cM. Thus, if a marker allele is found to be associated with disease susceptibility, a disease susceptibility locus is likely to be nearby. It is for this reason that genetic association is of interest to investigators mapping disease genes.

However, if mating in the population is nonrandom, then association may persist between unlinked alleles. Imagine a population that is stratified into

From: *Methods in Molecular Biology: vol. 195: Quantitative Trait Loci: Methods and Protocols.*
Edited by: N. J. Camp and A. Cox © Humana Press, Inc., Totowa, NJ

two groups. Mating only occurs between individuals who come from the same group and has done so for a number of generations. As a result, some alleles will be more frequent in one group than in the other. If a disease is more frequent in one of the groups, then any allele that is also more frequent in that group will be associated to some degree with disease status. However, such an allele is not necessarily linked to any disease-predisposing loci and will not be of help in mapping such loci. The extent of such stratification is difficult to quantify, and so it is important for tests of association to protect against such effects.

1.2. The Transmission/Disequilibrium Test

Methods for detecting association between marker alleles and disease status were first applied to dichotomous traits for which people could be described as either 'affected' or 'unaffected.' Two groups of individuals are collected: one consisting of those with the disease in question (cases) and the other consisting of those without the disease (controls). The individuals are then genotyped at a number of genetic markers and the allelic (or genotypic) frequencies in the case and control groups are compared. Any allele (or genotype) that has a significantly higher frequency in the case group compared with the control group is said to be associated with disease status (see Chapter 1).

However, the choice of appropriate controls is problematic. Unobservable ethnic differences between cases and controls, as described, can lead to 'spurious' association. Researchers are interested in association that is the result of proximity between a marker and a disease-susceptibility locus so that they are able to locate the causative mutation. Association between linked loci is known as 'linkage disequilibrium.'

One solution is to use parental data to provide a 'pseudocontrol,' as proposed by Rubinstein et al. (*1*). The principal behind the method is to genotype an affected individual together with his/her parents. The affected individual provides the case genotype, whereas the two untransmitted alleles from the parents provide the control genotype. Various methods have been based on this idea, but the most popular of these is the transmission/disequilibrium test (TDT).

The TDT analyzes the frequency with which alleles are transmitted from heterozygous parents to affected offspring. If the alleles being studied are unassociated with disease, then they will have an equal probability of transmission (0.5 from a heterozygous parent). The test was first proposed by Terwilliger and Ott (*2*), but was named the TDT by Spielman et al. (*3*), who recognized that only by conditioning on parental genotypes could you ensure that you would detect association resulting from linkage but not stratification. The TDT is a simultaneous test of both linkage and association and is, therefore, unaffected by alleles that are associated with but not linked to the disease-susceptibility locus. The TDT is simple to apply. The number of times an allele is transmitted from a heterozygous parent to an affected offspring is counted. The number of times the allele is transmitted is denoted by b and the number of times it is not transmitted is denoted by c.

The TDT statistic is $\dfrac{(b-c)^2}{(b+c)}$. This should follow a χ_1^2 distribution under the null hypothesis of no linkage and/or association. A significant deviation from this is evidence that the allele is associated with the disease. Data on transmissions from homozygous parents are discarded.

The original test as outlined by Spielman et al. (*3*) has a number of limitations: (1) It can only be applied to a single locus at a time. (2) That locus must be diallelic. Both of these problems can be overcome by testing every allele at every locus separately and accounting for multiple testing by a Bonferroni correction, although this is suboptimal. (3) Only one affected child from each nuclear family can be used in the analysis. If more than two offspring are included, the test is no longer valid for association, although it remains valid for linkage (*4*). (4) Only nuclear families in which both parents have been typed can be used. If either of the parents is missing, the results may be biased (*5*). Most of these problems have since been tackled and the TDT has been extended to include families with missing parents (*6,7*) and multiplex families (*8*) and to deal with multiple alleles (*9,10*) and multiple loci (*11,12*) more effectively.

The limitation of most interest to us here is that the TDT was originally designed for use with dichotomous traits. Various methods have been developed for applying TDT-style analyses to quantitative traits and the most significant of these are covered in the following section. It should be borne in mind that the aforementioned limitations of the original TDT persist for several of the methods described. In particular, no one has, as yet, described a quantitative TDT that is suitable for multilocus data. This is not such a problem when the loci are unlinked, but when markers are close enough to be in disequilibrium with each other, correction by the Bonferroni method, which assumes independence of the data, may be suboptimal.

2. Methods

2.1. Allison

The first adaptations of the TDT designed specifically for the analysis of quantitative traits were made by Allison (*13*). Allison introduced five different tests, named TDT_{Q1}–TDT_{Q5}, designed specifically to deal with nuclear families (trios) consisting of two parents and an offspring, as in the TDT. However, here, the offspring is affected not by a binary trait but by a trait that is measured quantitatively. All five tests assume that the locus being studied is diallelic so that if the locus has more than two alleles, each should be tested in turn against the remaining alleles. In calculating power, it is assumed that there is random mating, that Hardy–Weinberg equilibrium holds, and that the marker locus is the quantitative trait locus (QTL) itself. The standard assumption of no genotyping or phenotyping errors is also made.

The first four tests (TDT_{Q1}–TDT_{Q4}) require that one of the parents is heterozygous for the putative disease allele and the other homozygous. If this is not the case, then the validity of the tests will be compromised by the nonindependence of the observations. If data are missing on either of the parents, bias can result, as is found in the classical TDT (5).

2.1.1. TDT_{Q1}

When applying TDT_{Q1}, the families are divided into two groups according to which of the two alleles is transmitted from the heterozygous parent. The mean trait value in the two groups is compared using a t-test. It is assumed that the trait value (or, rather, the residuals) is Normally distributed (by invoking the Central Limit Theorem).

2.1.2. TDT_{Q2}

For TDT_{Q2}, the sample is again dichotomized according to which of the two alleles is transmitted from the heterozygous parent. Upper and lower threshold values (Z_U and Z_L) are chosen, such that $Z_U \geq Z_L$. Those individuals with a trait value above Z_U are placed in one category and those with a trait value below Z_L are placed in another category. The remainder are discarded. The data are summarized in a 2×2 table of counts, with the rows indicating whether the trait value is above Z_U or below Z_L and the columns indicating which allele has been transmitted from the heterozygous parent. Pearson's chi-squared test of independence is then performed to detect an association between trait value and allele transmitted. This is not strictly a test of whether transmission probabilities deviate from 0.5. It assumes that the residual distribution is Normal within each genotype.

2.1.3. TDT_{Q3}

TDT_{Q3} is a combination of TDT_{Q1} and TDT_{Q2}. It is assumed that the sample is large enough that the Central Limit Theorem holds. Only families in which the offspring has a trait value either above Z_U or below Z_L are selected. The test is then performed as for TDT_{Q1}.

TDT_{Q1} and TDT_{Q3} are t-tests and, as such, are identical to testing the significance of regressing the trait value on the transmission status from the heterozygous parent.

2.1.4. TDT$_{Q4}$

TDT$_{Q4}$ selects only those offspring whose trait value is either lower than Z_L or higher than Z_U and tests whether the probability of transmission from the heterozygous parent is equal to 0.5 in both quadrants.

2.1.5. TDT$_{Q5}$

The last of the five tests presented by Allison (*13*), and the only one that maintains consistently good power under all modes of inheritance, is TDT$_{Q5}$. TDT$_{Q5}$, as with the previous four tests, uses information from nuclear families (trios) consisting of two parents and one offspring with a quantitatively measured trait. However, TDT$_{Q5}$ uses data from all heterozygous parents rather than using only families with a single heterozygous parent. Only those families where the offspring has a trait value either greater than Z_U or less than Z_L are used. The allele of interest is denoted by 'a' and the other allele (or alleles) is denoted by 'A.' Thus, parental mating types can be categorized as either (1) Aa × AA, (2) Aa × Aa, or (3) Aa × aa. The number of 'a' alleles (0, 1, or 2) in the offspring is denoted by X. The trait value is then regressed on the mating type (1, 2, or 3) and the R^2 for the regression is found. R^2 is the proportion of the total variance of the trait value that is explained by the model and is denoted by R_1^2. Then X and X^2 are added to the model, and the R^2 calculated for this regression and is denoted by R_2^2. The joint additive and dominant effects of the locus under investigation can be tested by comparing R_1^2 and R_2^2 using the statistic

$$\frac{(R_2^2 - R_1^2)/2}{(1 - R_2^2)/(n - 5)} \tag{1}$$

where n is the number of nuclear family trios used. Under the null hypothesis, this should follow an $F_{2,n-5}$-distribution.

TDT$_{Q5}$ has the obvious advantage over the earlier tests in that families with two heterozygous parents, as well as those with only one, can be used. Furthermore, by using a regression method incorporating parental genotypes, the alleles transmitted from homozygous parents are taken into account. As an extension to this, Allison suggested including covariates such as ethnic background, age, and the trait values of the parents, or including interactions such as gene × gene, gene × environment, or transmission status × sex of parent (i.e., imprinting). The inclusion of covariates, when they are known and believed to interact with the trait value, will almost always increase power.

2.1.6. Power

Allison (*13*) shows that these methods have greater efficiency than the Haseman–Elston (*14*) and Extreme-Discordant-Sib-Pairs (*15*) methods, both of which are sib-pair linkage tests. However, the same problems as with Risch and Merikangas' work (16) regarding power calculations arise, because power is calculated under the assumption that the marker is the trait locus and that the mode of inheritance is additive. The former assumption is ideal for the TDT, which can lose much power when the marker is not in complete linkage disequilibrium with the trait locus (17). The ideal model of inheritance for the TDT is multiplicative and the additive model is very close to this. Under alternative modes of inheritance, Allison's tests may not compare so well to the sib-pair linkage methods, as was shown by Camp for the TDT (18,19).

Page and Amos (20) demonstrate that when there is no admixture, it is more powerful to compare trait values between those with and without a particular genotype/allele, ignoring the parents. However, when there is enough admixture to cause a reasonable amount of non-linkage-based disequilibrium, the false-positive rate of such tests is inflated and Allison's TDT_{Q1}–TDT_{Q4} will be more powerful. Of Allison's first four tests, Page and Amos (20) found that TDT_{Q3} was the most powerful [as did Allison (13)]. Unfortunately, Page and Amos (20) did not compare TDT_{Q5}, which Allison (13) found to be consistently the most powerful, because of difficulties in implementing the method.

2.1.7. Limitations

No advice is given regarding the threshold values of Z_U and Z_L to be used, although Allison selected them so that the top and bottom 10% of the trait distribution were included. It should be noted that the selection of extreme values is inadvisable when there are a number of genes that influence the trait value. Allison's tests (13) are straightforward in both concept and application. However, four are limited by using only families with one heterozygous parent. The fifth test offers a far more flexible approach to analyzing the data, although it still has limitations, such as only using diallelic loci. TDT_{Q1} has been extended by Xiong et al. (21) [clarified by Wang and Cohen (22)] to utilize multiallelic markers and families with more than one heterozygous parent. The extension has greater power than the original TDT_{Q1} (as it uses more of the data), but remains less flexible than TDT_{Q5}, as it cannot incorporate covariates and may even be less powerful.

2.2. Rabinowitz

The method presented by Rabinowitz (23) is similar to Allison's TDT_{Q5} (13). However, it requires no parametric assumptions about the distribution of the trait value and is applicable to multiallelic loci. Rabinowitz describes his method as being a test of association between marker alleles and trait values, which is modified by taking parental information into account, thereby avoiding spurious association caused by the population structure. Furthermore, the method allows the incorporation of covariates such as environmental factors.

Let the trait value of the jth child in the ith family be Q_{ij}. Initially, a single allele is considered with indicator variable Y_{ijM} equal to 1 if the allele is transmitted maternally to the jth child in the ith family and 0 if it is not transmitted. Y_{ijP} is equivalent to Y_{ijM} for paternally transmitted alleles. $Q_{..}$ represents the average trait value taken over all children in all families. Y^*_{iM} takes the value 1 if the mother of the ith family is heterozygous for the allele under investigation. Y^*_{iP} takes the value 1 if the father of the ith family is heterozygous for the allele under investigation. Then, the statistic

$$T = \sum_{i=1}^{n} \sum_{j=1}^{m_1} \left(Q_{ij} - Q_{..} \right) \left[Y^*_{iM} \left(Y_{ijM} - \frac{1}{2} \right) + Y^*_{iP} \left(Y_{ijP} - \frac{1}{2} \right) \right] \tag{2}$$

is a measure of the association between the trait and the allele under investigation. If there is no association, the expected value of this is zero, and if there is association, the expected value will deviate from zero. The statistic will not be influenced by association arising from population admixture or stratification because it uses only transmissions from heterozygous parents, as in the TDT.

The variance of the statistic is

$$\sigma^2 = \frac{1}{4} \sum_{i=1}^{n} \sum_{j=i}^{m_i} \left(Q_{ij} - Q_{..} \right)^2 (Y^*_{iM} + Y^*_{iP}) \tag{3}$$

If the marker has only two alleles, the test is simple. T^2/σ^2 will have a χ^2_1 distribution under the null hypothesis. Under the alternative hypothesis, that there is both linkage and association between the trait and the marker, the test statistic will deviate significantly from this distribution.

When the locus has multiple alleles, there are two possibilities for extending the test. The first is to test each allele in turn and use the value of the one with the highest score. Multiple testing is accounted for either by calculating the exact p-value through simulation or by applying the Bonferroni correction. Although the Bonferroni correction is simpler, it will lead to a more conservative test.

The second method for analyzing multiple alleles is to amalgamate the tests for each allele into a single test of all the alleles by taking into account the covariance between the tests. Let there be k alleles at the locus. Then, let Z^*_{iabM} equal 1 if the mother of family i has alleles a and b and let Z^*_{iabF} equal 1 if the father of family i has alleles a and b ($a, b=1, \ldots, k$). Then, the covariance between the test statistics for alleles a and b will be

$$\text{Cov}(a, b) = \frac{1}{4} \sum_{i=1}^{n} \sum_{j=i}^{m_i} (Q_{ij} - Q_{..})^2 (-Z^*_{iabM} - Z^*_{iabF}) \tag{4}$$

and let

$$S = \sum_{b=1}^{k-1} \sum_{a=1}^{k-1} \frac{T_a T_b}{\text{Cov}(a, b)} \tag{5}$$

where T_a is test statistic T applied to allele a and T_b is test statistic T applied to allele b. In large samples, S will have a χ^2_{k-1}-distribution under the null hypothesis of no linkage and no association. Deviations of S from 0, suggestive of both linkage and association, can be tested for significance in the usual way.

Covariates, such as environmental factors, can be accounted for by regressing the quantitative trait on the covariates. The fitted value for the jth child in the ith family, $\hat{Q}_{ij}$, then replaces Q_{ij} in the equations. This removes the component of variability in the traits that is explained by the covariates.

It should be noted that, as with previous tests, the transmissions to several individuals in the same sibship are not independent. Thus, the test will be valid for linkage, but not for association, when multiplex families are included in the analysis.

The test has been extended by Monks et al. (*24*) to be a valid test for association as well as linkage when analyzing nuclear families with multiple offspring. This is achieved by averaging the Rabinowitz statistic within each family so that each contributes a single score.

2.3. Allison et al. (25)—Sib QTDT

The SibTDT (*26*) is a variant of the TDT that deals with the situation in which parental data are unavailable. Allison et al. (*25*) have developed a similar sibling-based version of the quantitative TDT. An association between genotype and trait value is still valid regardless of population structure if sibship effects are controlled for, as this is equivalent to controlling for parental genotype. The data required for this test are sibships, each with a minimum of two individuals. Sibships in which all siblings have either the same trait value (which is not possible for truly continuous values) or the same genotype cannot be used, as these effects cannot be separated from the sibship effect and such families will add no information to the study.

Two methods are proposed by Allison et al. (*25*). The first is to fit a mixed-effects model and the second to use a permutation test.

2.3.1. The Mixed-Effect Model

Using the first method, we denote the phenotype of the kth sibling with the ith genotype in the jth sibship by Y_{ijk}. The marker locus is assumed to have m alleles and, therefore, $m(m + 1)/2$ possible genotypes. The genotype is modeled as a fixed factor A with $m(m + 1)/2$ levels and the sibship is modeled as a random factor with J levels (where J is the number of sibships). Therefore, the following two-factor mixed-effects model is fitted:

$$Y_{ijk} = \mu + \alpha_i + \beta_j + (\alpha\beta)_{ij} + e_{ijk} \tag{6}$$

where $i=1, \ldots, m(m + 1)/2, j=1, \ldots, J$, and $k=1, \ldots, n_{ij}$ (number of siblings in the jth sibship with the ith genotype). The effect sizes for α_i are for the fixed-genotype factor A, β_j are for the random sibship factor B, and the interaction effects $\alpha\beta_{ij}$ are also random. Therefore, genotypic effects are tested conditionally on sibship, because this is random. The model is tested using an ANOVA-based F-test.

2.3.2. The Permutation Test

The second method is a permutation test. The theory underlying this test is that if the trait value is independent of the genotype, then the mean trait value for each of the alleles should be the same. Thus, if the trait values are randomly reassigned to different individuals, the average trait value for each allele should not be significantly different. Here, because there may be a sibship effect due to population structure, trait values are only permuted within sibships. The mean of the ith allele observed in the jth sibship, μ_{ij}, averaged over all permutations is then

$$\mu_{ij} = \frac{1}{K_j} \sum_{k=1}^{K_j} Y_{jk} \sum_{k=1}^{K_j} N_{ijk} \tag{7}$$

There are K_j siblings in the jth sibship (and, therefore, K_j possible permutations) and N_{ijk} copies of the ith allele in the kth child of the jth sibship, Y_{jk} is the trait value of the kth sibling in the jth sibship. The variance of the trait value for the ith allele in the jth sibship, V_{ij}, is

$$
\begin{aligned}
V_{ij} = {}& \frac{1}{K_j} \sum_{k=1}^{K_j} Y_{jk}^2 \sum_{k=1}^{K_j} N_{ijk}^2 \\
& + \frac{1}{K_j(K_j - 1)} \left[\left(\sum_{k=1}^{K_j} Y_{jk} \right)^2 - \sum_{k=1}^{K_j} Y_{jk}^2 \right] \left[\left(\sum_{k=1}^{K_j} N_{ijk} \right)^2 \right. \\
& \left. - \sum_{k=1}^{K_j} N_{ijk}^2 \right] - \mu_{ij}^2
\end{aligned} \tag{8}
$$

Thus, the statistic

$$
S = \frac{m-1}{m} \sum_{i=1}^{m} \frac{\left[\sum_{j=1}^{J} \left(\sum_{k=1}^{K_j} Y_{jk} N_{ijk} - \mu_{ij} \right) \right]^2}{\sum_{j=1}^{J} V_{ij}}
\tag{9}
$$

can be approximated by a χ^2_{m-1}-distribution under the null hypothesis of no linkage and no association. Deviation from this is suggestive of both linkage and association.

2.3.3. Power

Allison et al.'s (**25**) power calculations showed both methods to have adequate power for reasonable sample sizes, even when the gene explains only 10% of the variance. They found that the larger the sibship size, the greater the power, but that this increase in power is mainly in going from sib pairs to sib trios; beyond sib trios, the power to be gained is marginal. The authors also investigated sampling only those sibships that were phenotypically either highly concordant or discordant; siblings had either very similar trait values or very dissimilar trait values. Analyzing this subset of the full dataset was found to increase power substantially. The similarity of the trait values was measured using the Mahalanobis distance (**27**, p. 234).

The sibling-based quantitative TDT was compared with one of Allison's (**13**) quantitative TDTs (which one is not specified). Simulations showed the sibling-based quantitative TDT to be the more powerful test. This may be because although the same number of individuals is genotyped for each test, fewer of the observations will be informative when parents are used. Alternatively, a family trio provides one known phenotype (from the offspring) and one unknown (from the untransmitted parental alleles), whereas three siblings provide three phenotypes, and so provide more information.

The permutation method was found in simulations to have relatively higher power when the effect of the trait locus was purely additive. When the trait included a dominance component (e.g., a dominant or recessive mode of inheritance), then the mixed-effects method had relatively higher power.

Both methods lose power as the number of alleles at the locus being tested increases. However, the permutation method is less affected by this, probably because it is concerned with allelic effects, whereas the mixed-effects method concentrates on genotypic effects.

2.4. Abecasis et al. (**28**)

Fulker et al. (**29**) developed a method for analyzing sib-pair data by partitioning the association into orthogonal within- and between-family components.

This has been extended by Abecasis et al. (*28*) to a test for analyzing quantitative traits in nuclear families of any size, with or without parental information. The basic model is designed with a diallelic marker locus in mind.

As in **ref. 29**, the trait is assumed to have a multivariate Normal distribution and effects are tested by use of a likelihood ratio test. The mean of the multivariate Normal distribution is modeled linearly and can be thought of as representing association. The variance is modeled using variance components methods (as described in Chapter 4) and can be thought of as representing linkage (see **ref. 29** for more about this concept).

2.4.1. The Association Aspect

First, we present the mean/linear/association part of the model. μ is the phenotypic mean over all individuals, y_{ij} is the trait value of the jth offspring in the ith family, m_{ij} is the number of copies of the allele being studied, and $g_{ij} = m_{ij}-1$. n_{-i} is the number of siblings in the ith subship:

$$b_i = \frac{\sum_j g_{ij}}{n_i} \tag{10}$$

If parental genotypes are unknown,

$$b_i = \frac{g_{iF} + g_{iM}}{2} \tag{11}$$

If parental genotypes are known, where g_{iF} is the genotype score analogous to g_{ij} in the father and g_{iM} in the mother, and $w_{ij} = g_{ij}-b_i$

The fitted model is of the following form:

$$\hat{y}_{ij} = \mu + \beta_b b_i + \beta_w w_{ij} \tag{12}$$

b_i represents the between-family component and w_{ij} represents the within-family component. Positive values of w_{ij} indicate that a child inherits more copies of the allele than would be expected given their family, whereas negative values indicate the inheritance of fewer copies than expected.

Abecasis et al. (*28*) showed that, as suggested by Fulker et al. (*29*), the β_w coefficient is an unbiased estimator of the additive genetic component a. Any 'spurious' association arising from population admixture is accounted for by β_b. β_b is equal to a when there is either no stratification or the phenotypic mean in every stratum is zero.

When the family units are larger than simple nuclear family trios (e.g., when there are extra siblings), then the variance must also be modeled, otherwise the model is invalid. This is because the transmissions, in this case, will no longer be independent.

2.4.2. The Linkage Aspect

The variance–covariance matrix is modeled in the usual way (see Chapter 4) and is decomposed into factors such as residual environmental variance, additive genetic variance, and so forth. When modeling association with the variance components fitted (as is required for extended families), residual variance, additive genetic variance, and polygenic variance should always be modeled, because the assumption in modeling association is that there is a polygenic effect and that this may be the result of a locus linked to the marker being tested.

2.4.3. Significance and Power

This method was demonstrated by the authors to have type 1 error rates close to their nominal values. These were unaffected by population structure, linked major loci, or additional sibling resemblance. Unsurprisingly, the error rates were most accurate for larger sample sizes.

Power is dependent on the level of disequilibrium and, when parents are unavailable, on the number of siblings in each family. The total number of genotypes required is smaller when parents are not used.

2.4.4. Testing for an Additive Genetic Component

The test of the within-family-association parameter β_w is equivalent to the test proposed by Rabinowitz (*23*). If β_w is not significant in the model, then this implies that there is no additive genetic component to the disease.

2.4.5. Extensions

The model can be extended to multiallelic loci by including separate between- and within-family components for every allele but one (because the presence or absence of the final allele is accounted for by the other alleles). As with all linear models, the incorporation of covariates such as environmental effects is possible.

Abecasis et al. (*28*) also presented a permutation test that is of use if multivariate Normality assumptions are violated; for instance, if the sample size is small or the trait value skewed. Otherwise, the permutation method has no advantage over the variance–components method. Dominance can also be included.

The method has the advantage of using all data on nuclear families, including those with missing parents. The linear model used is intuitively appealing, because it separates the association into the orthogonal components of between-family and within-family effects. The model is the most flexible of those presented here, as it can incorporate factors such as covariates and dominance easily. It allows the use of multiplex families, and, because it is a likelihood-based method, estimation of the additive genetic component is possible.

3. Interpretation

All of the tests described, when applied to the appropriate data, should be valid as tests of association that are robust to population stratification.

3.1. Allison (13)

Most of the tests suggested by Allison require only a simple comparison of a statistic against a standard distribution from a book of statistical tables. A p-value for the observed value of the statistic can then be found.

TDT_{Q5} is more complicated and requires analysis-of-variance (ANOVA) techniques. The test can be performed using the **QTDT** package described in **Subheading 4.**

It should be noted that all of Allison's tests (*13*) are valid only for simple nuclear family data, as is the case with the classical TDT. TDT_{Q1-Q4} can only use nuclear families in which one parent is heterozygous and one homozygous. TDT_{Q5} can use nuclear families in which one or both parents are heterozygous. Allison's model includes two regression coefficients (X and X^2), which should fit any genetic model. However, because the transmissions from parents are treated as independent events, the tests assume implicitly that the trait follows a multiplicative mode of inheritance. This will not affect the validity of the test, but will mean that it is most powerful when the trait being studied is, indeed, multiplicative.

3.2. Rabinowitz

Rabinowitz's test (*23*) can, like most of Allison's tests (*13*), be calculated by hand, but it is quite onerous. It can, instead, be implemented using the **QTDT** package described in **Subheading 4.**

The test models the mode of inheritance as additive, which is a fairly standard technique in modeling quantitative traits. No allowance is made for including dominance effects in the model. The test is designed to handle multiallelic loci; however, the test is not valid for multiplex families unless the extension of Monks et al. (*24*) is used.

3.3. Allison et al.—Sib-QTDT

This model is designed to be applied to data on sibships and assumes that sibships are independent (i.e., unrelated). Only full siblings can be used; half-sibs and monozygous twins are inappropriate.

The first test presented by Allison et al. (*25*) is an ANOVA-based F-test, which can be carried out using a standard statistical package such as SAS, SPSS, or Stata. The second test involves the calculation of a statistic that can be done by hand (although this is arduous for large datasets) and compared against a χ^2-distribution.

If the number of individuals in each sibship is unbalanced, then statistical inferences can be complex.

3.4. Abecasis et al. (28)

The model is a multivariate Normal distribution that can be fitted using the **QTDT** package. The model is compared under the null and alternative (full) hypotheses. If the latter model provides a significantly better fit, then the alternative hypothesis is accepted. Otherwise, the alternative hypothesis is rejected.

Thus, the best-fit model can be built up, as in a stepwise regression, by testing parameters one-by-one and adding them if they significantly improve the model.

The multivariate Normal distribution is expressed in terms of a mean and a variance–covariance matrix. When used by either Abecasis et al. (*28*) or Fulker et al. (*27*), the mean term can be thought of as representing association and the variance term as representing linkage.

Thus, if you want to test only for linkage, you would model only variance components. If you wanted to test only for association, you would fit only the means part of the model. If the family data consist of simple TDT trios (for Abecasis et al.'s method; **ref. 28**), just the linear (means) part of the model need be fitted. In this case, testing the within-family component of variance for significance is equivalent to a test of association that is robust to stratification.

If the families are larger than this, then transmissions are not independent of one another. In this case, the variance of the multivariate Normal distribution must also be modeled for the test to be valid. Again, the test for association is of the within-family component, but with the variance component already in the model. Residual environmental variance, polygenic variance, and an additive component of variance are included, because the test of association assumes both a polygenic effect and that one of the markers tested may be in the vicinity of an additive major locus.

Further parameters such as covariates, imprinting, dominance, and so forth may be tested for by adding them one by one, again as in a stepwise regression.

4. Software

A single program will be described in detail here (**QTDT**). Note that, in this section, program or file names are highlighted in bold and commands are shown in italics. **QTDT** is a package developed by Gonçalo Abecasis and is available free of charge. Details of how to download the package as well as on-line instructions for its use can be found at http://www.well.ox.ac.uk/asthma/ QTDT/. Executable versions of **QTDT** are offered for Linux (x86), SunOS, DecAlpha, and Silicon Graphics. The C++ source code is also available.

QTDT is a user-friendly package that implements several of the methods mentioned in this chapter as well as a few that are not covered. The methods implemented by **QTDT** are those of Abecasis et al. (*28*), Allison TDT$_{Q5}$; **ref. 13**), and Rabinowitz (*23*) (all described earlier) as well as Fulker et al. (*29*) and Monks et al. (*24*) (neither of which have been described in detail here). The package also includes a test for stratification. As a result, **QTDT** can analyze sib-pair, nuclear family, or extended family data, depending on which method is implemented.

QTDT requires several files containing data and an instruction typed in the command line. Results are then outputted to the screen, and parameter estimates are outputted to a file, **regress.tbl.**

4.1. Files

4.1.1. Pedigree File

Each line in the pedigree file contains information on a single individual. The file contains genotype data, trait values, and potential covariates as well as information on the parentage of every individual, a personal ID, a family ID, and their sex. Entries are separated by spaces or tabs. Each column contains a different piece of information. The types of information that can be included in a column are summarized in **Table 1.** For each type of data, 'Coding' indicates what form the data has to take. 'Missing value indicator' indicates how missing values should be represented (some data must be included and are marked 'values are required'). The first five columns must always contain family ID, personal ID, father ID, mother ID, sex in that order.

Figure 1 is an example of a pedigree file. Here, the columns are family ID, personal ID, father ID, mother ID, sex, trait value, marker genotype (with alleles delimited with a forward slash, /), and covariate. Note that the file finishes with the line 'end'. This is not a requirement, but is good practice. See **Note 1** for hints on entering data in the pedigree file.

If there are any pairs of twins in the study, this must be entered in the 'zygosity' column. Monozygous twins are entered in the zygosity column of the pedigree file as MZ and dizygous twins as DZ. All nontwins are entered as 0. If there is more than one set of twins with the same parents, the pairs are coded using integers in the zygosity column. To differentiate between monozygous and dizygous twins when they are numbered, monozygotes are always coded using odd numbers and dizygotes using even numbers.

Figure 2 is an example of twin coding. Here, there is a pair of dizygous twins in family 1. In family 2, individuals 4 and 5 are monozygous twins and individuals 6 and 7 are dizygous twins.

4.1.2. Data File

The data file is a companion to the pedigree file and indicates the type of data represented in each of the columns in the pedigree file. Each line of the data file relates to a column of the pedigree file and contains two items. The

Table 1
Types of Data That Can Be Included in the Pedigree File

Column type	Information	Coding	Missing value indicator
Family ID	Each family has a unique identifier.	Alphanumeric characters only	Values are required. No missing values accepted.
Personal ID	Each individual within a family has a unique identifier.	Alphanumeric characters only	Values are required. No missing values accepted.
Father/mother ID	One column will contain the mother ID and one the father ID. Either both or neither parents should be included.	The personal ID of the father/mother must exist.	0 or x
Sex	The sex of the individual	Male=1 or M Female=2 or F	0 or x
Marker genotype	Marker genotype should be entered as two numbers separated by a tab, space, or foreward slash	Integer values only	0 or x
Trait value	One or more trait values may be entered.	Real numbers only	x or user specified in command line
Covariate	One or more covariate values may be entered.	Real numbers only	x or user-specified in command line
Zygosity	This indicates twin status if there are twins in the study.	Monozygotes=MZ; dizygotes=DZ; Non-twins=0 (see later for more info on this)	Required if twins are present
Affection status	This denotes a binary phenotype that will be ignored by **QTDT.**	Integer only	Ignored by **QTDT,** so unimportant

1	1	0	0	1	3.4	1/1	15
1	2	0	0	2	2.7	1/2	12
1	3	1	2	1	5.8	1/2	9
2	1	0	0	1	4.3	1/1	3
2	2	0	0	2	5.4	1/2	12
2	3	1	2	2	4.4	1/1	9
2	4	1	2	1	6.5	1/1	8

end

Fig. 1. Example pedigree file, without twin data.

1	1	x	x	1	0	1/2	160
1	2	x	x	2	0	1/2	130
1	3	1	2	1	DZ	1/2	145
1	4	1	2	1	DZ	1/2	112
2	1	x	x	1	0	1/2	134
2	2	x	x	2	0	1/2	178
2	3	1	2	1	0	1/2	123
2	4	1	2	2	1	1/2	189
2	5	1	2	2	1	1/2	106
2	6	1	2	1	2	1/2	163
2	7	1	2	1	2	1/2	120

end

Fig. 2. Pedigree file with twin coding.

T   trait1

M   marker1

C   covariate1

Fig. 3. Data file used in conjunction with pedigree file from Fig. 1.

first is a code specifying what data type is in the column and the second is a column name. The first five columns are always family ID, personal ID, father ID, mother ID, and sex, in that order, and are, therefore, not mentioned in the data file. The codes used for the remaining columns are as follows:

    M = marker genotype

    T = trait value

    C = covariate

    Z = zygosity

    A = affection status

  $S[n]$ = skip column

The 'skip column' entry is used if a column is to be ignored in the analysis. If more than one consecutive column is to be ignored, the subscript n is used. For example, to skip two columns, use $S2$.

The pedigree file from **Fig. 1** would have the data file illustrated in **Fig. 3**. The names can be anything you want. See **Note 2** Section 6.2 for hints on labeling the columns in the data file.

4.1.3. IBD File

The third file used by **QTDT** is the IBD file. For every pair of individuals in a family, this file contains an estimate of the probability that their markers are identical by descent (IBD).

QTDT has a basic facility that can calculate **IBD** probabilities when both parents have been genotyped, in which case, the IBD file is not needed. If there is any missing data, the IBD file is required.

The IBD probabilities are calculated using either **GENEHUNTER 2** or **Simwalk2.** Both of these programs can be downloaded free of charge. The **QTDT** package includes the programs *prelude* and *finale*. *prelude* prepares the data in a form that can be read by **GENEHUNTER 2** or **Simwalk2** and *finale* takes the output from either **Simwalk2** or **GENEHUNTER 2** and converts it to an IBD file named **qtdt.ibd** that can be used by **QTDT.** It is recommended that the name of the IBD file be changed in order to avoid confusion with other IBD files you may have created. The commands for running *prelude, finale,* **GENEHUNTER 2,** and **Simwalk2** are given in **Subheading 4.2.**

The IBD file will have the format:

$$\langle family1 \rangle \; \langle person1 \rangle \; \langle person2 \rangle \; \langle marker1 \rangle \; \langle z0 \rangle \; \langle z1 \rangle \; \langle z2 \rangle$$

where z0, z1, and z2 are the probabilities that zero, one, and two alleles, respectively, are shared between person1 and person2 of family1 at marker1.

If other markers are used, the IBD probabilities for each are recorded on separate lines. See **Note 3** for hints on naming files.

4.2. Command Line

There are three uses of the command line in the **QTDT** package. One is to run the **QTDT** analysis, one is to provide summary statistics on the data, and the other (previously mentioned) is to prepare the IBD file. Each follows the same format. The name of the program to be run is entered first, followed by the names of the files to be used, and, finally, which options are required in the analysis (such as covariates and variance components). All are entered in a single line.

4.2.1. Summary Statistics

The summary statistics are produced using the command *pedstats.* The names of the data and the pedigree files to be analyzed must also be included in the command line. The IBD file may also be included. Assuming the data, pedigree, and IBD files are named **file.dat, file.ped** and **file.ibd,** respectively, the command would be

$$pedstats\ -d\ file.dat\ -p\ file.ped\ -i\ file.ibd$$

$-d$ indicates the data file used, $-p$ the pedigree file used, and $-i$ the IBD file used. The code used for missing values can be indicated by $-x$ (e.g., $-x$ -99.999 if this is the code used in the pedigree file for missing trait values or covariates).

The output from this is written to the screen and summarizes the number of families, the total number of individuals in the pedigree file, the range of family sizes, and the range of number of generations in the families. It shows the number of people typed for whom information exists at each marker locus and for the trait values. The mean and variance of the trait values are also given. The number of individuals for whom IBD probabilities have been calculated is listed and will equal zero if the IBD file has not been included in the *pedstats* command.

4.2.2. Preparing the IBD File

When the data include missing or untyped parents, **QTDT** is unable to calculate IBD probabilities. Instead, they must be calculated using either **GENEHUNTER2** or **Simwalk2.**

The input files are prepared using *prelude,* the IBD probabilities are calculated using either **GENEHUNTER2** or **Simwalk2,** and then the output from these is converted using *finale* into a form compatible with **QTDT.**

prelude uses the data and pedigree files and requires the recombination fraction between the marker loci as well as an indicator of which individuals will be included when estimating allelic frequencies. This is written as *prelude −d file.dat −p file.ped −t 0.0001 −aa*

where **file.dat** is the data file, **file.ped** is the pedigree file, and 0.0001 is the recombination fraction between the markers. The −a option indicates which individuals should be used to estimate allelic frequencies:

−*aa* = use all individuals;
−*ae* = assume alleles are equally frequent;
−*af* = use only founder alleles.

If there are more than two markers and these are not evenly spaced, then the recombination fraction will not be the same for all of them. For **Simwalk2,** you must edit section 000015 of **BATCH2.DAT.** For **GENEHUNTER2** you must edit the USE command in the file **genehunter.in**

Once *prelude* has prepared the files, you run either **Simwalk2** or **GENEHUNTER 2.** To create the IBD file using **Simwalk2** type:

simwalk

followed by

finale IBD-01.*

To create the IBD file using **GENEHUNTER 2** type:

gh < genehunter.in

followed by

finale genehunter.in

Here, *gh* and *simwalk* are the executable commands for **GENEHUNTER 2** and **Simwalk2,** respectively. These may vary. If you use a different command to run **GENEHUNTER 2,** such as *gh.sol,* that should be used instead.

Regardless of whether **GENEHUNTER 2** or **Simwalk2** is used, *finale* writes the IBD file to **qtdt.ibd.**

Simwalk2 is recommended if the families in the pedigree file are large. For small families, as are likely to be used in TDT-type analyses, **GENEHUNTER 2** is recommended because it runs more quickly.

4.2.3. Running **QTDT**

The most basic command for running **QTDT** is

qtdt −d file.dat −p file.ped

where **file.dat** is the data file and **file.ped** is the pedigree file. If this command is run using the same **file.dat** and **file.ped** files described earlier, the output to the screen from **QTDT** looks like the following:

```
QTDT - Quantitative TDT 2.1.11
(c) 1998-2000 Goncalo Abecasis (goncalo@well.ox.ac.uk)

This program implements tests described by
Abecasis et al, Am J Hum Genet 66:279-292 (2000)
Allison, in Am J Hum Genet 60:676-690 (1997) [TDTQ5]
Fulker et al, in Am J Hum Genet 64:259-267 (1999)
Monks et al, ASHG meeting (1998)
Rabinowitz, in Hum Hered 47:342-350 (1997)

The following parameters are in effect:
                QTDT Data File:        file.dat (-dname)
            QTDT Pedigree File:         file.ped (-pname)
          QTDT IBD Status File:       qtdt.ibd (-iname)
            Missing Value Code:        -99.999 (-xname)
                    Covariates:  USER SPECIFIED (-c{p|s|u|-})
             Association Model:       ORTHOGONAL (-a[a|f|m|o|p|r|t|w|-])
          Full Model Variances:    NOT MODELLED (-v{e|c|n|t|g|a|d|-})
          Null Model Variances:    NOT MODELLED (-w{e|c|n|t|g|a|d|-})
    Genetic Dominance Parameter:            OFF (-g[+|-])
       Parent of Origin Effects:           NONE (-o[f|t|m|p|-])
        Monte-Carlo Permutations:            0 (-m9999)
             Numeric Minimizer: NELDER AND MEAD (-n[n|p])
             First Allele Only:            OFF (-1[+|-])


Online documentation http://www.well.ox.ac.uk/asthma/QTDT
Comments, bugs: goncalo@well.ox.ac.uk

The following models will be evaluated. . .
  NULL MODEL
     Means = Mu + covariate + B
  FULL MODEL
     Means = Mu + covariate + B + W
Testing trait:                         trait1
===============================================
Testing marker:                        marker1
-----------------------------------------------


 Allele  df(0)   Rsq(0)   df(T)    Rsq(T)       F      p
   1 :   *** not tested***                          (3 probands)
   2 :   *** not tested***                          (3 probands)
```

As you can see, a number of options not specified in the command line are used here, because they are set as defaults. For instance, it is assumed that the IBD file, if it exists, is called **qtdt.ibd,** that the model used is 'Orthogonal'

(*28*), and that the numeric minimizer used is that of 'Nelder and Mead' (see later for more information about this).

To avoid mistakes, it is always best to specify exactly what you want your model to contain, without relying on default values.

Table 2 illustrates the summary of options if a description of the model is fitted. The null model fits a mean term, followed by the covariate in the pedigree file, then the between-family component of association. The alternative model is the same but adds a within-family component of association.

If the within-family component is significant, this suggests that there is an association between the trait value and the marker allele being analyzed, over and above any simple familial effect, caused by common environment or stratification, for instance. The effect of the marker on the trait value (if there is one) is assumed to be additive. A dominant component can be added using the $-g$ option.

After the model description, the results of the analysis are shown. In the example, the dataset is too small to test for any effects (only three probands; *see* **Fig. 1**), so no results are given.

4.2.3.1. Overview of QTDT Options

The various options that can be specified in the QTDT command line are given in **Table 2.** Default values are indicated in **bold.** The Command column indicates what should be entered in the command line. The Description column gives a brief description of the parameter. The Coding options column gives all the possible options that can be used in the command line, with a brief description of each. For instance,

$$qtdt -d\ file.dat -p\ file.ped -x -99.999 -af -cs -we -veg$$

will use the Fulker method (*29*), with missing covariate and trait values represented by −99.999. The data file used will be **file.dat** and the pedigree file used will be **file.ped.** Sex will be included as a covariate in the model of association. A variance components model with environmental and polygenic components will be tested against one that includes only environmental components. Thus, the significance of the polygenic components is tested for. By default, the IBD file used will be **qtdt.ibd** (if it exists) and no dominance parameter or parent of origin effect will be included. All alleles will be tested and *p*-values will be calculated assuming Normality (as opposed to using Monte Carlo methods). The variance components model will be minimized using Nelder and Mead's method.

The different options that can be included in the command line are now described more fully.

Table 2
QTDT Options

Command	Description	Coding options
-*d* data file	The name of the data file used	Any name
-*p* pedigree file	The name of the pedigree file used	Any name
-*i* IBD file	The name of the IBD file used	Any name
-*x* missing data	The code used for missing trait or covariate values	Any real number
-*a*[model]	The model used	-*aa* (Allison TDT$_{Q5}$; **ref. 13**) -*af* (Fulker, **ref. 29**) -*am* (Monks, **ref. 24**) -***ao*** (Abecasis, **ref. 28**) -*ap* (test for stratification) -*ar* (Rabinowitz, **ref. 23**) -*at* (test ignoring stratification) -*aw* (use within-family component only) -*a* (no association modelled)
-*c*[covariate]	The covariates included in the model	-*cp* (parental phenotypes) -*cs* (sex) -***cu*** (user-specified) -*c*- (no covariates)
-*w*[components]	The variance components included in the null model	-*we* (environmental) -*wc* (common family environment) -*wn* (nuclear family environment) -*wt* (shared twin environment) -*wg* (polygenic) -*wa* (major gene additive effect) -*wd* (major gene dominance effect) -**w**- (none)
-*v*[components]	The variance components included in the alternative model	-*ve*, -*vc*, -*vn*, -*vt*, -*vg*, -*va*, -*vd*, -**v**- (all as specified for -*w*)
-*n*[minimizer]	The numeric minimisation strategy used for solving variance components	-***nn*** (Nelder and Mead) -*np* (Powell)
-*m*[permutations]	Number of Monte-Carlo permutations used to get an empirical p-value	Any positive integer (default is ***0***)
-*g*[+/−]	Include a dominance parameter	-*g*+ (include dominance parameter) -***g***− (do not include dominance parameter)
-*o*[option]	Parent-of-origin effects	-*of* (models maternal/paternal separately) -*ot* (tests for maternal/paternal difference) -*om* (test only maternally inherited alleles) -*op* (test only paternally inherited alleles) -***o***− (none)
-*l*[+/−]	Test only first allele at loci	−*l*+ (include only first allele) −***l***− (include all alleles)

4.2.3.2. VARIANCE COMPONENTS (−w/v).

Linear models such as those of Allison (*13*) are not valid when there are multiple offspring in a family. This is because the linear model requires that all of the data are independent. In order to model the nonindependence between members of the same family, variance components are used. Variance components are specified using the −*w* command followed by the command appropriate to the type of variance component being modeled.

The components of variance that can be included in the model using **QTDT,** together with their codes, are as follows:

-*we* represents the environmental effect unique to each individual. This fulfills the same role as a residual error term and is fitted using the identity matrix.

-*wg* represents a polygenic effect caused by loci other than those that have been typed. It is modeled as a function of the degree of relatedness between family members and is fitted using the kinship matrix.

-*wa* represents the additive effect of linkage to a major gene. It is fitted using the $\hat{\pi}$ measure from the IBD matrix.

-*wd* represents the dominance effect of linkage to a major gene. It is fitted using the probability that two individuals share two alleles.

-*wt* represents the environment shared by twins but not other relatives.

-*wc* represents the common environmental effects shared by all members of a family.

-*wn* represents the environmental effect shared by all members of a nuclear family.

When the significances of individual components of variance are of interest, two separate models are compared. One includes the component of interest and one does not. This can be done in a single command line by specifying the null hypothesis in the -*w* command and the alternative hypothesis in the -*v* command. The options for -*v* are the same as those for -*w*.

To compare variance components it is best to exclude the components of the linear model. For example, to compare a model with just the environmental variance component with one that also includes the polygenic component, the following command can be used to test for heritability:

qtdt −d file.dat −p file.ped −a −c −we −veg

The results compare a model with only the environmental variance component fitted to one with the polygenic variance component added. The association is not modeled. Testing for stratification is done in a similar manner with the command:

qtdt −d file.dat −p file.ped −ap −wega

4.2.3.3. MODELING ASSOCIATION (−a).

The model used is specified using the -*a* command. Care must be taken to ensure that the remaining options, in particular the variance components, are set in accordance with the description of the test in the original article. For instance, Allison's TDT_{Q5} (*13*) does not include variance components, whereas Abecasis et al.'s Orthogonal test (*28*) and Fulker et al.'s test (*29*) both require variance components.

The tests indicated by *–aa, –af, –am, –ao,* and *–ar* are as described in the relevant articles. The others are as follows:

-*ap* implements a test for stratification based on the Orthogonal model (*28*), comparing the within- and between-family components of association. This requires variance components.

-*aw* indicates that only the within family component is to be included in the model.

-*at* is a test for association that evaluates the total information available. It should only be used when you can be certain that there is no stratification. It is not a TDT. Variance components are required for this.

-*a-* instructs **QTDT** not to model association. This is used when only components of variance are of interest (e.g., in estimating heritability).

4.2.3.4. COVARIATES (*–c*).

The covariates to be included in the model are specified using the -*c* command. If sex is to be included as a covariate, then -*cs* is used. If parental phenotypes are included as a covariate, then -*cp* is used. Any covariates listed in the pedigree file are included by default, if the -*c* command is not used, but the instruction to do this is -*cu.* If you do not want the covariants in the pedigree file included, then you must specify this with the command -*c-,* which means that no covariates are used. Multiple covariates can be included by, for instance, using -*csp* to indicate that both sex and parental phenotypes should be used as covariates. In this case, the covariates in the pedigree file would not be used.

If the significance of a covariate in the model is of interest, then the model can be fitted twice—once with the covariate and once without. The likelihoods of the two models are then compared to test the significance of the covariate. Twice the log likelihood difference should have a χ_1^2-distribution if the covariate has no influence on the trait. Significant deviation from this indicates that the covariate is important.

4.2.3.5. DOMINANCE PARAMETER (*–g*).

This adds a dominant component to the model of association. The command is -*g* or -*g+.*

4.2.3.6. MONTE CARLO METHOD (*–m*).

The method used by **QTDT** for calculating *p*-values depends on the data having a multivariate normal distribution. If this assumption is violated (for instance, if the samples are small or the data have been selected for extreme trait values), Normality assumptions may be violated. In this case, it is wise to calculate *p*-values using Monte Carlo permutations because these make no distributional assumptions. The permutations condition on the trait distribution, linkage, and familiality. Bear in mind that the Monte Carlo permutations may take some time to run.

-m1000 instructs **QTDT** to run 1000 permutations to calculate *p*-values. Any number of permutations can be implemented.

If a significant result is found using **QTDT,** it is always worth recalculating the *p*-values using Monte Carlo permutations to be sure that the results have not been biased by non-Normality of the data.

4.2.3.7. MINIMIZATION STRATEGY (-n).

-n specifies the numerical minimization strategy employed in fitting models that include variance components. The choice is either to use Nelder and Mead's method (*-nn*) or Powell's (*-np*). The default is to use Nelder and Mead's method. Although the two methods are different, there is little to choose between them. The interested reader may find out more about them in **ref. 30.**

4.2.3.8. PARENT-OF-ORIGIN EFFECT (-o).

The *-o* option allows for testing of parent-of-origin effects (imprinting). If these are shown to be significant, maternally and paternally inherited alleles can be fitted as separate components in the model, also using the *-o* option.

-ot tests whether there is a difference between maternally and paternally derived alleles; for example,

$$qtdt\ -d\ file.dat\ -p\ file.ped\ -ao\ -ot$$

If a difference is found, you can include either *-of*, which models maternally and paternally inherited alleles separately, or *-om/-op*, which includes only data from maternally/paternally inherited alleles

4.2.3.9. DIALLELIC MARKERS (-1).

If the markers used are all diallelic (e.g., SNPs), then the results from the two alleles at a locus will be identical. If this is this case, you can specify that only one marker at each locus be analyzed by implementing the option *-1* or *-1+*. This will reduce the output from **QTDT** as well as possibly speeding up the program.

4.3. Hints on Model Fitting

If the data consist solely of simple nuclear family trios, then either the method of Allison (*13*) or Abecasis et al. (*28*) is recommended. If any of the families are larger than this (either multiplex sibships or multigenerational families) then variance components must be modeled to take account of this. This can be done using the method of Abecasis et al. (*31*) [or Fulker et al. (*29*) if only siblings are present].

The command lines and model description in the output for the various methods are given below. The data files used here are the example files provided with **QTDT.** The **trios** files contain information on nuclear family trios and the **sibs** files contain data on sib pairs with unknown parents. Note that when using the **sibs** data, variance components must always be used because the sibling data will be correlated.

4.3.1. Allison (*13*)

> *qtdt -d trios.dat -p trios.ped -aa*

```
NULL MODEL
   Means = Aa*AA + Aa*Aa + Aa*aa
FULL MODEL
   Means = Aa*AA + Aa*Aa + Aa*aa + X
```

4.3.2. Fulker (*29*)

> *qtdt -d sibs.dat -p sibs.ped -i sibs.ibd -af -wega*

```
NULL MODEL
    Means = Mu + Covariate + B
Variances = Ve + Vg + Va
 FULL MODEL
    Means = Mu + Covariate + B + W
Variances = Ve + Vg + Va
```

4.3.3. Monks (*24*)

> *qtdt -d trios.dat -p trios.ped -am*

```
 Genotype = Conditional on Parental Alleles
Phenotype = Mu
Rab = (observed - Expected Genotype) * (Observed -
Expected Phenotype)
```

4.3.4. Abecasis (*28*)

> *qtdt -d trios.dat -p trios.ped -i trios.ibd -ao -wega*

```
NULL MODEL
    Means = Mu + B
Variances = Ve + Vg + Va
 FULL MODEL
    Means = Mu + B + W
Variances = Ve + Vg + Va
```

4.3.5. Rabinowitz (**23**)

> *qtdt -d trios.dat -p trios.ped -ar*

```
Genotype = Conditional on Parental Alleles
Phenotype = Mu
Rab = (Observed − Expected Genotype) * (Observed −
Expected Phenotype)
```

4.3.6. Stratification

> *qtdt -d trios.dat -p trios.ped -i trios.ibd -ap -wega*

```
NULL MODEL
    Means = Mu + X
Variances = Ve + Vg + Va
 FULL MODEL
    Means = Mu + X + W
Variances = Ve + Vg + Va
```

5. Worked Example

The worked example given here uses the data of Keavney et al. (**31**). The data concern the level of circulating angiotensin-I converting enzyme (ACE) and the influence on this of 10-diallelic-marker loci spanning 26 kb of the ACE gene. The markers used are T-5991C, A-5466C, T-3892C, A-240T, T-93C, T1237C, G2215A, I/D G2350A, and 4656(CT)$_{3/2}$. The data have previously been analyzed using the **QTDT** package by Abecasis et al. (**31**).

The dataset consists of 666 individuals plus some ungenotyped parents (who are included so that sibships will be recognized; *see* **Note 1**). Some of the families contain data on multiple siblings and are multigenerational, so variance components must be used in the analysis to account for the nonindependence of the transmissions. The best method to use is that of Abecasis et al. (**31**).

5.1. Files

5.1.1. Pedigree File

The pedigree file consists of the usual first five columns followed by 10 marker genotypes and the trait value (ACE). The first few lines of the pedigree file, **ace.ped**, are as follows:

```
1  1  0 0   1  0 0   0 0   2 2   2 2   2 2   0 0   1 2   1 2   1 2   1 2   −0.395
1  2  0 0   2  1 1   1 1   1 1   1 1   1 1   1 2   1 2   1 2   1 2   1 2   −1.788
1  3  1 2   1  0 0   1 2   1 2   1 2   1 2   0 0   2 2   1 1   1 1   1 1   −0.873
1  4  0 0   1  1 1   1 1   1 2   1 1   1 1   1 2   1 2   1 2   1 2   1 2   −0.477
1  5  1 2   2  1 2   1 2   1 2   1 2   1 2   1 2   1 2   1 2   1 2   1 2   −0.897
1  6  1 2   2  1 2   0 0   1 2   1 2   1 2   2 2   1 2   1 2   1 2   1 2   −0.486
1  7  1 2   2  1 2   1 2   1 2   1 2   1 2   1 2   1 2   1 2   1 2   1 2   −0.520
1  8  1 2   2  1 2   1 2   1 2   1 2   1 2   2 2   1 2   1 2   1 2   1 2   −0.863
1  9  4 5   2  1 2   1 2   1 2   1 2   1 2   1 2   1 2   1 2   1 2   1 2    0.337
1 10  4 5   2  1 1   1 1   1 1   1 1   1 1   1 1   2 2   1 1   1 1   1 1   −1.308
```

5.1.2. Data File

The data file, **ace.dat,** is as follows:

```
M T-5491C
M A-5466C
M T-3892C
M A-240T
M T-93C
M T1237C
M G2215A
M ID
M G2350A
M 4656CT
T ACE
```

Note that this lists 10 markers and a trait value. No covariates are included.

5.2. Command Line

5.2.1. Preliminary Analysis

The data are summarized using the command

pedstats −d ace.dat −p ace.ped

The output printed to the screen starts with the copyright details followed by a summary of the model used. Next the data are described:

```
PEDIGREE STRUCTURE
==================
Families:    83
Individuals: 666 (221 founders, 445 nonfounders)
Family Size: 4 to 18
Generations: 2 to 4


QUANTITATIVE TRAIT STATISTICS
=============================
            [Count]      [Founder]       Mean     Var
       ACE  405  60.8%    87  39.4%      0.000   0.998
     Total  405  60.8%    87  39.4%

MARKER GENOTYPE STATISTICS
==========================
            [Count]      [Founder]      Hetero    IBD
   T-5491C  541  81.2%   112  50.7%     44.2%     0/83 families
   A-5466C  536  80.5%   108  48.9%     45.5%     0/83 families
   T-3892C  538  80.8%   110  49.8%     52.6%     0/83 families
    A-240T  550  82.6%   113  51.1%     44.4%     0/83 families
     T-93C  540  81.1%   111  50.2%     44.1%     0/83 families
    T1237C  526  79.0%   108  48.9%     52.1%     0/83 families
    G2215A  518  77.8%   103  46.6%     54.1%     0/83 families
        ID  551  82.7%   112  50.7%     54.1%     0/83 families
    G2350A  509  76.4%   105  47.5%     53.4%     0/83 families
    4656CT  540  81.1%   112  50.7%     55.9%     0/83 families
     Total 5349  80.3%  1094  49.5%     50.0%
```

This tells us that the data consist of 83 families of between 2 and 4 generations. There are a total of 666 individuals, of whom 405 have known trait values. The average trait value among these is 0.000 and the sample variance is 0.998. Following this is information about the markers. Listed for each marker are the number of people who have been genotyped (the total number and the number who are founders), the percentage who are heterozygous, and the percentage for whom IBD probabilities have been calculated. Because we have not included an IBD file in the **pedstats** command, the IBD column records 0/83 for every marker.

5.2.2. Preparing the IBD File

Next, we must produce the IBD file to be used in the analysis. The recombination fraction across the region is 0.00026. The probability of a recombination occurring in this region is so small that we can assume the markers are equidistant. Therefore, θ is approximated to 0.00003. We prepare the data using **prelude** and then calculate IBD probabilities using **GENEHUNTER 2:**

$$prelude\ -d\ ace.dat\ -p\ ace.ped\ -t0.00003$$
$$gh < genehunter.in$$

This returns the problem

```
analyzing pedigree 22...
WARNING: due to computation time and memory constraints, individual
9 has been dropped from the analysis.
using non-originals:   10 7 12 13 14 15 16 17 3 4 5 6
FAILED: 1048577x8      bytes             total bytes alloced=-
574024788
Can't get enough memory for this scan
*** error *** possible memory fault/out of memory/software problem ***
```

because **GENEHUNTER 2** cannot deal with large pedigrees. Instead, we must use **Simwalk2,** which is slower, but can cope with larger families. On a Sun Ultra 10 Workstation, this takes 8 h, 20 min.

The IBD file, **qtdt.ibd** is then prepared using the command

$$finale\ IBD\text{-}01.*$$

The resulting IBD file, which we rename **ace.ibd,** is 28161 lines long. The first few lines of this are as follows:

```
1  2  1   T-5491C  1.000  0.000  0.000
1  2  1   A-5466C  1.000  0.000  0.000
1  2  1   T-3892C  1.000  0.000  0.000
1  2  1    A-240T  1.000  0.000  0.000
1  2  1     T-93C  1.000  0.000  0.000
1  2  1    T1237C  1.000  0.000  0.000
```

5.2.3. Running QTDT

5.2.3.1. HERITABILITY.

Next, we test for the heritability of the trait, although it is unlikely that the dataset would have been collected without already having evidence of heritability. The test for heritability does not require marker data; it simply tests for a polygenic component of the trait variance and does not model association (-*a*-):

>*qtdt −d ace.dat −p ace.ped −i ace.ibd −a− −we −veg*

The model is described in the output

```
The following models will be evaluated . . .
  NULL MODEL
      Means = Mu
  Variances = Ve

  FULL MODEL
      Means = Mu
  Variances = Ve + Vg
```

followed by the test for the polygenic component of variance:

```
Testing trait:                        ACE
==========================================

Allele   df(0)  LnLk(0)  df(V)  LnLk(V)  ChiSq       P
   1 :     403   573.67    402   544.77  57.80  0.0000  (405 probands)
```

The parameter estimates are given in **regress.tbl.** The estimate of 'residual' nonshared environmental variance is 0.333 and the estimate of the polygenic component of variance is 0.669. Thus, the polygenic heritability of the trait is estimated as $0.669/(0.333+0.669) = 0.667$. In other words, about two-thirds of the total variance can be explained by a polygenic component, suggesting that the trait is highly heritable.

5.2.3.2. VARIANCE COMPONENTS (-w/v).

Next, we test for the significance of a QTL additive component of variance (i.e., evidence for a major gene), again without modeling association:

qtdt −d ace.dat −p ace.ped −i ace.ibd −a− −weg −vega

This is equivalent to testing each marker locus for linkage to an additive major gene influencing the trait. The results for the first two loci are as follows:

```
Testing trait:                              ACE

=========================================

Testing marker:                             T-5491C

-----------------------------------------

Allele   df(0)  LnLk(0)  df(V)   LnLk(V)  ChiSq          p
   1 :     402   544.77    401    528.22  33.09    0.0000  (405 probands)
Testing marker:                             A-5466C

-----------------------------------------

Allele   df(0)  LnLk(0)  df(V)   LnLk(V)  ChiSq          P
   1 :     402   544.77    401    528.22  33.09    0.0000  (405 probands)
```

The results for the remaining eight loci are just as significant (all p-values < 0.0001), suggesting that all are strongly linked to a major additive trait susceptibility locus. These likelihoods can be converted to a LOD score using the formula LOD=(lnLk0-LnLk1)/($\log_e 10$), where LnLk0 is the log likelihood under the null hypothesis and LnLk1 is the log likelihood under the alternative hypothesis. So, the LOD score for marker T-5491C is (544.77–528.22)/(ln 10) = 7.19.

With the QTL additive component of variance included, we can also estimate the (narrow) heritability as a result of a single locus. This is calculated for every locus. In this case, because the loci are all very close, the estimated coefficients of variance are the same at each one. The estimates, given in **regress.tbl,** are 0.384 for the residual environmental variance, 0.001 for the polygenic component, and 0.559 for the additive component. Thus, the heritability resulting from a single locus is 0.559/(0.384 + 0.001 + 0.559) = 0.592, indicating that about three-fifths of the total variance is accounted for by a single locus. Note that when the additive genetic component of variance is fitted, the polygenic component virtually disappears, suggesting that a single trait locus may be responsible.

We may also test for the significance of components of variance resulting from a dominant linked locus, a shared nuclear-family effect, and a shared complete-family effect. The commands for these are respectively as follows:

> *qtdt -d ace.dat -p ace.ped -i ace.ibd -a- -wega -vegad*
> *qtdt -d ace.dat -p ace.ped -i ace.ibd -a- -wega -vegan*
> *qtdt -d ace.dat -p ace.ped -i ace.ibd -a- -wega -vegac*

However, none are found to be significant.

5.2.3.3. MODELING ASSOCIATION (-a).

Next, we model the association. Note that because our data consist of more than simple nuclear families, we must include variance components even if these effects are not found to be significant in the previous tests. If we are testing for association, we believe that there is a polygenic effect and that this may map to the locus where our markers are located; hence, our model must include the variance components −wega in the null model. Note that the tests of variance are less powerful than the tests of association, so it is possible for an effect to be a significant component of the mean but not a significant component of variance.

We use the orthogonal test of Abecasis et al. (*28*) and include the −*1* term because all of the markers are diallelic:

>*qtdt -d ace.dat -p ace.ped -i ace.ibd -ao -wega -1*

```
The following models will be evaluated . . .
  NULL MODEL
      Means = Mu + B
  Variances = Ve + Vg + Va

  FULL MODEL
      Means = Mu + B + W
  Variances = Ve + Vg + Va
```

This confirms that the between-family component of association is automatically fitted and it is the within-family component that is being tested for significance, because it is robust to stratification.

```
Testing trait:                          ACE
================================================
Testing marker:                         T-5491C
------------------------------------------------
Allele  df(0)  LnLk(0)  df(T)  LnLk(T)  ChiSq      P
   1 :   304   390.29   303    367.57   45.42  0.0000  (189/309 probands)

Testing marker:                         A-5466C
------------------------------------------------
Allele  df(0)  LnLk(0)  df(T)  LnLk(T)  ChiSq      P
   1 :   305   393.68   304    372.86   41.64  0.0000  (193/310 probands)
```

The first two markers are highly significant, as are the other eight (all *p*-values < 0.0001), suggesting strong association with the trait allele. If we were to model the association and then test for linkage (*qtdt -d ace.dat -p ace.ped -i ace.ibd -ao -weg -vega -1*), we would find that there was now little evidence for linkage. This is because when fitted in this order, only linkage that has not been explained by association can be detected. In an extreme case, if the marker allele were the trait allele or in complete disequilibrium with it, there would be no evidence at all of linkage once association had been fitted. See **ref. *29*** for a fuller explanation of this.

If we fit association and then test for linkage, the χ^2 values for the consecutive markers are 5.16, 3.73, 4.13, 1.59, 1.75, 1.77, 0.20, 0.01, 0.02, and 1.17. The two markers with the lowest χ^2 values here (I/D and G2350A) had the highest χ^2-values when testing for association after fitting the means, suggesting that it is these two that are in the greatest linkage disequilibrium with the trait allele.

5.2.3.4. COVARIATES (-c).

We return to the model with association fitted after linkage. In order to test for covariates, we fit the current model both with and without the covariate and look at the difference in log likelihoods, which are given in the output. Here, there are no covariates declared in the pedigree file, so we can test only for sex and parental phenotype as covariates using respectively

qtdt -d ace.dat -p ace.ped -i ace.ibd -ao -wega -cs −1

and

qtdt -d ace.dat -p ace.ped -i ace.ibd -ao -wega -cp −1

compared to

qtdt -d ace.dat-p ace.ped -i ace.ibd -ao -wega −1

The log likelihoods for each marker under the null and alternative hypotheses are given in the output from **QTDT**. Hence, from our current model, without any covariates fitted, the log likelihood under the alternative (full) model, which includes the within-family component, is 367.57 (on 303 degrees of freedom [d.f.]) for marker T-5491C and 372.86 (on 304 d.f.) for marker A-5466C. These values can be seen in the above output. If we include sex as a covariate, these log likelihoods become 367.57 (on 302 d.f.) and 372.86 (on 303 d.f.). Twice the log likelihood difference between the models with and without the covariate included is 0.00 for both markers. This is, of course, not significant compared to a χ_1^2-distribution. The degrees of freedom of the χ_1^2-distribution are equal to the difference in degrees of freedom between the two models.

However, when parental phenotype is included as a covariate, the likelihoods for the same two markers under the alternative hypothesis are 95.08 (on 81 d.f.) and 94.06 (on 80 d.f.). The log likelihood difference between each of these and the model without any covariates is 272.49 (222 d.f.) for marker T-5491C and 278.8 (224 d.f.) for marker A-5466C. These are tested against a χ_{222}^2- and a χ_{224}^2-distribution, respectively, giving *p*-values of 0.012 and 0.007. Similar *p*-values are found for the other eight loci, providing strong evidence that parental phenotype is an important covariate. This may be caused by a further genetic effect that is unexplained by the model.

5.2.3.5. DOMINANCE PARAMETER (-g).

Before a dominance component of association is tested, it must be included in the variance components model. Therefore, we compare the two models *qtdt -d ace.dat -p ace.ped -i ace.ibd -ao -wegad −1*

and

qtdt -d ace.dat -p ace.ped -i ace.ibd -ao -wegad −g −1

and compare the alternative (full) likelihoods of the two models. Once again, twice the log likelihood difference is compared against a χ^2-distribution. Here, the χ^2-distribution has two degrees of freedom because both within- and between-family dominance components are added.

We tested for a dominance effect, but this was not significant at the 5% level at any of the 10 loci. Thus, we include parental phenotype as a covariate but do not model dominance in our model.

Therefore our complete model to test for association is

qtdt -d ace.dat -p ace.ped -i ace.ibd -ao -wega -cp −1

which gives p-values of less than 0.0001 for every marker.

5.2.3.6. MONTE CARLO METHOD (-m).

Just to be sure that this is not caused by non-Normality of the data, we ran the test again, calculating p-values using 10,000 Monte Carlo simulations:

qtdt -d ace.dat -p ace.ped -i ace.ibd -ao -wega -cp −m10000 -1

This takes 11.5 h on a Sun Ultra 10 Workstation (1000 simulations takes 75 min). The empirical p-values produced are 0.0001, 0.0004, 0.0001, 0.0003, 0.0004, <0.0001, <0.0001, <0.0001, <0.0001, and <0.0001. This agrees well with the analytical p-values (which are all less than 0.0001) and supports the earlier evidence that it is the eighth and ninth markers (I/D and G2350A) that are likely to be closest to the trait locus.

We can find parameter estimates in the file **regress.tbl.** Under the alternative (full) hypothesis (which includes the within-family component of association), the data for the first marker (T-5991C) look as follows:

```
FULL HYPOTHESIS
---------------
Family #1 var-covar matrix terms [3]...[[Ve]][[Vg]][[Va]]
Family #1 regression matrix...
       [linear] =
       [6 × 5]      Mu father_y mother_y      B      W
            1.10   1.000   −0.477   −0.897   0.500   0.500
            1.5    1.000   −0.395   −1.788   0.000   0.000
            1.6    1.000   −0.395   −1.788   0.000   0.000
            1.7    1.000   −0.395   −1.788   0.000   0.000
            1.8    1.000   −0.395   −1.788   0.000   0.000
            1.9    1.000   −0.477   −0.897   0.500  −0.500
```

```
Some useful information...
               df : 81
  log(likelihood) : 95.08
        variances :    0.315    0.200    0.000
            means :    0.105    0.267    0.226    -0.387    -0.916
```

Thus, the estimate of the between-family association parameter is −0.387 and the within-family parameter is −0.916 at marker T-5991C. If there was no stratification, these should be equal. However, because they are not, we estimate the additive effect of this allele to be −0.916. Note that if **QTDT** analyzed both alleles, the estimate of the additive effect of the other allele would be 0.916. This is true for all diallelic loci. Instead, we just take the modulus of these to give us the estimated additive genetic effect of each of the alleles: 0.916, 0.853, 0.833, 0.895, 0.897, 0.903, 1.110, 1.029, 1.115, and 0.992. The greatest effect is seen at the eighth, ninth, and tenth loci, suggesting, once again, that the trait-susceptibility locus is in this region. The decrease in additive genetic effect away from this is indicative of a decay in linkage disequilibrium between the marker loci and the trait locus as the distance between them increases.

Despite finding a difference between the within- and between-family association parameters, if we test for stratification, (*qtdt -d trios.dat -p trios.ped -i trios.ibd -ap −wega*), we find no significant evidence at any of the loci. This may be because, as has been previously mentioned, tests for significance of variance components are less powerful than tests of the components of association. Thus, even when we find no significant evidence of stratification, it may still be an effect that we should protect against.

6. Notes

1. Hints on creating the pedigree file. Two individuals are indicated to be siblings by having the same mother and father IDs. These IDs must correspond to two individuals in the pedigree. Therefore, mothers and fathers of siblings should always be given a line each, with their personal ID, family ID and sex, even if no other information about them (genotype, trait, etc.) exists; otherwise, the data on the siblings will be lost.

    Data entry must be performed carefully as mistakes such as assigning the wrong sex to the parents or both parents being entered with same personal ID will not be picked up on by **QTDT.** Similarly, entering the wrong family ID for an individual will go unnoticed.

2. Hints on creating the data file. The data types in the data file are assigned sequentially to the columns in the pedigree file. Therefore, if a column is not listed in the data file, the last column in the pedigree file will be ignored. However, if there are too many columns listed in the data file, **QTDT** will give an error message when run.

3. Suggestions for naming files. **QTDT** uses default file names for the pedigree, data, and IBD files. These are **qtdt.ped, qtdt.dat,** and **qtdt.ibd,** respectively. If file names

are not specified, these are the ones that are used. It is sensible not to use the default file names in order to avoid confusion. This is particularly important if you are running several analyses, so that the correct data, pedigree and IBD files are used in each analysis.

Acknowledgments

Many thanks to Gonçalo Abecasis for advice on the use of his QTDT package. Thanks also to Bernard Keavney, Martin Farrall, and Colin McKenzie for providing the ACE dataset used in the worked example.

References

1. Rubinstein, P., Walker, M., Carpenter, C., Carrier, C., Krassner, J., Falk, C., et al. (1981) Genetics of HLA disease associations. The use of the haplotype relative risk (HRR) and the "haplo-delta (Dh) estimates in juveniles diabetes from three racial groups. *Hum. Immunol.* **3(4),** 384.
2. Terwilliger, J. D. and Ott, J. (1992) A haplotype-based 'haplotype relative risk' approach to detecting allelic associations. *Hum. Heredity* **42,** 337–346.
3. Spielman R. S., McGinnis R. E., and Ewens W. J. (1993) Transmission test for linkage disequilibrium: the insulin region and insulin-dependent diabetes mellitus (IDDM). *Am. J. Hum. Genet.* **52,** 506–516.
4. Spielman R. S. and Ewens W. J. (1996) The TDT and other family-based tests for linkage disequilibrium and association. *Am. J. Hum. Genet.* **59,** 983–989.
5. Curtis, D. and Sham, P. C. (1995) A note on the application of the transmission disequilibrium test when a parent is missing. *Am. J. Hum. Genet.* **56,** 811–812.
6. Clayton, D. (1999) A generalization of the transmission/disequilibrium test for uncertain-haplotype transmission. *Am. J. Hum. Genet.* **65(4),** 1170–1177.
7. Cervino, A. C. L. and Hill, A. V. S. (2000) Comparison of tests for association and linkage in incomplete families. *Am. J. Hum. Genet.* **67(1),** 120–132.
8. Martin, E. R., Kaplan, N. L., and Weir, B. S. (1997) Tests for linkage and association in nuclear families. *Am. J. Hum. Genet.* **61,** 439–448.
9. Sham, P. C. and Curtis, D. (1995) An extended transmission/disequilibrium test (TDT) for multi-allele marker loci. *Ann. Hum. Genet.* **59(3),** 323–336.
10. Morris, A. P., Curnow, R. N., and Whittaker, J. C. (1997) Randomization tests of disease-marker associations. *Ann. Hum. Genet.* **61(4),** 335–350.
11. Lazzeroni, L. C. and Lange, K. (1998) A conditional inference framework for extending the transmission/disequilibrium test. *Hum. Heredity* **48(2),** 67–81.
12. Terwilliger, J. D. (1995) A powerful likelihood method for the analysis of linkage disequilibrium between trait and one or more polymorphic marker loci. *Am. J. Hum. Genet.* **56(3),** 777–787.
13. Allison, D. B. (1997) Transmission-disequilibrium tests for quantitative traits. *Am. J. Hum. Genet.* **60,** 676–690.
14. Haseman, J. K. and Elston, R. C. (1972) The investigation of linkage between a quantitative trait and a marker locus. *Behav. Genet.* **2,** 3–19.

15. Risch, N. J., and Zhang, H. P. (1996) Mapping quantitative trait loci with extreme discordant sib pairs: sampling considerations. *Am. J. Hum. Genet.* **58,** 836–843.

16. Risch, N. and Merikangas, K. (1996) The future of genetic studies of complex human diseases. *Science* **273,** 1516–1517.

17. Müller-Mhysok, B. and Abel, L. (1997) Genetic analysis of complex diseases. *Science* **275,** 1328–1329.

18. Camp, N. J. (1997) Genomewide transmission/disequilibrium testing—consideration of the genotype relative risks at disease loci. *Am. J. Hum. Genet.* **61,** 1424–1430.

19. Camp, N. J. (1999) Genomewide transmission/disequilibrium testing: a correction. *Am. J. Hum. Genet.* **64,** 1485–1487.

20. Page, G. P. and Amos, C. I. (1999) Comparison of linkage-disequilibrium methods for localization of genes influencing quantitative traits in humans. *Am. J. Hum. Genet.* **64,** 1194–1205.

21. Xiong, M. M., Krushkal, J., and Boerwinkle, E. (1998) TDT statistics for mapping quantitative trait loci. *Ann. Hum. Genet.* **62,** 431–452.

22. Wang, J. and Cohen, J. (1999) A correction to TDT statistics for mapping quantitative trait loci. *Ann. Hum. Genet.* **63,** 469.

23. Rabinowitz, D. (1997) A transmission disequilibrium test for quantitative trait loci. *Hum. Heredity* **47,** 342–350.

24. Monks, S. A. and Kaplan, N. L. (1998) Removing the sampling restrictions from family-based tests of association for a quantitative trait locus. *Am. J. Hum. Genet.* **66,** 576–592.

25. Allison, D. B., Heo, M., Kaplan, N., and Martin, E. R. (1999) Sibling-based tests of linkage and association for quantitative traits. *Am. J. Hum. Genet.* **64,** 1754–1764.

26. Spielman, R. S. and Ewens, W. J. (1998) A sibship test for linkage in the presence of association: the sib transmission/disequilibrium test. *Am. J. Hum. Genet.* **62,** 450–458.

27. Krzanowski, W. J. (1998) *Principles of Multivariate Analysis.* Oxford Science, Oxford.

28. Abecasis, G. R., Cardon, L. R., and Cookson, W. O. C. (2000) A general test of association for quantitative traits in nuclear families. *Am. J. Hum. Genet.* **66,** 279–292.

29. Fulker, D. W., Cherny, S. S., Sham, P. C., and Hewitt, J. K. (1999) Combined linkage and association analysis for quantitative traits. *Am. J. Hum. Genet.* **64,** 259–267.

30. Press, W. H., Teukolsky, S. A., Vetterling, W. T., and Flannery, B. P. (1992) *Numerical Recipes in C: The Art of Scientific Computing,* 2nd ed. Cambridge University Press, Cambridge.

31. Keavney, B., McKenzie, C. A., Connell, J. M. C., Julier, C., Ratcliffe, P. J., Sobel, E., et al. (1998) Measured haplotype analysis of the angiotensin-I converting enzyme gene. *Hum. Mol. Genet.* **7(11),** 1745–1751.

32. Abecasis, G. R., Cookson, W. O. C., and Cardon, L. R. (2000) Pedigree tests of transmission disequilibrium. *Eur. J. Hum. Genet.* **8,** 545–551.

6

Joint Linkage and Segregation Analysis Using Markov Chain Monte Carlo Methods

Ellen M. Wijsman

1. Introduction

Complex genetic traits are some of the most challenging in human studies. Such traits, which are characterized by genetic and etiologic heterogeneity, typically show evidence of familial influences, but do not follow simple Mendelian patterns of inheritance. Of interest in this chapter are complex traits that are measured on a scale that permits analysis as quantitative traits. A few examples are Alzheimer's disease (where age at onset is the continuous trait), various lipid levels, learning disabilities, and hypertension. The goal is to map quantitative trait loci (QTLs) that contribute to such traits.

Although there are a number of widely used approaches to QTL mapping, all have limitations. Model-free methods may be restricted to specific pedigree structures. They are also inefficient in comparison to methods that both accurately specify the trait mode of inheritance and can be applied to pedigrees of arbitrary structure (*1*). On the other hand, because of the need for computational tractability, traditional model-based log odds (LOD) score methods are based on overly simplistic mode-of-inheritance models. There may be loss of power in application to multilocus traits because of the inherent misfit between the assumed monogenic model and the underlying true mode of inheritance (*2*). In considering analytic approaches, there is also a trade-off between the size of pedigrees and the number of markers that can be handled in analysis. There are no exact methods that are computationally tractable for analysis with large numbers of markers on large pedigrees. However, studies of simulated complex traits have clearly shown the advantages, in some situations, of use of both multipoint analyses and large pedigrees (*1*). Finally, none of these methods are

From: *Methods in Molecular Biology: vol. 195: Quantitative Trait Loci: Methods and Protocols.*
Edited by: N. J. Camp and A. Cox © Humana Press, Inc., Totowa, NJ

computationally tractable for simultaneous analysis of the multiple genomic regions that may be typical of QTLs.

Markov chain Monte Carlo (MCMC) provides an approach to achieving a number of analytic goals that are otherwise difficult to achieve. With newly developed MCMC approaches, it is possible to perform linkage analysis with any number of marker loci, multiple-trait loci, and multiple genomic segments. At the same time, these approaches allow the use of pedigrees of arbitrary size and complexity. In addition to mapping the loci, Bayesian reversible-jump MCMC approaches (*3*) allow one to estimate the number of loci and associated individual-locus model parameters as well as covariate effects in a joint linkage and oligogenic segregation analysis. This is particularly useful when the possibility of multiple contributing loci is a possibility, but the number is unknown, as is usually the case in QTL analyses, so that it is advantageous to be able to estimate the number of contributing loci, rather than to have to fix this number *a priori*. The compromise made in order to achieve these goals lies in the overall approach, which is based on statistical sampling rather than exact enumeration of all possible underlying but unobserved genotypes.

The basic principles of MCMC in QTL mapping are based on several interrelated ideas. First, there are situations for which exact computation is infeasible or impractical because of issues such as combinatorial problems. Second, it is, in principle, possible to use statistical sampling methods to obtain realizations of possible unobserved genotypes, haplotypes, and other unobserved traits (latent variables) from the underlying sample space instead of enumerating all possibilities. These realizations can then be used to obtain desired parameter estimates. Finally, an efficient way to obtain realizations of the latent variables is to generate a series of correlated samples, each compatible with the observed data and derived from the previous sample. This is an efficient way to confine the realizations to those with positive probability, which may be a tiny subset of all that could be enumerated in the absence of data on the pedigrees.

Several caveats must be noted. First, these methods are under active development. Efficiency is being improved and capabilities for handling different types of data are being added to existing analytic approaches. Details about current implementations will quickly become outdated and incorrect, including details about computer programs and related file formats. Therefore, in what follows, technical details describing the algorithms used in the implementations are purposely kept to a minimum. Similarly, all details associated with program use should be checked against current program documentation. Second, unlike methods that have a long history of use and evaluation, MCMC methods have not yet been thoroughly evaluated to determine situations in which they give erroneous or misleading conclusions, although they have worked well in a number of simulated (*4,5*) and real data situations (*6,7*). Finally, for approaches based on a Bayesian framework, the interpretation of the results is not yet well understood relative to more traditional mapping methods in human genetics. A small amount of guidance will be given here, but, again, this is unlikely to provide the final word in using these methods for analysis of real data.

2. Methods

2.1. Genetic Models

We will focus heavily here on the Bayesian MCMC approach implemented initially by Heath (**4**) in the program Loki. Loki has also been extended to certain types of censored trait (**6**). The basic linear model used in MCMC analysis of oligogenic models has a number of components. The user must specify which components to consider in an analysis and which variables in a dataset fulfill the roles for the components included in the model. We can schematically describe the trait model as follows:

$$y_j = \mu + \sum_{i=1}^{n} Q_{ji} + \sum_{i=1}^{s} \beta_i C_{ji} + \sum_{i=1}^{k} G_{ji} + e_j \qquad (1)$$

In this linear model y_j is the observed phenotype for individual j, μ is the overall baseline, or mean, quantitative trait level against which all other effects are measured, and e_j is an error term assumed to be distributed as $N(0, V_e)$ where V_e is the environmental, or residual, variance. There are k diallelic QTLs which contribute to the phenotype, where k is a parameter that varies over iterations in the MCMC analysis and G_{ij} is the value of the genotypic effect of the ith locus in individual j. The ith QTL is characterized by an allele frequency, p_i, along with three genotype means expressed as deviations from μ. Following the nomenclature in Falconer (**8**), if we refer to alleles 1 and 2 at QTL locus i, for individual j these genotypic deviations are $-a_i$ if j's genotype is the 1/1 homozygote, d_i for the 1/2 heterozygote, and a_i for the 2/2 homozygote. We will refer to these deviations as the *genotypic effects* for QTL i. If markers are included in the model, for the ith QTL, there is also a location, λ_i, on the genetic map. This location may be either an unlinked location or may be on the specified part of the genetic map.

The model, shown in Eq. (1), also includes a fixed number of covariates, which may exist in two forms. The first is the usual type of continuous or discrete measured covariate, C_{ji}, such as age, sex, stratum, or other such factor. There may be any fixed number, s, of such covariates. The second type of covariate, Q, is one (or more) "major-gene covariate"—a locus with a proven or hypothesized role on the phenotype of interest. Unlike the diallelic QTLs, which are modeled as described above, a major-gene covariate can have any prespecified number of genotypes. However, unlike the trait loci, the number, n, of such major gene covariates in the model is fixed.

Finally, in addition to the components of the model that describe the trait phenotype, one must consider the marker model. This model consists of the same components as are in all multipoint linkage analyses: marker allele frequencies, map locations, and a map function. The codominant markers needed for such analyses may have allele frequencies specified by the user, or estimated from the data as part of the analysis. Markers must have locations on a user-specified map with "known" intermarker distances, which may be either a sex-averaged or sex-specific map. Finally, for analyses with multiple linked loci, a map function is necessary. The Haldane map function (**9**) is almost always used for such analyses. The map/marker component of the model is combined with the trait component in the usual sort of computation, which can be described as

P(trait phenotypes | trait model, marker model, covariate data, marker data, pedigree relationships).

2.2. Assumptions

In using the model specified in Eq. (1) for data analysis, there are several assumptions.

2.2.1. Distributional Assumptions

The residual variance is distributed as $N(0, V_e)$ and is the same for all multilocus QTL genotypes.

2.2.2. Genetic Effect Assumptions

All effects are additive; for example, there is no epistasis or gene–environment interaction.

2.2.3. Population Assumptions

There is random mating among founders and the population is in Hardy–Weinberg equilibrium

2.2.4. Locus Assumptions

There is linkage equilibrium among loci.

2.3. Basics of the MCMC Approach in Human QTL Mapping

An MCMC analysis requires specifying prior, or proposal, distributions. For example, in human pedigrees, founder genotypes are often unobserved for marker loci, and the trait loci are never directly observed. For both types of loci, a proposal distribution for founder genotypes must be specified. In each MCMC iteration, a possible genotype for each locus in each individual with missing genotype data is proposed, using prior distributions combined with genotypes on other pedigree members to determine proposal probabilities. For the markers, external information about marker allele frequencies, coupled with the assumptions of Hardy–Weinberg equilibrium within each locus, linkage equilibrium between loci, and Mendelian transmission probabilities, can be used to construct such a proposal distribution. In the absence of external allele frequency estimates, a uniform prior distribution on 0 to 1 for trait or marker allele frequencies may be assumed. Examples of other prior distributions that must be specified are (1) QTL locations, (2) the number of QTLs in the model, and (3) variance in the genotypic effects. It is important to note that although a proposal distribution is necessary, it need not perfectly reflect the true distribution. However, as for any MCMC approach, it is useful for this distribution to approximate the true distribution reasonably well because if the approximation is good, proposed states from the prior distribution will have relatively high probability in the true, but unknown, distribution, and thus will be frequently accepted during the acceptance/rejection step.

Clearly, for a given analysis, there is likely to be more knowledge about some prior distributions than others. In the absence of any information on QTL map location, it is not unreasonable to use a uniform prior distribution on gene location. Two examples of possible prior distributions on number of QTLs in the model are (1) a uniform distribution on 0 to K loci, where K is a maximum number of QTLs that must be specified by the user, or (2) a Poisson distribution with mean number, κ, per genome specified by the user [e.g., Poisson(κ)]. The Poisson distribution with a low κ will favor models with relatively few QTLs; the uniform distribution will give equal prior weight to all models having between 0 and K QTLs. When using the program Loki, the distribution of genotypic effects (both those of the homozygotes and heterozygote) is assumed to be distributed as $N(0, \tau)$, where τ, in turn, is determined by one of several functions of the user-specified variable, τ_β combined with V_e. Generally, firm information about the number of QTLs and τ is unavailable, so some care to evaluate assumptions about the magnitude of these parameters is well advised during data analysis (*see* **Subheading 5.**).

Markov Chain Monte Carlo analysis involves many iterations. An iteration is one cycle through the whole process of potentially sampling a new value for the latent variables on each individual in the dataset. In Bayesian QTL mapping, an iteration therefore refers to one cycle in which all missing or unobserved genotypes at all loci in the model are sampled, gene frequencies, and genotypic effects are estimated for each QTL in the model, QTL gene locations are possibly changed, the number of QTLs in the model may be changed, and all covariate effects and the overall baseline mean are recomputed. The values of the latent variables in each of these iterations may be used for parameter estimation. Each iteration involves two basic steps, which are repeated for each variable or set of variables in the model. First, a new value for the missing value of the variable is proposed from its prior distribution. Second, this value is either accepted or not, using an acceptance/rejection step. If the proposal is rejected, the value for the variable remains unchanged over its value in the previous iteration. The two steps may be carried out separately with a Metropolis–Hastings acceptance/rejection step (*10*) following the proposal step. Alternatively, the special case of the Gibbs sampler (*11*) may be used, where the two steps are combined. If the proposal distribution approximates the true distribution reasonably well, the proposal states will frequently be accepted. If the sampler mixes well (see below), this process will guarantee that the samples obtained eventually will be drawn from the correct equilibrium distribution (*12*) and will give rise to good estimates of parameters of interest.

In order for the MCMC process to provide useful estimates, it is necessary for the sampler to successfully move around the sample space. In other words, it must propose and accept possible genotypes (and other latent variables) from the entire possible sample space. This process is often referred to as "mixing." A sampler that mixes well moves frequently from one part of the sample space to another. However, it may be desirable that it remains in a part of the sample space for long enough that convergence to a local maximum is possible. Samplers that can efficiently produce realizations of data on pedigrees are difficult to design. This is an area that has seen steady improvement, and current implementations are likely to continue to be replaced as better approaches are discovered. Samplers that have been implemented include the following: (1) those that resample a single genotype at a single locus in a single individual at one time (single site samplers); (2) those that resample data for all loci at one time for a single individual (meiosis samplers); (3) those that resample data on all individuals, but at only one locus at one time (locus samplers); and (4) combinations of these (hybrid samplers).

Finally, depending on the starting configuration, it may take some time for the sampler to begin to propose values for the latent variables that have the highest probability. Burn-in refers to initial iterations of the MCMC process that are used to get the sampler into this part of the sample space. Parameter values from these initial iterations may be quite different than those obtained once the process has settled into the equilibrium distribution. Therefore, some investigators prefer to ignore the results of the early iterations.

2.4. Covariates and Missing Data

There are currently two types of covariate that can be incorporated into the model: major-gene covariates and all other types. A major-gene covariate is a measured locus for which genotype data are available on some individuals and for which there is some reason to believe that different genotypes may have differential effects on the quantitative trait level. One reason for treating a gene as a covariate is that unlike the QTLs with unmeasured genotypes in the model, for a major-gene covariate there is no assumption that the locus is diallelic. For example, APOE, with three alleles, is well known to have an effect on Alzheimer's disease age at onset (*13*), with effects that are genotype-specific and which differ among genotypes. In the context of a major-gene covariate, the effect of each APOE genotype on age at onset can be estimated (*14*), but in the context of a QTL in the model, the locus would have to be modeled as a diallelic locus. The reason that a distinction needs to be made between major-gene covariates and other covariates relates to the issue of missing covariate data. Missing genotypes for a gene can be sampled from the genotype distribution, conditional on the observed genotypic data on the sampled individuals, the pedigree relationships, and the known (or estimated) allele frequencies. Thus, missing data on a major-gene covariate is easy to handle. For other covariates, it is not always obvious what distribution to use to sample values for missing covariate data. Thus, for major-gene covariates, missing data are allowed in analysis with the program Loki, whereas for other covariates, missing data are not currently allowed on anyone with observed quantitative trait data.

2.5. Use of MCMC Samples

A MCMC linkage analysis produces a sequence of realizations for all of the latent variables in the model. It is up to the analyst to use these realizations to derive estimates for parameters of interest. For most parameters, this will involve using an ancillary program to extract part of the output file and to reformat it for use in a standard statistical and/or graphical analysis package. It is generally well advised to examine results graphically as well as through computation of standard summary statistics: Some distributions are routinely multimodal (e.g., QTL allele frequencies) so that simple summaries, such as the mean over all iterations, can be quite misleading. Analysis of the MCMC realizations can be used both as diagnostic indicators of whether or not the MCMC process has "mixed well," as well as for obtaining estimates of parameters of interest.

Although many graphs are useful for displaying certain results of an MCMC linkage analysis, the following are particularly useful. In the context of a linkage analysis, a scatter plot of QTL "size" as a function of location on a chromosome is highly informative for conveying a picture of both the QTL location, as well its size. Here, size is the square root of the additive genetic variance of the QTL, and each point in the graph represents size versus location in one MCMC iteration. A surface plot can be used as an alternative and gives a nice representation of the relative number of QTL placements in a particular region. If a simpler plot is desired, the number (or proportion) of iterations in which a QTL is placed into a particular small map interval can be displayed with a histogram. Similarly, a histogram gives a picture of the posterior distribution of number of QTLs.

2.6. Diagnostics

A major issue when using MCMC methods is determining when the parameter estimates have converged and when the sampler has appropriately visited various parts of the sample space. Various diagnostics are therefore important. Similar to the ongoing work toward developing better samplers, there is ongoing work toward identifying useful diagnostics. Again, a number of types of graph have proved useful for evaluating the quality of an analysis run. Although it is difficult to demonstrate that mixing has been good, in some cases it is easy to determine if mixing was poor and the run should be discarded. Several features need to be demonstrated, and failure of any of these is indicative of problems in the analysis. First, parameter estimates should stabilize: μ and V_e should stabilize, as should the number of QTLs in the model. The value for each of these variables graphed against iteration number should always be examined. For μ and V_e, a scatter plot is effective. For the number of QTLs, it is more effective to use lines to connect the points in successive iterations. All plots should show variability from iteration to iteration, but there should be no overall drift in the parameter values, and estimates of V_e should not fall below the measurement error. Second, there should be evidence of successful mixing. Variation in the number of QTLs in the model over iterations, without the number hitting a high upper bound, is some evidence of good mixing. Evidence that estimates for λ_i for the ith QTL are confined to a small genomic region over many iterations, but also move far away from this region and return multiple times, is also indicative of good mixing. A scatter plot of QTL location (on a particular chromosome) against MCMC iteration is useful for evaluating this latter issue. It is important to note that lack of movement between possible models indicates that the sampler is not mixing, so that although stable parameter values are desired, there should also be evidence that the parameter values change between iterations. Finally, results from separate runs with different random seeds should give similar results and parameter estimates.

2.7. Bayesian Aspects

There are both advantages and disadvantages to the Bayesian approach for QTL mapping. A major advantage is that it allows variation in the number of QTLs in the model without the investigator needing to prespecify this number. With a Bayesian approach, this number is a variable, which can be estimated, rather than a fixed parameter based on an assumption about the unknown number of contributing QTLs. There are also some disadvantages to the Bayesian approach. First, it is necessary to provide a prior distribution on the number of QTLs and on other unknown parameters of the model. Both of these require specifications of unknown parameter values. Second, the genetic model for a particular QTL may "flip" from one iteration to the next, just as in traditional segregation analyses, so that the first allele, allele "1," in one iteration refers to the rarer of the two alleles, and in another iteration, it refers to the more common allele. In addition, the stochastic nature of the process means that parameter estimates will vary from iteration to iteration, unlike in traditional linkage and segregation analysis. This makes it difficult to identify the models that are identical because of symmetry. Finally, because the increase and decrease in number of QTLs in the model is achieved by splitting and combining QTLs, individuals QTLs are not identifiable from one iteration to the next. It can, therefore, be difficult to extract meaningful distributions of model parameters such as gene frequency and genotype effects for any specific QTL.

Another issue is that the outcome of the analysis is not given in terms of more familiar LOD scores or p-values. A Bayesian analysis produces estimates of posterior distributions of parameter values. For example, the observed frequency with which a QTL is placed into a particular map interval provides an estimate of the posterior probability that there is a QTL linked within that interval. Similarly, the observed fraction of iterations with i QTLs, $i = 1 \ldots \kappa$, provides an estimate of the posterior probability distribution of the number of QTLs contributing to the phenotype. These posterior distributions need not be unimodal.

3. Interpretation

Analysis and interpretation of results is different from more traditional analyses for three reasons. First, it requires a different framework for interpretation than for more traditional analyses. Second, there are many questions that may be addressed by using results of such an analysis; it is up to the user to decide exactly what to do with the resulting output, and there is no single way to use the results. Third, it requires considerable use of ancillary programs to process the output files and to produce summary statistics and graphical displays to analyze the very large output files. Choice of analysis and graphing programs for this purpose is up to the user, as long as they can handle very large files. All graphs and summary analyses performed in the example in **Subheading 5.** were done with the freely available program gnuplot, which works very well for this purpose. At this point, there are also relatively few accompanying ancillary programs to preprocess the output files from MCMC analyses. Users of MCMC programs can expect to produce some of their own such programs in order to extract desired results from the output files.

3.1. Posterior Distributions

The results of a Bayesian analysis are in the form of posterior distributions of parameter values, which then may be further interpreted. For linkage analysis, an estimate of the posterior distribution of trait gene locations, or the posterior probability of linkage, is generally the parameter of greatest interest. The fraction of all iterations in which a QTL is placed in a particular interval, or the fraction of iterations in which at least one QTL is placed in an interval, provides an estimate of the posterior probability of linkage in that interval. However, unlike interpretation of a traditional LOD score (*15*), or a *p*-value from a model-free test, there is no easy comparison of results with those expected under the null hypothesis of the absence of linkage. Currently there is also no good calibration of results obtained with more familiar statistical measures such as LOD scores or *p*-values. Interpretation of linkage signals may be facilitated by considering the risk ratio, q_1/q_0, of the posterior probability, q_1, to prior probability, q_0, of linkage within a particular interval, or the odds ratio, $[q_1/(1-q_1)]/[q_0/(1-q_0)]$. Both of these ratios have, at various times, been called Bayes' factors. Such ratios can be computed for each interval between two markers on a map, or as a moving average of such a ratio over a series of fixed-width intervals, plotted at the center of the interval under consideration. Either the prior probability of QTL placements in an interval that is based on the expected mean number, κ, of QTLs can be used, or one that is based on the observed mean number of QTLs estimated per iteration can be used (the empirical Bayes' estimate of κ). The prior probability of at least one QTL placement per interval of length υ can be computed as $1-\exp(-\upsilon\kappa/L)$ for a total genome length of L cM. Limited experience suggests that a ratio of 100 : 1 or greater (or a $\log_{10}$ ratio of 2 or more) for posterior to prior probabilities is very strong evidence of linkage and may be comparable in some situations to a LOD score of 3–4. Similarly, a ratio that is considerably below 1 provides exclusionary evidence. However, the two statistics are not strictly comparable. Most importantly, a LOD score can increase without bound as the size of a dataset increases, whereas the ratio of posterior to prior probability is bounded by $1/q_0$.

It is also possible to obtain posterior distributions of parameters other than linkage locations. For example, the fraction of iterations in which there is at least one QTL in the model provides an estimate of the probability that there is at least one gene of sizable effect. Similarly, the posterior distribution of the QTL size can be computed from the results of the MCMC iterations, as can the posterior distribution of covariate effects. Individual QTLs may not always be identifiable in all MCMC implementations. This creates some complications in analyzing and summarizing the parameter values of individual QTLs. Because allele frequencies may "flip" between the rare and common allele, it is incorrect to simply summarize the allele frequency by averaging over all iterations of the QTL with the largest size. To examine the models for the individual QTLs, it is necessary to display the distribution of results rather than to simply compute summary statistics. The graphical results will expose multimodality, which might otherwise be missed. For example, a plot of allele frequency estimates for the QTL with the largest size will generally be at least bimodal, and it may be multimodal if the rank of QTL size varies over iterations.

3.2. Diagnostics

Diagnostic graphs are also helpful for the interpretation of the mixing characteristics of a MCMC analysis. Scatter plots effectively show μ, V_e, and QTL location as a function of MCMC iteration. A location by iteration scatter plot is useful for determining whether or not there is evidence that QTLs are both attracted to a particular location, but also sometimes leave this location. It is also important to look at the number of QTLs in the model as a function of iteration. An effective plot for this purpose is to use lines rather than dots because then each vertical line indicates a change in the model dimensionality, whereas horizontal lines represent a series of iterations with a fixed number of QTLs. If desired, a similar plot can be made for the number of QTLs placed on a particular chromosome. The size of QTLs as a function of location on a chromosome can provide additional evidence about the mapped QTL: A signal representing a real gene will generally show a tight cluster of points of moderate or large size on a scatter plot rather than the ubiquitous, essentially uniformly placed QTLs with small size, which are characteristic of the normal background noise of such an analysis.

4. Software

Very few MCMC software packages are currently available for distribution for use in human QTL mapping. Again, as are the underlying methods, the software implementing the methods is under constant development, so it is likely that additional programs and program modifications will become available in the future. Similarly, currently available programs are rapidly evolving.

Loki (*4*) is academically produced and freely available at website http://www.stat.washington.edu/thompson/Genepi/Loki.shtml. Loki currently runs under Digital UNIX, Linux, and Sun/Solaris operating systems. Input file formats are flexible and are based on a key-word syntax. An ancillary program, *prep*, first prepares files for analysis, using information supplied in a user-defined input file. A second user-defined input file, together with the output files from *prep*, then provides input to Loki. A final ancillary program, *loki_ext*, is available for extraction of results for QTLs placed on specific chromosomes from the single output file from Loki, loki.out. Data can be in a single file or distributed in any number of different files. The alphanumeric IDs of individuals need to be unique in the entire dataset, but otherwise have no restrictions. The program deduces the pedigree structures of possibly multiple and/or complex pedigrees from the information supplied in this file. Pedigrees may be arbitrarily large or small, simple, or complex. The maximum pedigree size and complexity is largely defined by the patience of the analyst rather than any intrinsic limitation. Because of the flexibility of the input format (program documentation is over 20 pages long), an exhaustive description of file formats is not possible here. Instead, examples of the necessary files are given in the worked example.

GAP is a commercial package; the website for information on ordering the package is at website http://icarus2.hsc.usc.edu/epicenter/gap.html. It is available for UNIX (Solaris), PC Windows 3.1, Windows 95, and Windows NT. Pedigrees may be large or small. A useful plotting program for processing MCMC output files is Gnuplot. Gnuplot is available for all platforms under which MCMC linkage analysis programs will run and is freely available from http://www.gnuplot.org. All graphs presented in the demonstration analysis in **Subheading 5.** were made with Gnuplot.

5. Example

5.1. The Data

The example here is a simulated dataset consisting of three simple-structure pedigrees, of size 100, 50, and 50 individuals, respectively. In each pedigree, the number of siblings per sibship was two in generations 2 and 3 and four in generations 4 and later. All children in generations 2 and 3 married and had children. In generation 4 and later, only two siblings in each sibship married and reproduced. In the pedigree of size 100, there were 5 generations in which all eligible marriages yielded offspring, plus a sixth generation with 6 additional sibships of size 4. The two pedigrees of size 50 consisted of 4 generations in which all marriages yielded offspring, plus a fifth generation in which there were 4 additional sibships of size 4. In all three pedigrees, all individuals in the oldest three generations were assumed to be missing all phenotypic and marker data (e.g., deceased). In the largest pedigree, three additional individuals were assumed to be unavailable in generation 4—all of whom were members of sibships in generation 4 and who themselves had offspring. With the exception of the deceased individuals, all other individuals were assumed to have complete marker and trait data.

A two-locus model, with loci on different chromosomes, was simulated on these pedigrees with salient features of these two loci given in **Table 1**. Locus 1 was large, locus 2 was more modest in size, and, together, the two loci accounted for 74% of the total trait variance. In addition, in this simulation $\mu=500$ and $V_e=80$. Ten markers with four equally frequent alleles were uniformly spaced at 10-cM intervals on each 110-cM chromosome, starting at 10 cM on each chromosome map.

Table 1
Characteristics of Loci Used for Simulated Dataset

Locus	Chromosome	Position (cM)	p	Genotypic effects 1 / 1	1 / 2	2 / 2	V_g	V_g/V_t
1	1	55	0.4	−13.2	−8.2	16.8	161.76	0.53
2	2	73	0.3	−11.9	−6.9	8.1	64.89	0.21

Note: V_g = contribution of single locus to variance; V_t = total phenotypic variance.

5.2. Sample Analysis with Loki

The first analysis runs established useful parameter values for prior distributions. Using these values for the prior distributions, the second analysis runs were single-chromosome analyses. These were followed with longer multiple-chromosome linkage analyses. User-specified input files for *prep* and Loki are summarized in **Tables 2** and **3**. The examples in **Tables 2** and **3** are for runs involving marker data on *both* chromosomes 1 and 2; for runs involving only one of the two chromosomes and for those involving no marker data, the corresponding lines that specify map positions and linkage groups in the analysis were removed by adding a comment symbol (#) to the beginning of the line.

Initial segregation analysis runs first established values for κ, the value of the parameter in the assumed Poisson distribution on number of QTLs, and for the prior variance of genotype effects, parameterized here simply as τ_β. The segregation analysis (which included no markers in the analyses) specified $\kappa=1$, but varied the value for τ_β, starting with $\tau_\beta = 2$ and successively doubling the value, using runs of length 50,000 iterations. The average number of QTLs per iteration increased and then decreased with increasing τ_β (**Fig. 1**), indicating that a value for τ_β of about 64 maximizes the acceptance rate of QTLs. This indicates good fit of the model to the data through a high acceptance rate of proposed QTLs. The mean number of QTLs per iteration in all of the runs other than those with low τ_β was also about 2 (2.4 in the run for $\tau_\beta = 64$), suggesting use of $\kappa=2$ may provide a better fit to the model than $\kappa=1$ as used in the initial analyses.

Initial linkage analyses were performed for each chromosome in turn, using all 10 markers on that chromosome, $\tau_\beta =64$, a Poisson prior distribution with $\kappa=2$, and 100,000 MCMC iterations. Follow-up analyses were done using all 10 markers on each of *both* chromosomes 1 and 2 in a simultaneous analysis, with 200,000 MCMC iterations. In order to illustrate what happens when prior distributions are less than ideal, a few analyses with different values of κ and τ_β were also performed. For the purpose of plotting and summarizing the results,

Table 2
Example of Two-Chromosome Input File for the Program prep

Command[a]	Explanation
FILE "ped.dat", id, father, mother, sx, . . . , exqtl	Input file, variables names
PEDIGREE id, father, mother	Variable names describing pedigree triplets
SEX sx 1,2	Codes for sex
FILE "ch1.dat", id, a1a, a1b, a2a, a2b, ..., a10a, a10b	File name for chromosome 1 markers, ID, marker allele variable names
FILE "ch2.dat", id, b1a, b1b, b2a, b2b, ..., b10a, b10b	File name for chromosome 2 markers, etc.
MISSING "0"	General missing data code in this dataset
MISSING "-999" exqtl	Missing data code for quantitative trait exqtl
MARKER LOCUS d1mrk1 [a1a,a1b]	Name of marker d1mrk1, with marker allele variable names
(etc. for each marker on both chromosomes)	
MARKER LOCUS d2mrk10 [b10a, b10b]	Last marker
LINK "Chromosome 1", d1mrk1, d1mrk2, ..., d1mrk10	List of markers on chromosome 1
LINK "Chromosome 2", d2mrk1, d2mrk2, ..., d2mrk10	List of markers on chromosome 2
TRAIT LOCUS QTL	Type of trait locus to consider in analysis
MODEL exqtl=QTL	Model to use in analysis
LOG "example.log"	Output log file

[a]Capitalized words are reserved key words. Variable names must not use these reserved words.

the ancillary program *loki_ext* was used to extract information relevant to each chromosome using the syntax

loki_ext loki.out 1 > on1.out

to extract into the file "on1.out" information about QTLs placed on the 1st linkage group, as defined at the beginning of the file loki.out. For the single-chromosome analyses, **Fig. 2** shows clear evidence for QTLs on both chromosomes. These plots also give some idea of both the map location and the size of each QTL, showing the somewhat smaller size of QTL 2 compared to QTL

Table 3
Example of Two-Chromosome Input File for Program Loki

Command	Explanation
ITERATIONS 200000	Number of iterations in a run
START OUTPUT 1	Iteration to start recording results
OUTPUT FREQUENCY 1	Output results every iteration
TRAIT LOCI 0, 10	Range of allowable number of trait loci
SET TAU BETA 64.0	Prior on function of variance of genotype effects
SET TAU MODE 1	Variance on trait loci effects is τ_β
TRAIT LOCI MEAN 2	Use Poisson prior with mean 2
POSITION d1mrk1 10.0	Map location (cM) of d1mrk1 on chromosome 1
(etc. for each marker)	
POSITION d2mrk10 100.0	Map location (cM) of d2mrk10 on chromosome 2
MAP "Chromosome 1" 0.0, 110.0	Total range of map on chromosome 1 to consider
MAP "Chromosome 2" 0.0, 110.0	Total range of map on chromosome 2 to consider
TOTAL MAP 3000	Total size of genome (cM) in analysis

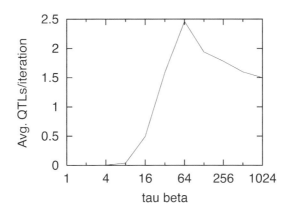

Fig. 1. Average number of QTLs per iteration as a function of the value of τ_β in segregation analysis runs of 50,000 iterations, assuming that the number of QTLs is distributed as Poisson(1).

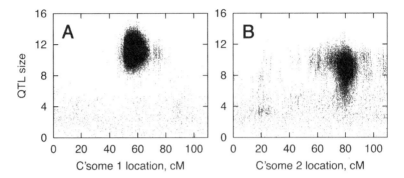

Fig. 2. QTL size versus map location. Size is the square root of the genetic variance of the linked QTL. Each dot represents the size and location of a QTL in a single MCMC iteration in single chromosome analyses on (a) chromosome 1 and (b) chromosome 2.

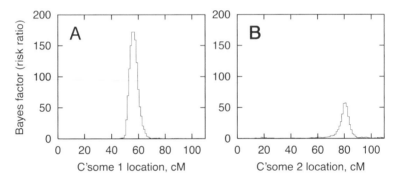

Fig. 3. Bayes factor risk ratios for single chromosome runs for (a) chromosome 1 and (b) chromosome 2, computed with the empirical Bayes estimate for the number of QTLs from the associated run.

1. Alternative histograms (**Fig. 3**) give a clearer picture of gene location and make comparison of strength of signals on different chromosomes easier than comparison of scatter plots. Similar results were obtained for the joint two-chromosome analysis, but results are not shown. **Fig. 4** gives a picture of the posterior distribution of number of QTLs identified in two different runs: a single-chromosome analysis of chromosome 1 and a joint analysis of chromosomes 1 and 2. The corresponding mean (and standard deviation) of the number of QTLs was 2.2 (0.9), 1.9 (1.1), and 2.4 (0.9) from the single-chromosome analyses of chromosomes 1 and 2 and the joint chromosome analysis, respectively. Finally, **Fig. 5** shows the posterior distribution for allele frequencies of

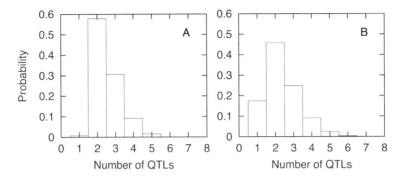

Fig. 4. Distribution of number of QTLs obtained from **(a)** single-chromosome analysis with chromosome 1 and **(b)** two-chromosome analysis using both chromosomes 1 and 2.

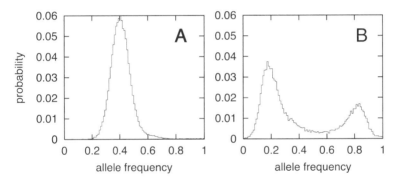

Fig. 5. Distribution of QTL allele frequencies among iterations from single-chromosome analyses for QTLs mapping to **(a)** chromosome 1 and **(b)** chromosome 2.

all QTLs mapping to chromosomes 1 and 2 in the single-chromosome analyses. This figure illustrates two things: the typical bimodality of the allele frequency distribution that is observed for the QTL on chromosome 2 in **Fig. 5b**, and a more unimodal distribution in **Fig. 5a**, which is discussed more later in this section. Similar plots could be generated for other parameters in the model (e.g., for V_e, the overall mean, variance contribution of the linked QTL, etc.).

Diagnostic plots were also routinely generated. The results in **Fig. 6** show map location as a function of MCMC iteration for the single-chromosome analyses. The strong signal on chromosome 1 is apparent, as is the weaker signal on chromosome 2. The signal on chromosome 2, in particular, illustrates a desirable property of the analysis: The evidence for a QTL near 80 cM

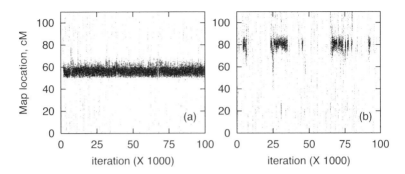

Fig. 6. Single-chromosome runs for map location as a function of iteration for (**a**) chromosome 1 and (**b**) chromosome 2. Each dot represents the location of one QTL in a particular iteration.

remains steady for a period of iterations, then disappears and reappears several times, indicating that there is attraction to this location, yet at the same time that the sampler is mixing. The signal on chromosome 1 (**Fig. 6a**) is actually too steady, indicating difficulty in moving around the parameter space. Two graphs provide evidence for this. First, the contrast in the unimodal versus bimodal distributions of allele frequencies in **Fig. 5** is evidence that in this single-chromosome run the sampler is not moving around the trait-model space (other runs showed more evidence of mixing). Second, the very low number of iterations in which there were fewer than two QTLs (**Fig. 4a** vs **Fig. 4b**) suggests that the single chromosome-1 run is somewhat aberrant compared to other runs. Failure to mix between the two phases of the QTL model is not particularly problematic here because the two parts of the parameter space are equivalent, but possible implications for interpretation should be kept in mind, particularly concerning trait model parameter estimates.

Use of other values of τ_β and κ illustrates the importance of using a fairly long run even for exploratory analyses. For example, for $\kappa=1$ and $\tau_\beta=64$, the evidence for a gene on chromosome 1 did not start to appear until approx 30,000 iterations. For $\tau_\beta = 100$ and $\kappa=1$, 50,000 iterations passed before QTLs began to be placed near the chromosome-1 QTL location. Both of these signals would have been missed if a very short initial run length had been used. The effect of this initial failure to place QTLs on chromosome 1 can also be seen for the run in **Fig. 7**, which shows number of QTLs as a function of iteration for a less ideal run in which $\kappa=1$ and $\tau_\beta=64$: The plot of number of QTLs as a function of iteration shows a distinct increase in number of QTLs once the localization to chromosome 1 became apparent. Both the initial approx 30,000 and the later iterations appeared to have reached a steady state, but at two

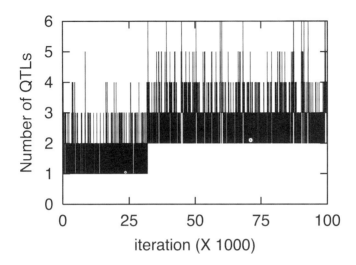

Fig. 7. Number of QTLs in the model as a function of iteration, for a run in which κ=1 and τ$_β$=64. Vertical lines represent shifts in the dimensionality of the model (i.e., changes in the number of QTLs in the model).

different mean number of QTLs. This illustrates the danger of depending on only one measure to conclude that the equilibrium distribution has been achieved. However, despite the fact that the burn-in stage lasted longer for these runs with less ideal prior distributions, resulting parameter distributions for the QTLs mapping to these chromosomes were unchanged over those found with the more ideal parameter values. Diagnostic scatter plots of the overall mean and V_e as a function of MCMC iteration for the runs with τ$_β$ =64 and κ=2 showed stable values, similar to results in **Fig. 6**, and are not shown.

6. Notes

1. Choosing initial parameters. It is important to determine that there is a peak in the number of QTLs when exploring possible values for prior distributions. If the number of QTLs simply increases with increasing or decreasing the value of τ$_β$, this indicates a problem with the data and/or model. It is also important to plot V_e as well as the number of QTLs: if V_e approaches 0, this is also indicative of problems with the model and/or data since V_e should be at least as large as the variance associated with measurement error of the trait phenotype.
2. Bounding parameter values. A reasonably large but not excessive upper bound (10–15) on the number of QTLs should normally be adequate. If the number of QTLs in the model consistently reaches the upper bound even when this is set increasingly higher, this is indicative of problems with the data and/or model. V_e can also be bounded so that it is not allowed to go to zero. This is often necessary

when analyzing censored data, such as age-of-onset data. Possible solutions include further exploration of prior distributions to find more suitable distributions, as well as careful investigation of analysis files to make sure that phenotype codes are appropriately assigned.

3. Number of alleles for a major-gene covariate. Although a major gene covariate can have more than three genotypes, it is important to avoid specifying models with very large numbers of genotypes because most datasets will then have insufficient data to estimate the genotype-specific effects. Because the number of genotypes increases quickly with the number of alleles, this means that for practical purposes, depending on the size of the dataset, major-gene effects can be estimated for loci with perhaps up to five to six alleles, but not usually many more, unless some sort of allele pooling can be justified. When a plot of the posterior distribution of genotype effect is very flat, this indicates that there is insufficient data to estimate the genotype effect.

4. Length and number of runs. The number of iterations (run length) needs to increase with the total number of loci in the model, including both trait and marker loci. Parameter estimates from analyses that are based on only a few marker intervals generally stabilize within fewer iterations than do estimates in analyses with many marker intervals. The amount of CPU time per MCMC iteration will also be lower for models with fewer rather than many loci. The number of iterations needed and the time needed for an analysis are both approximately linear in the number of genes in the analysis.

In addition to the complexity of the model, the run length depends on the type of phenotypic data and on the purpose of the run. Quantitative traits that are not subject to censoring, such as cholesterol levels, tend to be more informative than are traits subjected to censoring, such as age at onset of a disease. More informative, uncensored traits are less sensitive than are censored traits to poor choices of prior distributions on the parameter values, which reduces the length of the runs needed, both because the burn-in period is shorter and because there is less problem with poor mixing. The purpose of the run also affects the choice of run length. For an initial analysis—either to evaluate choice of prior distributions or to obtain initial evidence in a genome screen for which there is some evidence for linkage—the runs may be considerably shorter than for later analyses that focus on areas showing evidence of linkage. For example, exploratory runs with an uncensored quantitative trait and analyses one chromosome at a time on a 10-cM map can usually be done reliably with 50,000 iterations, whereas 100,000 may be needed for initial analyses with a censored trait. For final analyses, the uncensored trait may require 100,000–200,000 iterations, whereas the censored trait may require 200,000–500,000 iterations.

A small number of long runs is better than many short runs. The early part of the run that involves burn-in produces relatively poor parameter estimates. Use of many short runs involves a much larger fraction of iterations involved in the burn-in phase than does use of a smaller number of long runs with the same total number of iterations. Averaging over several short runs involves averaging these poor estimates, which generally will not give a good overall estimate. In principle, a single very long run provides the best parameter estimates. However, because there is always the possibility that a particular run is aberrant, experience suggests that three to five long runs is the best pragmatic choice for allocating total number of MCMC iterations.

5. Many vs. single chromosomes. It is most efficient to initially perform a series of analyses with individual chromosomes and to follow up on these analyses with a multichromosome analysis of the subset of chromosomes with some evidence of linkage. In principle, it is possible to perform simultaneous analyses with any number of chromosomes, including the whole genome. However, this is impractical because of the large number of iterations needed to explore all genomic regions adequately. A more practical approach is to analyze each chromosome in turn and to follow up with a longer joint analysis of the small number of chromosomes with the strongest linkage signals in a final analysis.

6. Maps. Some comments are needed on ideal characteristics of maps used for analysis. Generally, equally spaced multiallelic markers with approximately equivalent heterozygosity work best. A 10-cM marker spacing seems to be ideal for a first-pass screen. If markers are unevenly spaced, sometimes weak but false signals may be observed in the larger intermarker intervals. Weak but false signals also often occur at the ends of the chromosomes, where there is less total meiotic information. One solution is to add markers to the larger intervals midway between the flanking markers or to the end of the chromosome, when such markers are available. False signals generally disappear upon inclusion of additional markers in such intervals, although care needs to be taken to ensure a good quality map, both in distance and marker order, when additional markers are added to such analyses. A 20-cM map is a bit too loose; many weak positive signals may result because the looser map results in fewer rejections of proposed gene placements, requiring considerable work in follow-up. Very closely spaced markers (e.g., 1 cM) can produce problems with mixing; whether this is because the map is inaccurately estimated or because of intrinsic problems with the samplers is unknown. One trick that can be tried in this context is to inflate the map around those markers. Also, for regions with a very tight marker spacing, male and female maps often differ considerably from each other; this also can affect the mixing properties in an analysis based on a sex-averaged map. The solution is to reanalyze the data with sex-specific maps.

7. Missing data. Missing data is not generally a problem for markers or for the quantitative trait under analysis. However, it is important to avoid the situation when there are multiple pedigrees in the analysis *and* that there is no overlap among groups of pedigrees for the markers typed. Not all markers need to be typed on all pedigrees.

   Missing covariate data can be a problem, except for missing data on major-gene covariates. If there is a small amount of missing covariate data on individuals who otherwise provide phenotypic information, there are two choices: either delete the trait data on individuals with missing covariates or use an external data imputation method to "fill-in" the missing covariate data.

8. Problems—detection and fixing. One problem that sometimes occurs, particularly in the analysis of censored traits, is that the number of QTLs consistently hits a high upper boundary or generally continues to increase while the residual variance

goes to 0. This is symptomatic of problems with the data and/or choice of prior distribution for some of the parameters in the model. A problem with the data that could produce this effect would be in a study where age at onset was the response variable and only males get the disease, but females were coded as unaffected with observed age as censoring age (e.g., prostate cancer). In this situation, a model with a few genes of large variance contributions will fit the data poorly, favoring models with genes contributing small amounts to the variance, thus driving up the estimated number of QTLs. The solution is to make sure that individuals who *cannot* have the disease are coded as unknown for disease status. If the data coding is not the source of the problem, then it is possible that the prior distribution on one or more model parameters such as τ_β is poorly chosen. If the problem exists only when there are markers in the analysis, but disappears when markers are removed from the analysis, there could be problems with either marker genotypes or the marker map, or again, the proposal distributions. Finally, if none of these solutions fixes the problem, it is possible to bound the residual variance so that it cannot go to zero, in which case, generally, the number of QTLs is also prevented from increasing without bound.

9. Program bugs. Problems with the data need to be fixed before an analysis can be performed. Loki will list genotype incompatibilities for individuals with accompanying parents. In version 2.2, there is a bug in this procedure such that the parents are reversed in this listing (i.e., the father is listed as the mother, and vise versa).

There is also a bug in use of sex as a covariate. If sex is to be used as a covariate, sex must be coded as a 1,0 (male, female) numeric indicator. The results will be incorrect if a character notation is used for sex.

Acknowledgment

This work was supported by grant GM 46255 from the National Institutes of Health.

References

1. Wijsman, E.M. and Amos, C. (1997) Genetic analysis of simulated oligogenic traits in nuclear and extended pedigrees: summary of GAW10 contributions. *Genet. Epidemiol.* **14**, 719–735.

2. Schork, N.J., Boehnke, M., Terwilliger, J.D., and Ott, J. (1993) Two-trait-locus linkage analysis: a powerful strategy for mapping complex genetic traits. *Am. J. Hum. Genet.* **53**, 1127–1136.

3. Green, P.J. (1995) Reversible jump Markov chain Monte Carlo computation and Bayesian model determination. *Biometrika* **82**, 711–732.

4. Heath, S.C. (1997) Markov chain Monte Carlo segregation and linkage analysis for oligogenic models. *Am. J. Hum. Genet.* **61**, 748–760.

5. Heath, S.C., Snow, G.L., Thompson, E.A., Tseng, C., and Wijsman, E.M. (1997) MCMC segregation and linkage analysis. *Genet. Epidemiol.* **14**, 1011–1016.

6. Daw, E.W., Heath, S.C., and Wijsman, E.M. (1999) Multipoint oligogenic analysis

of age-at-onset data with applications to Alzheimer's disease pedigrees. *Am. J. Hum. Genet.* **64**, 839–851.

7. Yuan, B., Neuman, R., Duan, S., Weber, J., Kwok, P., Saccone, N., et al. (2000) Linkage of a gene for familial hypobetalipoproteinemia to chromosome 3p21.1–22. *Am. J. Hum. Genet.* **66**, 1699–1704.

8. Falconer, D.S. (1995) *Introduction to Quantitative Genetics*. Longman, Scientific and Technical, Harlow, UK.

9. Haldane, J.B.S. (1919) The combination of linkage values, and the calculation of distance between the loci of linked factors. *J. Genet.* **8**, 299–309.

10. Hastings, W.K. (1970) Monte Carlo sampling methods using Markov chains and their applications. *Biometrika* **57**, 97–109.

11. Geman, S. and Geman, D. (1984) Stochastic relaxation, Gibbs distributions and the Bayesian restoration of images. *IEEE Trans. Pattern Anal. Mach. Intell.* **6**, 721–741.

12. Gilks, W.R. (1996) *Markov Chain Monte Carlo in Practice*. Chapman & Hall, New York.

13. Corder, E.H., Lannfelt, L., Bogdanovic, N., Fratiglioni, L., and Mori, H. (1998) The role of APOE polymorphisms in late-onset dementias. *Cell. Mol. Life Sci.* **54**, 928–934.

14. Daw, E.W., Payami, H., Nemens, E.J., Nochlin, D., Bird, T.D., Schellengerg, G.D., et al. (2000) The number of trait loci in late-onset Alzheimer disease. *Am. J. Hum. Genet.* **66**, 196–204.

15. Morton, N.E. (1955) Sequential tests for the detection of linkage. *Am. J. Hum. Genet.* **7**, 277–318.

II

Mapping Quantitative Trait Loci in Rodents

7

Approaches to the Analysis of QTL Data in Mice, Using the Nonobese Diabetic Mouse as an Example

Heather J. Cordell

1. Introduction

One route to the identification of genes involved in human complex disease is to exploit an animal model such as the rodent model of human type 1 diabetes, the nonobese diabetic (NOD) mouse. Although the genes predisposing to disease in an animal model may not be identical to those in the human, the underlying genetic basis in terms of number of genes involved, interactions, and physiological disease processes may be similar between the species. In addition, major disease-susceptibility loci may lie in homologous regions of the human and animal genomes, so that identification of a locus in the animal model may point directly to a region of interest on the human genome. For instance, in type 1 diabetes, the major susceptibility locus, *IDDM1*, lies in the major histocompatibility complex (MHC) on human chromosome 6 in a region syntenic with the primary determinant of murine diabetes, *Idd1* on mouse chromosome 17 (*1*).

Historically, a number of statistical methods have been developed for the analysis of experimental cross-data in the context of plant or animal breeding. A variety of software packages exists for the implementation of these methods. Many of the statistical methods developed originally in an agricultural context can be applied to the problem of disease gene mapping in rodents. However, the focus of the approaches may be somewhat different as the aim of rodent studies is usually to identify loci in order to help focus human studies and/or gain understanding of disease mechanisms, rather than to improve fitness for agricultural applications. The nature of the phenotype of interest may also differ with rodent studies, often focusing on dichotomous or categorical traits (e.g.,

From: *Methods in Molecular Biology: vol. 195: Quantitative Trait Loci: Methods and Protocols.*
Edited by: N. J. Camp and A. Cox © Humana Press, Inc., Totowa, NJ

presence/absence of disease, different levels of severity, etc.) rather than on genuinely quantitative phenotypes.

There are a number of different breeding designs that are used for identifying quantitative trait loci (QTLs) using inbred lines. Many of the standard software packages allow analysis of a bewildering variety of different breeding schemes. For the purposes of this chapter, we will confine ourselves to the most popular designs that have been used in NOD mouse studies, namely the backcross (BC) design, the intercross (F2) design, and the congenic strain design. All of these designs start with two divergent inbred lines, P1 and P2 say, where P1 and P2 have been generated by selective breeding to be homozygous for different alleles at loci assumed to influence values of a particular quantitative trait. Animals from P1 may be assumed to have genotype BB and animals from P2 to have genotype NN, for instance, where N denotes a disease-susceptibility allele and B a resistance allele. A cross between these lines generates heterozygous filial (F1) offspring. In the BC design, the F1 is (back-)crossed to one of the parents, female F1 to male P2 say, generating offspring whose genotype is either NN or NB at each locus. In the F2 designs, two F1 individuals are crossed in order to generate offspring with genotype NN, NB, or BB. For the development of congenic strains, specific chromosome intervals from one inbred strain (e.g., P1) are introgressed onto the background of the recipient strain (e.g., P2) by repeated backcrossing. Allelically variable markers are used to guide the strain construction and to make sure that after several generations of backcrossing only the desired chromosome segment is of P1 origin. As an extension of this strategy, double congenic strains have also been developed, where a single strain possesses two well-defined congenic regions derived from two separate single congenic strains.

1.1. Summary of QTL Mapping Methods

Quantitative trait loci mapping can be considered at varying levels of complexity. At the simplest end is a simple test of association between trait values and the genotypes of individual marker loci. Examples of tests of this type include *t*-tests for equality of the means between the different genotype classes, analysis of variance, Wilcoxon rank-sum test (Mann–Whitney test), Kruskal–Wallis test, Kolmogorov–Smirnov test and various single-marker regression approaches (all of which may be found in standard statistical texts). Because the marker loci are tested individually, it is not generally required that they be mapped relative to one another. As an extension of these approaches, multiple-regression methods may be used (*2,3*), in which the genotypes at several markers are simultaneously used to predict the trait outcome.

A more sophisticated approach to QTL mapping is to use a method known as interval mapping (*4,5*). This method requires prior construction of a genetic marker map (although note that this map can usually be estimated from the data). Interval mapping evaluates the association between the trait values and a hypothetical QTL that may be positioned at multiple-analysis points between each pair of adjacent loci. The expected QTL genotype is estimated from the known genotypes of the flanking marker loci, taking into account their distance from the QTL.

A more complex approach is to use a method called either composite interval mapping (CIM) (*6–8*) or multiple QTL mapping (MQM) (*9*). Like simple interval mapping, CIM/MQM evaluates a QTL effect at multiple analysis points between each pair of adjacent marker loci. However, the method also includes effects at one or more (background) markers assumed to be linked to alternative QTLs in the region, which may increase the power for detection of the QTL of interest by reducing the overall residual genetic variation. Furthermore, inclusion of background markers which are linked to the interval containing the QTL being tested may help separate the effects of this QTL from the effects of other linked QTLs on the opposite sides of the background markers.

A further degree of complexity is achieved with the use of Bayesian methods for the evaluation of models with multiple QTLs (*10–13*). These methods are highly computationally intensive and may be prohibitively time-consuming. However, they do provide a way to model the effects of multiple QTLs with varying strengths at varying positions.

A final approach of interest, most suited to the situation where two or more QTLs have already been detected, is analysis of epistatic interactions between QTLs. Theoretically, analysis of epistasis can also be used to search for QTLs that have an epistatic effect but no detectable main effects. This topic is an area of current active research.

2. Methods

2.1. Single-Locus Associations

2.1.1. t-Tests

Suppose we have BC data where every marker locus has genotype NN or NB. One way of detecting QTLs is to perform, for each marker, a *t*-test for the equality of means in the two genotype groups:

$$t = \frac{y_1 - y_2}{\sqrt{(s^2(1/n_1 + 1/n_2)}} \tag{1}$$

where y_1 is the mean trait value among the n_1 animals with genotype NN, y_2 is the mean trait value among the n_2 animals with genotype NB, s^2 is the pooled variance,

$$s^2 = \frac{(n_1 - 1)s_1^2 + (n_2 - 1)s_2^2}{n_1 + n_2 - 2} \tag{2}$$

where s_1^2 and s_2^2 are the sample variances of the two groups. This test depends on the assumption that the population variances are the same in two groups; under the assumption of unequal variances, the approximate t-statistic is computed as

$$t' = \frac{y_1 - y_2}{\sqrt{w_1 + w_2}} \tag{3}$$

where $w_1 = s_1^2/n_1$ and $w_2 = s_2^2/n_2$. This test can be performed in a variety of standard statistical software and spreadsheet programs.

2.1.2. Analysis of Variance

An extension of the t-test for the situation where there are more than two genotype groups (e.g., an F2 design with groups NN, NB, and BB), assuming equal variances in each group, is to carry out a one-way analysis of variance (ANOVA). Let y_{ij} denote the phenotype value of the jth animal in group i. Suppose there are m groups and n_i animals in group i. The procedure partitions the total sum of squares

$$SS_{total} = \sum_i \sum_j (y_{ij} - y)^2 \tag{4}$$

into the between-group and within-group sums of squares (SS_b and SS_w, respectively):

$$SS_b = \sum_i (y_i - y)^2$$

and

$$SS_w = \sum_i \sum_j (y_{ij} - y_i)^2 \tag{5}$$

where y_i is the mean phenotype value in group i and y is the overall mean. To test the null hypothesis of no QTL effect, we use the F-statistic

$$F = \frac{SS_b / (m-1)}{SS_w / \sum_i (n_i-1)} \tag{6}$$

with $m-1$ and $\sum_i (n_i - 1)$ degrees of freedom. This test is also available in most standard statistical software and spreadsheet programs.

2.1.3. Nonparametric Statistics

An alternative to ANOVA is to use a nonparametric approach such as a Wilcoxon rank-sum test (two groups) or Kruskal–Wallis test (more than two groups) that performs the analysis on the rank scores of the trait phenotypes rather than on the phenotypes themselves. Another possibility is the Kolmogorov statistic, which compares the overall empirical distribution of phenotypes within each of the groups to that in the pooled data (all groups combined). All of these procedures are available in most standard statistical packages and may be available in some QTL mapping software packages.

2.1.4. Regression Techniques

The linear model underlying the ANOVA analysis can be written as follows:

$$y=b_0+b_1x_1+b_2x_2+\cdots+e \tag{7}$$

where for each animal, y is the trait value, the x_i correspond to coded genotype values (one for each genotype or marker contrast), the b_i are unknown fixed parameters to be estimated, and e is a random environmental effect assumed to be drawn from a Normal distribution. For instance, for BC data, we might have $y=b_0+b_1x_1+e$, where x_1 takes the value 1 is an animal has genotype NN at the marker locus being tested, and 0 otherwise.

The advantage of this formulation is that the problem is set up in the form of a regression equation, with the quantitative phenotype y being regressed on the predictor variable x_1. Standard statistical software packages for least squares regression can be used to estimate the b_0 and b_1: The QTL test corresponds to a test of whether $b_1=0$, with significance evaluated using a t-statistic. This procedure is also implemented in several QTL mapping software packages. An alternative to least squares regression is to use maximum likelihood (ML) estimation via the expectation–maximization (EM) algorithm, which is also implemented in several QTL mapping software packages. The ML method is generally slower than least squares regression but is easier to extend to more complicated situations such as the presence of missing or ambiguous marker data or non-Normally distributed environmental contributions. The regression approach is easy to generalize to multiple linear regression, in which more than one marker locus is included in the regression equation. For instance, for BC data, we might fit the model in terms of four separate marker loci:

$$y=b_0+b_1x_1+b_2x_2+b_3x_3+b_4x_4+e \tag{8}$$

If the loci are unlinked, this models four separate QTL effects linked to the four markers. For linked loci, we may fit a series of models with two adjacent loci included in the regression equation each time (*2,3*). The resulting parameter estimates and their significance can be used to estimate the location of QTLs in a way that approximates some of the more complicated interval mapping approaches outlined next.

2.2. Interval Mapping

A problem with single-locus association methods is that the QTL itself may lie some distance away from the marker being tested. By testing a single marker, it is not possible to differentiate, for instance, between a QTL of small effect, which is tightly linked to the marker, and a QTL of large effect, which is only loosely linked. This problem can be overcome by using multilocus marker genotypes to estimate the genotype at a hypothetical QTL that is positioned at a series of analysis points on the known marker map. For a given analysis point, the likelihood of the data, $L(x)$, can be calculated and maximized with respect to the underlying genetic parameters at the QTL (**4**). Suppose we wish to analyze BC data. As in the regression method, we assume a linear model:

$$y = b_0 + b_1 x_1^* + e \qquad (9)$$

where e is assumed to be Normally distributed with mean 0 and x_1^* takes the value 1 if an animal has genotype NN at the QTL, and 0 otherwise. Because the genotype at the QTL is not observed, the true value of x_1^* is unknown, but it can be inferred probabilistically from the genotypes at the flanking markers. The likelihood of the data depends on the probabilities that x_1^* takes the values 1 and 0 and on the unknown parameters b_0 and b_1. The likelihood can be maximized using the EM algorithm (**14**). The test statistic at each point is based on the likelihood ratio statistic:

$$LR = 2 \ln \frac{\max L(x)}{\max_{H0} L(x)} \qquad (10)$$

where $\max_{H0} L(x)$ is the maximum of the likelihood function under the null hypothesis of no segregating QTL or, equivalently, on the log odds (LOD) score:

$$LOD = \log_{10} \frac{\max L(x)}{\max_{H0} L(x)} = \frac{LR}{4.61} \qquad (11)$$

This analysis can be carried out using a number of QTL software packages (e.g., Mapmaker/QTL, QTL Cartographer, MapQTL). The analysis point with the highest LOD score is taken to be the estimated location of the putative QTL.

A problem with ML estimation is that it can be computationally demanding, particularly if the analysis is to be repeated thousands of times in order to generate simulation-based *p*-values or confidence intervals. Fortunately, a simple least squares regression approach, which is much quicker, has been shown to give an excellent approximation to the ML map for interval mapping (**15,16**). In this method, at every analysis point (assumed QTL position), the quantitative phenotype is regressed on variables that are functions of the conditional QTL genotype probabilities given the flanking marker genotypes, rather than explicitly maximizing the likelihood. This analysis can be carried out using standard statistical software or using a QTL software package such as Map Manager QT. The ML and regression approaches to interval mapping both assume that the quantitative trait follows a mixture (over different QTL genotypes) of Normal distributions. A nonparametric interval mapping approach that does not assume underlying Normality has also been developed (*17*). Alternatively, the regression and interval mapping approaches, together with the composite interval mapping procedures described next, are theoretically easy to extend to other exponential family distributions via the usual generalized linear model approach (*18*), although, to our knowledge, this has not been implemented in any program packages other than in the standard statistical packages.

2.3. Composite Interval Mapping

When a trait is caused by multiple QTLs, the strength of evidence for a QTL at a given position may be affected by the presence of other QTLs linked to this position. In fact, the positions of the likelihood peaks on a given chromosome may not necessarily correspond to the correct QTL positions. For instance, Martinez and Curnow (*16*) present a situation in which the effects of two linked QTLs combine to suggest evidence for a false QTL (a "ghost QTL") in between the two true QTLs. In order to address this problem, two methods that are virtually identical, composite interval mapping (CIM) (*6–8*) and multiple QTL mapping (MQM) (*9*) have been developed. The feature of these methods is to include genotypes at one or more background markers as cofactors or predictor variables in an otherwise standard interval mapping procedure using the model:

$$y = b_0 + b_1 x_1^* + b_2 x_2 + b_3 x_3 + \cdots + e \tag{12}$$

Here, x_1^* corresponds to the unobserved QTL genotype at the position being tested, whereas x_2, x_3, $\cdots$, correspond to observed marker genotypes at other positions. Inclusion of markers linked to the interval of interest can condition out effects resulting from other linked QTLs. Inclusion of unlinked markers can account for the residual variance resulting from unlinked QTLs, increasing the power to detect the QTL in the interval under consideration. A number of software packages are available for CIM/MQM analysis, including QTL Cartographer, MapQTL, and Map Manager QT.

2.4. Bayesian Methods

Another method for modeling the effects of multiple QTLs is to employ a Bayesian approach via MCMC techniques. In this type of analysis, the posterior probability of the number of QTLs and their positions and effects is evaluated conditional on the observed data using simulation and sampling from an ergodic Markov chain rather than by directly maximizing the (usually intractible) likelihood surface. Several different algorithms have been proposed (*10–13*). However, they are all highly computer intensive and may suffer from problems of convergence if not run for a sufficiently long period of time (it may also be difficult to tell whether or not the procedure has reached convergence).

2.5. Analysis of Epistasis

For a quantitative trait, epistasis or interaction between two loci occurs when the combined effect of the loci does not equal the sum of the individual effects. For instance, for a BC population, epistasis between two loci can be represented by the linear model.

$$y_{ij} = b_0 + b_1 x_1^* + b_2 x_2^* + b_3 x_1^* x_2^* \tag{13}$$

where x_1^* takes the value of 1 if an animal has genotype NN at the first QTL, and 0 otherwise, and x_2^* takes the value 1 if an animal has genotype NN at the second QTL, and 0 otherwise. QTL genotypes may need to be inferred from flanking marker genotypes or, alternatively, double congenic data can be used in which the genotypes at two specific QTL locations have already been fixed. The model is easy to fit using any standard statistical software. There is also a program Epistat (*19*) designed specifically for detection and analysis of epistasis.

3. Interpretation

3.1. Estimation of Significance Levels

Pointwise significance values (*p*-values) can be assigned to LR or LOD values using standard asymptotic statistical theory that predicts that the LR has a χ^2-distribution with degrees of freedom (df) equal to the additional number of estimated parameters under the alternative hypothesis. In a QTL analysis, a large number of tests for marker–trait associations are typically performed. Even if the significance level (*p*-value) for each test is set at a very low level, there is a high probability that the entire experiment (i.e., the whole collection of tests) will show a number of false positives. To correct for multiple independent tests, as would occur if every marker tested were on a different chromosome, we can use a Bonferroni correction, which multiples the *p*-value by the total number of tests performed. However, this procedure is very conservative if applied to multiple nonindependent tests.

In **refs. 4** and **20**, the authors investigate the relationship between the pointwise (i.e., at a single marker or location) significance level and the overall genomewide significance level. They propose stringent pointwise significance criteria to keep the overall genomewide type 1 error at a reasonable level.

Specifically, a LOD threshold of between 3 and 4 is proposed to correspond to an overall false-positive rate of 5% for experimental organisms such as the mouse. Another approach to correct for multiple testing in the dataset actually analyzed is to use a permutation procedure (*21*). In this procedure, the original analysis is repeated many times on datasets generated by randomly shuffling the original trait values of the individuals. Comparison of the original test statistic to those test statistics generated from the shuffled replicates allows an empirical *p*-value to be calculated. The only disadvantage with this approach is that many reshufflings and reanalyses may be required (e.g., 10,000 or more may be necessary to generate stable critical values for a *p*-value of 0.01). As an alternative to this rather computationally demanding procedure, tables of precalculated values have been generated by simulation (*22*) that can be used together with a simple formula to get the genomewide significance level for different types of experimental populations with any size of genome.

The above-mentioned procedures implicitly test the null hypothesis that there is no QTL linked to any of the regions being studied rather than any other null hypothesis such as the presence of one QTL but no additional QTLs. However, a modification of the permutation approach (*23*) can be used to construct tests for the presence of minor QTL effects while accounting for effects of known major QTLs. The choice of an appropriate null hypothesis for QTL mapping is not always clear; it has been argued (*24*) that single QTL models should be compared with an infinitesimal model rather than a no-QTL model, as we usually know that the heritability is nonzero.

3.2. Confidence Intervals

Often, the main point of a QTL analysis is simply to gain an idea of the pattern of significance across a chromosomal region. The analysis point with the highest LOD score is taken to be the location of the putative QTL, with an approximate 95% confidence interval or "one-LOD support interval" corresponding to locations where the LOD score is within one unit of its maximum value. It has been proposed (*25*) that support intervals should, in fact, be based on two-LOD differences in order to have a high probability of containing the QTL. A more robust procedure would be to use a resampling or bootstrap approach (*26*), in which confidence intervals are constructed by repeating the analysis a large number of times on datasets obtained by sampling observations with replacement from the original dataset.

3.3. Sample Size Requirements

The sample sizes required for detection of QTLs with specific effects may be calculated (*4,27*). The basic conclusion from previous studies is that relatively modest numbers of individuals (in the region of 100–200) and markers (around 20–100) are generally sufficient to detect QTLs in rodents (*27*).

3.4. Epistasis

The main problem when analyzing epistatic interactions is in the interpretation of the results. Lack of epistasis (e.g., when the coefficient b_3, in **Subheading 2.5.**, is found to equal 0) is often assumed to correspond to independence of effects at the two loci, implying that they may act on two separate causal pathways with regard to the trait. However, results are very dependent on scale (e.g., an epistatic interaction may exist when the phenotype is measured on the original scale but not when measured on some transformed scale such as the logarithm). Statistically, it is of interest to accurately describe the joint action of two QTLs. Epistasis may, therefore, be of more interest from a statistical modeling point of view than for its biological implications, which remain a topic of active research (*28*). There are situations in which QTLs may have an epistatic effect but no detectable main effects. In this case, analysis taking account of epistasis may allow identification of QTLs that would otherwise remain undetected.

4. Software

As previously mentioned, there is a bewildering variety of software available for analysis of experimental cross-data. A useful summary of the major program packages is given in **ref. *29***, together with a more detailed account of the package Map Manager QT. It is likely that for most people, the choice of software will be made on the basis of platform availability (Mac OS, Dos, UNIX, etc.) or convenience. For the worked example (**Subheading 5.**) we concentrated on programs that are available under UNIX, because these tend to be the simplest to describe in terms of input and output files and analysis steps required. Note that all of the programs come with between 13 and 180 pages of instruction in the form of a user manual; the reader is strongly advised to consult this document when using any of the programs, as it will give far more detailed instructions and hints on running the programs and interpreting the output than is possible in this short chapter.

For many, a crucial step will be the actual downloading of the programs. For most packages, this may be done through the World Wide Web or by anonymous ftp. Packages that are commercial rather than freely available may have different arrangements for obtaining the programs and organizing payment. As a guide, most of the packages have information or at least a contact address posted on their website (*see* **Table 1**). If a user is unfamiliar with the process of downloading and uncompressing and compiling programs, it is recommended that they consult their system administrator for help. Alternatively, they may be able to obtain an account on a system where the programs have already been set up (e.g., for academic users in the United Kingdom, the Human Genome Mapping Project [HGMP] Resource Centre offers access to many useful packages [see http://www.hgmp.mrc.ac.uk/ for details]).

Table 1 provides a list of programs that can be used for QTL analysis in inbred strains. Four of the programs are described in more detail in the worked example in the **Subheading 5.**; For details of the input/output files and so forth required by these programs, see **Subheading 5.**

5. Worked Example

For this example, we will use data derived from a backcross between the NOD mouse and C57BL/10-NOD.H2g7 (B10.H2g7), a diabetes-resistant strain. These data represent a modified and updated version of the data analyzed in **ref. 3**. The data consist of genotypes (heterozygous or homozygous) at 10 marker loci on each of two chromosomes for 305 mice. Each mouse also has a dichotomous phenotype according to whether it is affected or unaffected with diabetes and an ordinal categorical phenotype corresponding to the histology of the pancreas in terms of eight increasing levels (on a scale of 0–7) of severity of insulitis (an intermediate phenotype) in the pancreas. For the purposes of this analysis, we assume that the marker loci have already been mapped; if the relative positions of the markers are, in fact, not known, they may be estimated from the data using computer programs such as JoinMap described in Chapter 9.

5.1. Single-Locus Associations Using SAS

As mentioned earlier, many tests for single-locus association can be carried out using standard statistical packages or spreadsheet programs (e.g., Excel). To carry out some of these analyses using the statistical package SAS, we prepare an input command file which we will arbitrarily name npar.sas containing the following SAS commands:

```
DATA genetic;
INFILE "bc.dat";
INPUT ID J1 I1 H1 G1 F1 E1 D1 C1 B1 A1  A3 B3 C3 D3 E3 F3 G3 H3 I3 J3 DIAB
HIST;
PROC NPAR1WAY DATA=genetic ANOVA EDF WILCOXON;
     CLASS F1;
     VAR HIST;
     TITLE 'Grouped by F1';
     RUN;
ENDSAS;
```

This is not the place for a detailed tutorial on using the SAS statistical package, but for those unfamiliar with SAS, the first and second lines of this command

Table 1.
List of QTL Software and Availability

Name	Platform	Cost	URL	Design	Worked example
Standard statistical or spreadsheet packages (e.g., SAS, Splus, Excel)	UNIX, Dos, Mac	Yes	–	–	Yes
MAPMAKER/QTL	UNIX, Dos	No	http://www.genome.wi.mit.edu/ ftp/distribution/software/ mapmaker3	BC, F2, F3	Yes
QTL Cartographer	UNIX, Dos, Mac	No	http://statgen.ncsu.edu/qtlcart	BC, RI, others	Yes
Map Manager QT or QTX	Dos, Mac	No	http://mcbio.med.buffalo.edu/ mapmgr.html	BC, F2, RI, others	No
QGene™	Mac	Yes	qgene@clarityconnect.com	BC, F2, F3, DH, others	No
MapQTL™	SunOS, Dos, Mac, VMS	Yes	http://www.cpro.dlo.nl/cbw/	BC, F2, RI, DH, others	Yes
PLABQTL	Dos, AIX	No	http://www.unihohenheim.de/ ~ipspwww/soft.html	BC, F2, others	No
MQTL	SunOS, Dos	No	ftp://gnome.agrenv.mcgill.ca/pub/ genetics/software/MQTL/	BC, DH, RI	No
Multimapper	SunOS, Linux	No	http://www.RNI.Helsinki.FI/~mjs/	BC, F2	No
The QTL Cafe	Java-enabled browser	No	http://sun1.bham.ac.uk/g.g.seaton	BC, F2, DH, RI	No
Epistat	Dos	No	http://www.larklab.4biz.net/ epistat.htm	BC, RI	No

Note: Platform indicates the operating systems under which the program will run. URL indicates the Internet address for information about the software and, for those programs which are freely available, from where the software may be downloaded. Design indicates the type of population a program will analyze: BC=backcross; F2=intercross; F3=F3 intercross (by self-mating); RI=recombinant inbred; DH=doubled haploids derived from the gametes of an F1.

file tell the program to read data from an input file named bc.dat and store it as an object that we have arbitrarily named "genetic." The third line indicates that the data will be read in in the form of 23 columns, which we will name ID, J1, ..., DIAB, HIST. We will have previously prepared the input file bc.dat to consist of 305 lines of data, 1 line for each mouse, with columns corresponding to an ID, genotype (homozygous or heterozygous) for 10 loci on chromosome 1 (which we name J1–A1), genotype for 10 loci on chromosome 3 (which we name A3–J3), the disease status (DIAB), and quantitative trait value (HIST) corresponding to the histology of the pancreas. Having read in the data, lines 4–9 tell the program to perform a nonparametric analysis (hence, the choice of name of the command file) relating the quantitative trait value (HIST) to the genotype at locus F1.

The first and last few lines of the input data file bc.dat are shown as follows:

```
1 2 2 2 2 2 2 2 2 2 2  2 1 1 1 1 1 1 1 1 1 M 1 5
2 2 2 1 1 1 1 1 2 2 2  2 2 2 2 2 2 2 2 1 M 1 1
3 1 1 2 2 2 2 2 2 2 2  1 1 1 1 2 2 2 2 1 M 1 1
.
.
303 1 1 1 M 1 1 2 2 2 2  M 1 1 M 1 1 1 1 1 1 2 7
304 2 2 2 M 2 2 1 1 1 1  2 2 2 M 2 1 1 1 1 1 2 7
305 1 1 1 M 1 1 1 1 2 2  M M M M M M M M M M 2 7
```

The ID number for each animal goes from 1 to 305 for convenience. The genotype data (columns 2–21) takes the value 1 if an animal is homozygous and 2 if an animal is heterozygous at that marker locus. The penultimate column corresponds to disease status, with 1 corresponding to unaffected and 2 corresponding to affected. The final column corresponds to the "quantitative" trait, which, in this case, is actually an ordinal categorical variable taking values between 0 and 7. For all columns, we have used M to represent missing data.

The program can be run by typing "sas npar" at the UNIX prompt, assuming one is in the subdirectory containing the input files npar.sas and bc.dat. The program will write output to the files npar.log and npar.lst. The file npar.log gives information about the smooth running (or otherwise) of the program together with warning and error messages; note that, in this case, it will give an error message for every value of M that was read in, although the program will still run correctly and perform the analysis with missing values excluded.

The results of the analysis are in the output file npar.lst. The Wilcoxon command in the SAS code actually tells the program to perform a variety of nonparametric tests, including Wilcoxon and Kruskal–Wallis tests, as well as a standard analysis of variance. An example of part of the output is as follows:

```
N P A R 1 W A Y   P R O C E D U R E
Analysis of Variance for Variable HIST
Classified by Variable F1

F1    N       Mean          Among MS              Within MS
                            50.1993342            6.51604152
2     142     3.83802817
1     154     4.66233766    F Value               Prob > F
                            7.704                 0.0059


Kruskal-Wallis Test (Chi-Square Approximation)
CHISQ =  5.9693     DF =  1       Prob > CHISQ = 0.0146
```

We see that there are 142 animals with genotype 2 and 154 with genotype 1 at locus F1. The mean histology scores are 3.83 and 4.66 in the two genotype groups, suggesting that homozygotes have generally higher histology values than heterozygotes. The ANOVA suggests that this effect is significant, with a p-value of 0.0059, although note that this analysis may not be completely valid owing to the ordinal rather than strictly quantitative Normally distributed nature of the trait. The Kruskal–Wallis test, however, confirms the presence of a difference between the trait values in the two genotype groups at a p-value of 0.0146.

The analysis can be repeated for a different marker locus simply by replacing the variable F1 on lines 5 and 7 of the command file by the name of the required marker locus (e.g., A3). The results as output by SAS for the different loci are shown in **Table 2**. We see that the pattern of the results is quite similar for both the ANOVA and the Kruskal–Wallis analyses: Chromosome 1 shows significant evidence of linkage to a QTL across loci A1-F1 with the peak at locus C1, with some weaker evidence at loci I1 and J1; chromosome 3 shows broad evidence of linkage to a QTL across the whole region studied, with the peak at locus E3. Note that SAS does not provide accurate p-values below 0.0001 (e.g., the true p-value at A1 for a χ^2 of 16.892 on 1df is 3.96×10^{-5}.

SAS may be used for many other analyses of these data; in particular, the SAS procedures for simple linear and multiple regression and for logistic and ordinal logistic regression may be of interest. Such analyses may also be undertaken using other statistical or spreadsheet packages. It is recommended that these analyses only be undertaken by persons who are familiar with the relevant statistical package.

5.2. MapQTL

5.2.1. Single-Locus Associations

We will now confirm some of the results we found using SAS by analysing the same data using the QTL analysis package MapQTL. This package will

Table 2.
Kruskal–Wallis and ANOVA F-Statistics Output by SAS for Different Marker Loci

Marker locus	Kruskal–Wallis χ^2	SAS p-value	ANOVA F-statistic	SAS p-value
A1	16.892	0.0001	19.464	0.0001
B1	17.253	0.0001	20.226	0.0001
C1	17.849	0.0001	21.148	0.0001
D1	14.037	0.0002	16.727	0.0001
E1	10.146	0.0014	12.819	0.0004
F1	5.969	0.0146	7.704	0.0059
G1	1.656	0.1981	2.289	0.1319
H1	1.014	0.3141	1.369	0.2429
I1	4.370	0.0366	4.399	0.0368
J1	4.144	0.0418	4.295	0.0391
A3	23.270	0.0001	26.916	0.0001
B3	37.185	0.0001	44.358	0.0001
C3	39.088	0.0001	48.291	0.0001
D3	49.008	0.0001	61.720	0.0001
E3	54.684	0.0001	65.251	0.0001
F3	44.080	0.0001	52.696	0.0001
G3	43.296	0.0001	53.674	0.0001
H3	44.720	0.0001	54.121	0.0001
I3	27.200	0.0001	29.848	0.0001
J3	5.161	0.0231	5.536	0.0197

also calculate Kruskal–Wallis statistics across a region, but it has the advantage that it can also be used to undertake more complicated analyses such as simple interval mapping and MQM. To undertake an analysis using the UNIX version of MapQTL, three input files must be prepared: a locus genotype file with the file extension .loc, a map file with the file extension .map, and a quantitative data file with the extension .qua. (These files are described next and in more detail in the program manual.)

5.2.1.1. LOCUS GENOTYPE FILE

The first and last few lines of the locus genotype file are shown below. For convenience, because this is a backcross dataset, we name this file bc.loc. The file consists of a four-line header that tells the program to (arbitrarily) name this population NOD, that the data comes from a backcross (BC1) population, and that there are 305 individuals (mice) and genotype data on 20 loci. These values can be changed by altering the values on the right of the equal signs in the header. The header is followed by data consisting of the name of each marker locus followed by the genotypes of the 305 mice at that marker locus. The codes a, h, and u refer to homozygotes, heterozygotes, and missing data, respectively. Note that the order of the individuals must be identical over all loci in the file.

```
name = NOD
popt = BC1
nind = 305
nloc = 20

J1
h h a a a h a h h h h a h a h a a a h a a h h h a h a a h a a h a a a
a a a h h a a h a h a a h h h a a a a h a h a h a a a h a h h a h a h
h h a h h h h a a h a a h h a a h h h h a a h h h a a u u u u u u h u
h h a h a a a a a a a h h h h h a h a a a a a a h a a h h h a h h a
a a a a h a h a a a a h a a a a h h h a h a h h a a h h a h a h a a h
a a h a a a a u h a h h a a a a h a h h h h a h h h a a h a h a a a h a
h a h h a h h h h h h h a a a h h a h a h a h a h a a h a a a h a h h h h
h h a h h h a h a h a a a a h a h h a a h a a a h h h a h h h h a h h a
a a h a h h h h h h a a h h h a h a h a h a h a a h a
I1
h h a a a h a h h h h a h a h a a a h a a h h h a h a a h a a h a a a
a a a h h a a h a h a a h h h a a a a h a h a h a a a a a h a h h h a h a h
h h a h h h h a a h
.

.
J3
u u u u u u u u u u u u u u u u u u u u u u u u u h a a h a a h h a h
a h a h a a a h h h h h h a h h a a h a a a h h h a h a a h h a a a a h a
h u u h h a h h a a a h a h h a a a a a h a a h h h a a h h a h a h u
h a h a h a u a a a a a u h u h a a h u u u u u u u u u u u u u u u
u u u u u u u u u u u u u u u u u u u u u u u u u u u u u u u u u u u
u u u u u u u u u u u u u u u u u u u u u u u u u u a a a h a a a a a h h
a a h a h h a a a h h a a h h h h h h a a a a h a a h a a a a a h a a
a a a h a a h a h a h a a h h a a a a a a a h a a a a h a a h h a h a
a h a h a a a a u u u u a a a u u u u u u u u a a u
```

5.2.1.2. THE MAP FILE

The map file for these data, which we name bc.map, is as follows:

```
chrom 1
A1 0.0
B1 1.3
C1 19.1
```

```
D1 23.3
E1 29.7
F1 35.0
G1 35.5
H1 41.9
I1 65.8
J1 67.1

chrom 3
A3 0.0
B3 12.4
C3 26.1
D3 31.4
E3 38.9
F3 52.6
G3 56.8
H3 57.8
I3 81.7
J3 102.5
```

This file separates the marker loci into two linkage groups on separate chromosomes and gives their locations in cM (measured from some arbitrary starting location). Such information can be obtained using (for example) the JoinMap programs as described in Chapter 9.

5.2.1.3. THE PHENOTYPE FILE

The first and last few lines of the quantitative data file bc.qua are given below. This file consists of a three-line header, followed by the IDs and quantitative trait values for the 305 mice. None that the order of the individuals must correspond to the order used in the locus genotype file. The header defines two traits, which are then (line 4) given the names nr and hist. The first trait is, therefore, not a real trait, but a dummy trait corresponding to the ID numbers. Line 2 and 3 tell the program that there are 305 individuals and that the code for missing trait values in this file is M.

```
ntrt = 2
nind = 305
miss = M

nr hist
1       5
2       1
3       1
.
.
.
304     7
305     7
```

To run MapQTL, it is first necessary to tell the program the name of the directory in which the license file is stored. Suppose the license file is in the subdirectory /home/MAPQTL. Then, before running the program, you will need to type "setenv MQDIR /home/MAPQTL/" at the UNIX prompt. It may be convenient to set up things so that this command is executed automatically at login (see your system administrator for details).

The program itself can be started in the usual way, by typing the name of the executable program (usually mq) at the UNIX prompt. The program itself then asks you to type in the name of the relevant input files. The program asks you which trait number you wish to analyze, to which you should respond 2, and which analysis you wish to run, to which (for the time being) you should respond K for Kruskal–Wallis analysis. The program asks you which linkage groups you wish to analyse (respond ALL) and asks you for the name of an output file, to which hist.KW might be a good suggested response. If preferred, these preferences may be input at the start by typing mq l=bc.loc m=bc.map q=bc.qua t=2 k (type mq h to see a complete list of options for the command line).

5.2.1.4. OUTPUT FROM MAPQTL

A portion of the output file is shown below. In addition to some general information concerning the genotype and trait data, we see that the results from the Kruskal–Wallis analysis are identical to those obtained using SAS.

```
locus genotype file:                            bc.loc
  population name:                              NOD
  population type:                              BC1
  nr. of loci:                                  20
  nr. of genotyped individuals:       305  (9 without quant. data)
map file:                                       bc.map
  nr. of linkage groups:                        2
  analysing linkage groups:                     all
quantitative data file:                         bc.qua
  nr. of not-genotyped individuals:   0  (0 without quant. data)
  nr. of traits:                                2
  analysing trait nr. 2:                        hist
  population mean:                              4.26689
           variance:                6.64161  (unbiased:  6.66412)
           skewness:                          −0.293834
           kurtosis:                          −1.48918
performing Kruskal-Wallis analysis

(?) means: genotype data found outside genotype classes

significance levels: *:0.1 **:0.05 ***:0.01 ****:0.005 *****:0.001
******:0.0005  *******:0.0001
```

```
linkage group nr. 1 (1):
map    locus nr inf      K* (df)
-------------------------------
0.0    A1          296         16.892 (1) *******
1.3    B1          296         17.253 (1) *******
19.1   C1          294         17.849 (1) *******
23.3   D1          296         14.037 (1) ******
29.7   E1          296         10.146 (1) ****
35.0   F1          296          5.969 (1) **
35.5   G1          197          1.656 (1)
41.9   H1          296          1.014 (1)
65.8   I1          296          4.370 (1) **
67.1   J1          296          4.144 (1) **


linkage group nr. 2 (3):
map    locus nr inf      K* (df)
-------------------------------
0.0    A3          285         23.270 (1) *******
12.4   B3          291         37.185 (1) *******
26.1   C3          295         39.088 (1) *******
31.4   D3          278         49.008 (1) *******
38.9   E3          295         54.684 (1) *******
52.6   F3          292         44.080 (1) *******
56.8   G3          294         43.296 (1) *******
57.8   H3          295         44.720 (1) *******
81.7   I3          295         27.200 (1) *******
102.5  J3          181          5.161 (1) **
```

5.2.2. Simple Interval Mapping

5.2.2.1. SIMPLE INTERVAL MAPPING WITH MAPQTL

The same input files may be used for simple interval mapping with MapQTL. Exactly the same procedure is used, except that when asked which analysis you wish to use, you should reply i for interval mapping, for the name of the output file you might reply hist.IM, when asked to print either LOD score or deviance we suggest you reply L for LOD score, and when asked for the mapping step size we suggest you could reply 5 to calculate a LOD score every 5 cM, or 1 to generate a finer map at every cM.

5.2.2.2. OUTPUT FROM SIMPLE INTERVAL MAPPING

Selected portions of the output for a 5-cM screen are shown below. The different columns correspond to the map position and then, for each position, the LOD score, the number of iterations needed to reach convergence, the mean trait value among homozygotes, the mean trait value among heterozygotes, the residual variance after fitting a QTL at this position, the percentage variance

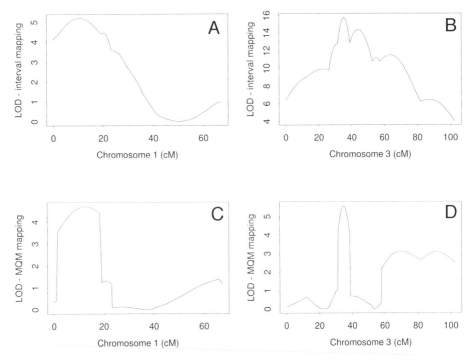

Fig. 1.

explained by the QTL, the estimated additive effect, and the position of the marker loci. The peak LODs occur at 11.3 cM on chromosome 1 and 36.4 cM on chromosome 3. Nevertheless, the overall significance remains quite high (LOD > 3) across broad regions of both chromosomes. A graphical representation of these results, this time for a 1-cM screen, is shown in **Fig. 1** (panels a and b).

```
linkage group nr. 1 (1):
map     lod     iter    mu_A     mu_H     var      %expl  add         locus
---------------------------------------------------------------------------
0.0     4.12    4       4.91783  3.63333  6.22921  6.2    1.28447     A1
1.3     4.28    4       4.92517  3.61745  6.21409  6.4    1.30772     B1
6.3     4.98    7       5.03394  3.50603  6.05799  8.8    1.52791
11.3    5.19    7       5.06427  3.47746  6.01213  9.5    1.58681
16.3    4.81    6       5.00494  3.54354  6.10774  8.0    1.46140
 .
65.8    0.95    4       3.96026  4.58621  6.54370  1.5    -0.625942   I1
67.1    0.93    4       3.95973  4.57823  6.54598  1.4    -0.618500   J1
```

```
linkage group nr. 2 (3):
map      lod     iter    mu_A    mu_H    var     %expl   add       locus
-------------------------------------------------------------------------
0.0      6.39    5       4.99142 3.38340 6.00149 9.6     1.60802   A3
5.0      7.84    6       5.11187 3.28492 5.81186 12.5    1.82695
.
.
.
31.4     12.76   5       5.27966 3.06021 5.41952 18.4    2.21944   D3
36.4     15.47   8       5.40069 2.78421 4.96056 25.3    2.61647
38.9     12.89   5       5.21571 2.99001 5.43008 18.2    2.22570   E3
.
.
102.5    4.06    7       4.91276 3.46732 6.12519 7.8     1.44544   J3
```

5.2.3. MQM and Restricted MQM Mapping

5.2.3.1. MQM USING MAPQTL

To undertake MQM mapping in MapQTL, an additional file must be prepared to tell MapQTL the names of the loci to be used as cofactors in the MQM analysis. The selection of cofactors is not trivial. Because in our initial analyses we found strongest evidence of linkage in the B1–C1 region on chromosome 1 and broad significance in the A3–I3 region on chromosome 3, we select the six markers B1, C1 (from chromosome 1) and A3, D3, E3, and I3 (from chromosome 3) as cofactors. We chose these markers to cover the regions of initial significance while limiting the total number of cofactors considered; markers B3 and C3 were not included because they are not in the region of highest significance, but A3 was included to account for any possible effects in this region of the chromosome. We, therefore, prepare an input file bc.cof:

```
ncof = 6

B1
C1

A3
D3
E3
I3
```

The program may be run as previously, with analysis option M for MQM mapping. This option includes all cofactors except when a cofactor is one of the flanking markers of the interval on which the QTL is fitted. An alternative analysis option is r for restricted MQM mapping, which uses only those cofactors not on the linkage group on which the QTL is being fitted. Because the broad spread of significance on chromosome 3 suggests there may be more than one QTL on this chromosome, we prefer the M option in order to condition out effects of additional QTLs on the same chromosome. The program will prompt you for the name of the cofactors file and whether you wish to generate a cofactor monitor output file (to which we suggest you reply none).

5.2.3.2. OUTPUT FOR MQM

Selected output from MQM mapping is shown below. A graphical representation of these results is shown in **Fig. 1** (panels c and d). Those loci that are cofactors are shown with an exclamation mark. We find that MQM mapping has again identified a QTL with a peak of linkage at 11.3 cM on chromosome 1, with the effect on chromosome 3 being separated out into two potential QTLs, one at around 36.4 cm and one in the 60- to 100-cM region.

```
linkage group nr. 1 (1):
map     lod     iter    mu_A    mu_H    var     %expl   add         locus
------------------------------------------------------------------------
0.0     0.36    4       4.30495 3.86622 4.71718 0.4     0.438727    A1
1.1     3.51    4       4.60304 3.55646 4.80072 4.1     1.04657     B1!
6.3     4.31    6       4.71014 3.45418 4.68309 5.9     1.25596
11.3    4.70    6       4.74314 3.42184 4.64253 6.5     1.32130
16.3    4.58    5       4.70608 3.45882 4.68994 5.8     1.24726
.

.
65.8    1.37    3       3.76907 4.43054 4.61438 1.5     -0.661470   I1
67.1    1.18    4       3.78936 4.40236 4.62755 1.3     -0.613003   J1


linkage group nr. 2 (3):
map     lod     iter    mu_A    mu_H    var     %expl   add         locus
------------------------------------------------------------------------
0.0     0.13    3       4.22266 3.94541 4.71317 0.1     0.277256    A3!
5.0     0.30    5       4.32250 3.84550 4.69860 0.3     0.476998
.

.
31.4    4.24    4       4.94470 3.26711 4.75937 5.0     1.67758     D3!
36.4    5.26    8       5.02883 3.10413 4.55218 8.1     1.92470
38.9    0.70    3       4.46320 3.70487 4.71317 0.7     0.758336    E3!
.

.
102.5   2.49    6       4.58291 3.59636 4.67658 3.5     0.986548    J3
```

Note that the results described here were obtained using MapQTL version 3.0. A later version, MapQTL version 4.0, has been developed that allows considerably more functionality (e.g., automatic selection of cofactors for MQM mapping and a permutation test for interval mapping). MapQTL version 4.0 is not available under the UNIX operating system, and for this reason, as well as in the interests of space, we do not include here results from analysis using MapQTL version 4.0.

5.3. MAPMAKER/QTL

5.3.1. Simple Interval Mapping

The simple interval mapping analysis performed earlier with MapQTL can also be undertaken with the program package MAPMAKER/QTL. This is a companion program to the package MAPMAKER/EXP and uses MAPMAKER/EXP to preprocess the data and, if required, to estimate positions of the marker loci before performing an interval mapping analysis. Note that both MAPMAKER programs, but MAPMAKER/EXP in particular, include options for more sophisticated analysis than can be described in this brief example. See the program manual for details.

5.3.1.1. INPUT FILES

To perform the analysis, two input files are required: a file of raw genotype and quantitative phenotype data with the file extension .raw, and a file of MAPMAKER/EXP commands with the extension .prep. In the following, we show the first and last few lines from our input file bc.raw. The file consists of a two-line header with the first line defining the type of cross and the second line indicating the number of animals (305), the number of marker loci (20), and the number of quantitative traits (1). After this comes each of the locus names preceded by an asterisk and the genotype data for that locus with codes a, h, and - for homozygotes, heterozygotes, and missing data, respectively. At the end of the marker data comes the quantitative phenotype data (hist) in the same format. Note that the order of the individuals must be identical over all loci and traits in the file.

```
data type f2 backcross
305 20 1

*J1
h h a a a h a h h h h a h a h a a a h a a h h h h a h a a h a a h a a a
a a a .
.
.
*I1
h h a a a h a h h h h a h a h a a a h a a h h h h a h a a h a a h a a a
a a a
.
.
```

```
*hist
5 1 1 4 6 1 6 5 4 2 1 1 4 5 4 6 5 2 0 1 1 6 6 2 2 4 1 2 0 0 1 2 4 2 0
4 1 1 2 3 2 1 6 1 3 0 5 3 2 5 5 6 5 1 5 3 1 5 4 2 3 0 0 0 5 0 1 4 5 1
1 2 5 3 1 4 .
.
7 7 7 7 7 7 7 7 7 7 7 7 7 7 7 7 7 7 7 7 7 7 7 7 7 7 7
```

The other input file is used for the preprocessing with MAPMAKER/EXP. The format of this file varies slightly depending on whether the user wishes to calculate a genetic map for the markers from the data themselves or to use a predefined map. An example of the required file bc.prep using the predefined map is as follows:

```
units cm
make chromosome chrom1 chrom3
seq A1 =1.3 B1 = 17.8 C1 =4.2 D1 =6.4 E1 =5.3 F1 =0.6 G1 =6.4 H1 =23.9 I1 =
1.3 J1
anchor chrom1
frame chrom1
seq A3 =12.4 B3 =13.7 C3 =5.3 D3 =7.5 E3 =13.7 F3 =4.2 G3 =1.0 H3 =23.9 I3 =
20.8 J3
anchor chrom3
frame chrom3
save
```

Line 1 defines the units of map distance to be in cM. Line 2 defines two chromosomes, which we name chrom1 and chrom3. Lines 3–5 and 6–8 define the positions of the loci on the two chromosomes. Note that intermarker distances are given rather than absolute distances from a fixed position. Note also that the distance between markers F1 and G1 has been set to equal 0.6 cM, as opposed to the true value, which should be 0.5 cM. This is because MAPMAKER/EXP automatically assumes distances less than or equal to 0.5 must be recombination fractions rather than map distances. Alternatively one could convert this interval (and/or any other of the intervals) to recombination fractions.

5.3.1.2. RUNNING MAPMAKER/EXP AND MAPMAKER/QTL

To process the files through MAPMAKER/EXP, type "mapmaker" at the UNIX prompt. This allows you to enter the program. Then type "photo photo exp.out" at the MAPMAKER/EXP prompt to save a record of your session to the file photoexp.out. Next, type "prepare data bc.raw" to process the raw data, and "q" and "yes" to exit and save.

MAPMAKER/EXP should now have generated a number of other files that will be used by the program MAPMAKER/QTL. To run this program, type "qtl" at the UNIX prompt and then "photo photoqtl.out" to save a record of the session. Now, type "load data bc" to read in the preprocessed data. Next, type the commands "seq [chrom1]," "scan," and "draw scan" to perform a simple interval mapping analysis on chromosome 1, and "seq [chrom3]," "scan," "draw scan," "q," and "yes" to do the same for chromosome 3 and exit the program.

5.3.1.3. OUTPUT FROM MAPMAKER/QTL

In your file directory, you should now find postscript (.ps) files, which provide a graphical representation of the results, and a record of your results in the file photoqtl.out. Some of this output is shown as follows (and a further example can be found in Chapter 10.

```
Sequence: [chrom1]
POS    WEIGHT   %VAR    LOG-LIKE
------------------------------ 10-9 1.3 cM
0.0   -1.285    6.2%    4.121    *********
------------------------------ 9-8 17.8 cM
0.0   -1.308    6.4%    4.277    **********
2.0   -1.410    7.5%    4.596    ***********
4.0   -1.494    8.4%    4.869    ************
6.0   -1.553    9.1%    5.071    *************
8.0   -1.583    9.4%    5.183    *************
10.0  -1.584    9.4%    5.195    *************
12.0  -1.556    9.1%    5.107    *************
14.0  -1.500    8.5%    4.926    ************
16.0  -1.416    7.5%    4.670    ***********
------------------------------ 8-7 4.2 cM
0.0   -1.326    6.6%    4.396    **********
2.0   -1.382    7.2%    4.375    **********
4.0   -1.227    5.7%    3.661    *******
------------------------------ 7-6 6.4 cM
0.0   -1.198    5.4%    3.557    *******
2.0   -1.230    5.7%    3.515    *******
4.0   -1.193    5.3%    3.269    ******
6.0   -1.085    4.4%    2.845    ****
------------------------------ 6-5 5.3 cM
0.0   -1.054    4.2%    2.743    ***
2.0   -1.001    3.8%    2.381    **
4.0   -0.907    3.1%    1.956
```

```
Sequence: [chrom3]
------------------------------- 11-12 12.4 cM
 0.0   -1.607    9.6%   6.382   ******************
 2.0   -1.717   11.0%   7.019   *********************
 4.0   -1.796   12.1%   7.581   ***********************
 6.0   -1.847   12.8%   8.054   *************************
 8.0   -1.875   13.2%   8.439   **************************
10.0   -1.885   13.3%   8.739   ***************************
12.0   -1.876   13.2%   8.956   ***************************
------------------------------- 12-13 13.7 cM
 0.0   -1.872   13.2%   8.990   ***************************
 2.0   -1.929   14.0%   9.291   *****************************
 4.0   -1.970   14.5%   9.536   ******************************
 6.0   -1.996   14.9%   9.721   ******************************
 8.0   -2.009   15.1%   9.842   *******************************
10.0   -2.006   15.0%   9.894   *******************************
12.0   -1.986   14.7%   9.864   *******************************
------------------------------- 13-14 5.3 cM
 0.0   -1.949   14.2%   9.763   *******************************
 2.0   -2.202   18.1%  11.700   ***************************************
 4.0   -2.254   19.0%  12.624   *******************************************
------------------------------- 14-15 7.5 cM
 0.0   -2.219   18.4%  12.751   *********************************************
 2.0   -2.574   24.6%  15.039   *********************************************
 4.0   -2.647   25.9%  15.715   *********************************************
 6.0   -2.523   23.5%  14.726   *********************************************
------------------------------- 15-16 13.7 cM
 0.0   -2.224   18.2%  12.857   *********************************************
 2.0   -2.413   21.5%  13.802   *********************************************
 4.0   -2.500   23.1%  14.260   *********************************************
 6.0   -2.525   23.5%  14.274   *********************************************
 8.0   -2.503   23.1%  13.882   *********************************************
10.0   -2.420   21.5%  13.096   *********************************************
12.0   -2.265   18.8%  11.934   ****************************************
------------------------------- 16-17 4.2 cM
 0.0   -2.063   15.6%  10.725   **************************************
 2.0   -2.146   16.8%  11.197   ***************************************
 4.0   -2.084   15.8%  10.844   **************************************
```

We find that the results for the LODs (column 4) are very similar to those obtained using MapQTL. Note that the results are divided into intervals flanked by the marker loci, which are identified on the far right of the output according to their position in the original raw data file (i.e., marker 10 corresponds to A1, marker 1 to J1, etc.).

5.4. QTL Cartographer

5.4.1. Single-Locus Associations

Many of the analyses performed using MapQTL and MAPMAKER/QTL can also be done using the program package QTL Cartographer. We start with some tests for single-locus association using a simple linear regression model. QTL Cartographer can accept input files either in the form of MAPMAKER/ EXP files or in an alternative format specific to QTL Cartographer. Note that if MAPMAKER/EXP files are used, the genotype and phenotype data are input into QTL Cartographer as the input raw data file for MAPMAKER/EXP, whereas the locus map data is input as the output map file from MAPMAKER/ EXP (i.e., MAPMAKER/EXP must first be used to generate this file).

5.4.1.1. INPUT FILES

In this example, we use the QTL Cartographer format input files. An example of part of the genotype and phenotype data file, which we shall call bccross.inp, is shown later in this section. The first line consists of a # followed by a large integer number chosen by the user to uniquely identify the file. We then have the command -filetype cross.inp, which helps the program identify the type of file it is reading. We then have lines starting with the commands -SampleSize, -Cross, -traits, and -otraits, which are followed by information as to the number of individuals, the type of cross (here, B1 stands for backcross), the number of quantitative traits to be analyzed and number of any other traits. The command -case should be followed by yes or no depending on whether the names of the marker systems are case sensitive. Note that any extraneous text after that required by a command is ignored. (See the program manual for more details.) Next, we have a translation table that allows the user to define the symbols used for marker values. The first two columns of the table should be identical to that given here; the third column can take any values specified by the user. Here, we have chosen to use the symbols a, h, - (for homozygous, heterozygous, and missing, respectively). We must also fill in values for the other possible genotypes, although in our data, these codes will never appear. Finally, we define the missing trait code to also be -.

Now, we come to the marker data, which is in a very similar format to that used by MapQTL and MAPMAKER/QTL. This is followed by the trait data. Note that the marker data must appear in between the two commands -start markers and -stop markers, whereas the trait data must appear in between the commands -start traits and -stop traits.

```
# 123456789 -filetype cross.inp
-SampleSize        305    is the sample size
-Cross    B1    is the type of cross
-traits        1   is the number of traits
-otraits       0   is the number of other traits
-case   yes
-TranslationTable
        AA      2     a
        Aa      1     h
        aa      0     x
        A-     12     y
        a-     10     z
        --     -1     -
-missingtrait -
-start markers
 J1
 h h a a a h a h h h h a h a h a a a h a a h h h a h a a h a a h a a a
 a a a h h a a h a h a a h h h a a a a h a h a h a a a h a h h h a h a h
 h h a h h h
 .

 .
 I1
 h h a a a h a h h h h a h a h a a a h a a h h h a h a a h a a h a a a
 a a a h h a a h a h a a h h h a a a a h a h a a a a a h a h h h a h a h
 h h a h h h
 .

 .
-stop markers
-start traits
 hist
 5 1 1 4 6 1 6 5 4 2 1 1 4 5 4 6 5 2 0 1 1 6 6 2 2 4 1 2 0 0 1 2 4 2 0
 4 1 1 2 3 2 1 6 1 3 0 5 3 2 5 5 6 5 1 5 3 1 5 4 2 3 0 0 0 5 0 1 4 5 1
 1 2 5 3 1 4 .
 .
 7 7 7 7 7 7 7 7 7 7 7 7 7 7 7 7 7 7 7 7 7 7 7 7 7 7
-stop traits
```

The second input file required by QTL Cartographer is a map data file, which we will call bcmap.inp. An example of this is given next. Again, we start with a line with # followed by a large file identifier, and the command bychromosome - filetype map.inp, which indicates how the map should be read in and the file type. We then have the command -type, which should be followed by the words "positions" or "intervals," depending on how the map distances are to be read in. The commands -function, -Units, -chromosomes, and -maximum define the mapping function, units of distance, number of chromosomes, and maximum number of markers per chromosome, respectively, whereas -named should be followed by yes or no depending on whether the markers have names. After this comes the actual map information, which should be fairly self-explanatory.

```
# 12345678 bychromosome -filetype map.inp
-type positions
-function     1 (1=haldane, 2=kosambi, 3=fixed)
-Units        cM where cM means centiMorgans
-chromosomes  2 the haploid number of chromosomes
-maximum     10 markers on any chromosome.
-named      yes markers will have names.


-start
-Chromosome chr1
A1 0.0
B1 1.3
C1 19.1
D1 23.3
E1 29.7
F1 35.0
G1 35.5
H1 41.9
I1 65.8
J1 67.1
-Chromosome chr3
A3 0.0
B3 12.4
C3 26.1
D3 31.4
E3 38.9
F3 52.6
G3 56.8
H3 57.8
I3 81.7
J3 102.5
-stop


-end
```

5.4.1.2. RUNNING QTL CARTOGRAPHER

The input files bcmap.inp and bccross.inp must be processed by QTL cartographer to produce its own .map and .cross output files. To do, this type "Rmap" at the UNIX prompt.

A list of different numbered menu options will be presented. Type "16" followed by "bc" to tell the program to change the file name stem to name all the files it creates from now on bc.ext, where ext stands for a file extension. Type "1" followed by "bcmap.inp" to tell the program to read the input file bcmap.inp, and then "0" to continue with these parameters, finish, and exit. There should now be a new file bc.map in your directory. To process the other input file, type "Rcross" at the UNIX prompt, followed by "1" and "bccross.inp" and then "0" to finish and exit. There should now be a new file bc.cro in your directory.

To perform the simple linear regression analysis, including a permutation test of significance, type "LRmapqtl" at the UNIX prompt, followed by "6" to choose the option to change the number of permutations, and then "10000" and "0" (this instructs the program to do 10,000 permutations, so this number should be lowered if it turns out to be too time-consuming). Results will be output to the file bc.1r. Selected results are shown in the following. As with our previous analyses, we find broad regions of significance on both chromosomes.

Chrom.	Marker	b0	b1	LR	$F(1,n-2)$	$Pr(F)$	
1	1	3.652	1.284	18.989	19.464	0.000	****
1	2	3.637	1.308	19.709	20.226	0.000	****
..							
2	9	3.371	1.598	29.172	30.412	0.000	****
2	10	4.107	0.236	0.387	0.385	0.535	

```
# Performed 10000 permutations of the phenotypes and genotypes
# Here are the comparisonwise counts of permuted test statistics

#Chrom Mark MarkerName Cnts Pval
     1    1        A1    1  0.00
     1    2        B1    0  0.00

     .
     .

     1    8        H1 2440  0.24
     1    9        I1  363  0.04
     1   10        J1  388  0.04
     2    1        A3    0  0.00
     2    2        B3    0  0.00

     .
     .

     2   10        J3 5410  0.54
```

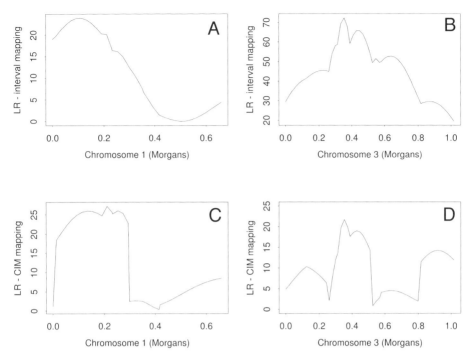

Fig. 2.

A stepwise regression analysis can be carried out using the commands SRmapqtl and 0 (results output to bc.sr) to identify the most influential markers. This analysis must be carried out if composite interval mapping with model 6 (*see* **Subheading 5.4.2.**) is to be performed later. In our data, this identified six important markers, with marker 5 on chromosome 2 (i.e., E3) and marker 3 on chromosome 1 (i.e., H1) as the most important.

5.4.2. Simple and Composite Interval Mapping

QTL Cartographer may be used to perform simple and composite interval mapping. For simple interval mapping, type "Zmapqtl," "2," (to choose the option to change the output file name), "bc.model3," and "0"; the results will be output to the file bc.model3, where model 3 corresponds to the interval mapping procedure of Lander and Botstein (*4*). The output is described in more detail in the program manual; the most important results are columns 3 and 4, which give the position and LR test statistics. A graphical representation of these results is shown in **Fig. 2** (panels a and b). The shape of the plot is found to be identical to that from MapQTL (*see* **Fig. 1**) or MAPMAKER/QTL, although the scale is different because MapQTL and MAPMAKER/QTL output LOD scores rather than LR statistics.

Composite interval mapping may be performed in QTL Cartographer using a variety of different models. Here, we use the recommended model 6. A prior analysis with SRmapqtl must have been performed in order to select the markers to control for the genetic background. To run the analysis, type "Zmapqtl," "2" (to choose the option to change the output file name), "bc.model6," "8" (to choose the option to change the model), "6" (to select model 6), and "0" to finish. The results are output to bc.model6. A graphical representation of these results is shown in **Fig. 2** (panels c and d). We find, again, that the peak of linkage on chromosome 1 remains, with the effect on chromosome 3 being separated out into two or possibly three potential QTLs. These results are similar to those from MapQTL, although there are some differences caused by the different ways of choosing markers as cofactors in the analysis.

6. Notes

1. User manuals. We have attempted in the course of the worked example to draw attention to some of the possible pitfalls one may encounter when using computer software for QTL analysis. However, it is important to carefully read the user manual for the program being used and pay attention, in particular, to required file formats, coding schemes, and whether or not the program is case sensitive. Beware of programs that overwrite files with the same name and always keep a copy of your raw data in a different directory. Many programs come with example or tutorial files and it is well worth working through an analysis with these before proceeding to analyze your own data.

2. Choosing the most relevant software package. A final recommendation may be given as to which software might be preferable to use in which circumstances. If only one QTL exists, the results from simple single-locus association and simple interval mapping analyses are likely to be very similar, with interval mapping having the advantage of giving a convenient graphical output for localizing the QTL. If more than one QTL exists, it makes sense to take account of this using a CIM/MQM approach. Because in practice we may not know how many QTLs there are, we would almost invariably recommend use of a package such as MapQTL or QTL Cartographer that allows implementation of both CIM/MQM methods and simpler approaches.

Acknowledgments

Support for Heather Cordell was provided by a Wellcome Trust Career Development Fellowship jointly funded by the Wellcome Trust and the Juvenile Diabetes Research Foundation. I thank John Whittaker and Aruna Bansal for their useful comments on this chapter and Johan van Ooijen and Ritsert Jansen for giving useful comments and making a version of the program MapQTL available.

References

1. Todd, J. A., Aitman, T. J., Cornall, R. J., Ghosh, S., Hall, J. R. S., Hearne, C. M., et al. (1991) Genetic analysis of autoimmune type 1 diabetes mellitus in mice. *Nature* **351,** 542–547.
2. Whittaker, J. C., Thompson, R. and Visscher, P. M. (1996) On the mapping of QTL by regression of phenotype on marker-type. *Heredity* **77,** 23–32.
3. Cordell, H. J., Todd, J. A., and Lathrop, G. M. (1998) Mapping multiple linked quantitative trait loci in non-obese diabetic mice using a stepwise regression strategy. *Genet. Res.* **71,** 51–64.
4. Lander, E. S. and Botstein, D. (1989) Mapping Mendelian factors underlying quantitative traits using RFLP linkage maps. *Genetics* **121,** 185–199.
5. Carbonell, E. A., Gerig, T. M., Balansard, E., and Asins, M. J. (1992) Interval mapping in the analysis of nonadditive quantitative trait loci. *Biometrics* **48,** 305–315.
6. Zeng, A.-B. (1993) Theoretical basis for separation of multiple linked gene effects in mapping quantitative trait loci. *Proc. Natl. Acad. Sci. USA* **90,** 10,972–10,976.
7. Zeng, Z.-B. (1994) Precision mapping of quantitative trait loci. *Genetics* **136,** 1457–1468.
8. Jiang, C. and Zeng, Z.-B. (1995) Multiple trait analysis of genetic mapping for quantitative trait loci. *Genetics* **142,** 305–311.
9. Jansen, R. C. (1993) Interval mapping of multiple quantitative trait loci. *Genetics* **135,** 205–211.
10. Jansen, R. C. (1996) A general Monte Carlo method for mapping multiple quantitative trait loci. *Genetics* **142,** 305–311.
11. Satagopan, J. M., Yandell, B. S., Newton, M. A., and Osborn, T. C. (1996) A Bayesian approach to detect quantitative trait loci using Markov chain Monte Carlo. *Genetics* **144,** 805–816.
12. Uimari, P., Thaller, G., and Hoeschele, I. (1996) The use of multiple markers in a Bayesian method for mapping quantitative trait loci. *Genetics* **143,** 1831–1842.
13. Sillanpaa, M. J. and Arjas, E. (1998) Bayesian mapping of multiple quantitative trait loci from incomplete inbred line cross data. *Genetics* **148,** 1373–1388.
14. Dempster, A. P., Laird, N. M., and Rubin, D. B. (1976) Maximum likelihood from incomplete data via the EM algorithm. *J. R. Statist. Soc. Ser. B* **39,** 1–38.
15. Haley, C. S. and Knott, S. A. (1992) A simple regression method for mapping quantitative trait loci in line crosses using flanking markers. *Heredity* **69,** 315–324.
16. Martinez, O. and Curnow, R. N. (1992) Estimating the locations and the sizes of the effects of quantitative trait loci using flanking markers. *Theor. Appl. Genet.* **85,** 480–488.
17. Kruglyak, L. and Lander E. (1995) A nonparametric approach for mapping quantitative trait loci. *Genetics* **139,** 1421–1428.
18. McCullagh, P. and Nelder, J. A. (1989) *Generalized Linear Models,* 2nd ed. Chapman & Hall, London.
19. Chase, K., Adler, F. R., and Lark, K. G. (1997) Epistat: a computer program for

identifying and testing interactions between pairs of quantitative trait loci. *Theor. Appl. Genet.* **94,** 724–730.

20. Lander, E. and Kruglyak, L. (1995) Genetic dissection of complex traits: guidelines for interpreting and reporting linkage results. *Nature Genet.* **11,** 241–247.

21. Churchill, G. A. and Doerge, R. W. (1994) Empirical threshold values for quantitative trait mapping. *Genetics* **138,** 963–971.

22. Van Ooijen, J. W. (1999) LOD significance thresholds for QTL analysis in experimental populations of diploid species. *Heredity* **83,** 613–624.

23. Doerge, R. W. and Churchill, G. A. (1996) Permutation tests for multiple loci affecting a quantitative character. *Genetics* **142,** 285–294.

24. Visscher, P. M., Haley, C. S., and Thompson, R. (1996) Marker-assisted introgression in backcross breeding programs. *Genetics* **144,** 1923–1932.

25. Van Ooijen, J. W. (1992) Accuracy of mapping quantitative trait loci in autogamous species. *Theor. Appl. Genet.* **84,** 803–811.

26. Visscher, P. M., Thompson, R., and Haley, C. S. (1996) Confidence intervals in QTL mapping by boot-strapping. *Genetics* **143,** 1013–1020.

27. Lynch, M. and Walsh, B. (1998) Mapping QTLs: Inbred line crosses, in *Genetics and Analysis of Quantitative Traits.* Sinauer, pp. 431–489.

28. Cordell, H. J., Todd, J. A., Hill, N. J., Lord, C. J., Lyons, P. A., Peterson, L. B., et al. (2001) Statistical modeling of interlocus interactions in a complex disease: rejection of the multiplicative model of epistasis in type 1 diabetes. *Genetics* **158,** 357–367.

29. Manly, K. F. and Olson, J. M. (1999) Overview of QTL mapping software and introduction to Map Manager QT. *Mammal. Genome* **10,** 327–334.

8

Experimental Designs for QTL Fine Mapping in Rodents

Anne Shalom and Ariel Darvasi

1. Introduction

1.1. Definition of Complex Traits and QTL

For a simple genetic trait, determined by a single gene, the Mendelian segregation of two or three phenotypes may be observed for the three possible genotypes at a specific locus.

For a complex trait, such a one-to-one relationship cannot be drawn between genotype and phenotype. Complex traits, such as neurobiological and behavioral phenotypes, are likely to be influenced by a large number of biochemical, physiological, and morphological processes, with nongenetic environmental factors also playing a major role. In humans, traits such as anxiety or depression may represent extremes of a continuum of Normally distributed phenotypical traits and are most aptly considered under a complex or polygenic model. Complex traits are often quantitative in nature or can be measured in a quantitative manner. In many instances, their genetic architecture is conveniently dissected under a quantitative model, in which the genetic factors analyzed are termed *quantitative trait loci* (QTL) (*1*).

1.2. Purpose of QTL Detection

Quantitative trait loci detection and mapping aims to uncover the genetic blueprint underlying a given complex trait, by identifying specific chromosomal segments, and ultimately specific genes, or regulatory elements, which influence the phenotypic expression of the trait. This represents one of the major challenges of genetics today and is being made possible only recently through the development of novel molecular and analytical technologies.

From: *Methods in Molecular Biology: vol. 195: Quantitative Trait Loci: Methods and Protocols.*
Edited by: N. J. Camp and A. Cox © Humana Press, Inc., Totowa, NJ

In the past few years, researchers have begun to be successful in detecting and locating QTLs that affect complex traits in humans, model organisms, and agricultural species (*2–21*). However, there has been less success in reducing the broad chromosomal regions thus identified down to regions narrow enough to allow positional cloning (*22–24*). Yet, as the number of genes identified through genome initiatives increases, the candidate gene approach is expected to become more useful as a parallel approach to the positional cloning strategy. In this scheme, functional gene mapping within a reduced chromosomal interval surrounding a QTL may be tested for association with the complex trait under study (*25–29*).

The existence of a large variety of inbred stocks in mouse, the abundance of genetic markers, the well-documented phenotypic variation between strains and its relatively easy manipulation make the mouse model most valuable for the analysis of complex traits (*30,31*). The importance and utility of the mouse for QTL analysis (*32,33*) as well as its physiological resemblance to other mammals (including humans) make it worthwhile to investigate mouse models of human behavior.

1.3. The Various Stages of QTL Analysis

It is important to note that QTL analysis is a multistage procedure and that different approaches are required at different stages of the process. Each of these stages presents its distinct refinements. In this chapter, we shall only briefly review the first two stages of QTL detection and mapping (analytical methods for these are covered in detail in Chapter 7). We will give particular attention in this chapter to the third stage: fine mapping.

1.3.1. Stage I: QTL Detection

The first stage, QTL detection, tests the hypothesis that a marker or a set of markers is linked to the QTL. A genomewide scan utilizing anonymous markers is the common strategy. Genetic analysis is carried out on a large experimental population segregating for both DNA markers and alleles of the QTL, so that marker(s) associated with the trait will indicate the existence of a QTL by detecting it on a specific chromosome.

1.3.2. Stage II: QTL Mapping

The second stage, commonly done with the same data, estimates the position of the QTL on the chromosome where the QTL was detected (estimation of map location). This procedure is conceptually different, involving parameter estimation (as opposed to hypothesis testing for the first stage). Unless the number of animals in the cross is very large or unless special efforts have been made to increase recombination frequency in the study population, the second stage usually provides only limited information as to the position of the gene (*34*).

1.3.3. Stage III: Fine Mapping

A third stage, fine mapping, is thus required in order to precisely position the gene to a limited chromosomal interval. At this stage of fine mapping, single QTLs are considered, rather than the genomewide analysis carried out for the first two stages. Various strategies and specialized segregating populations have been developed for efficient fine mapping (*35*) and are presented next.

1.3.4. Stage IV: Gene Cloning

The fourth stage in QTL mapping is the actual cloning of the genes. This stage involves the identification of the polymorphism(s) that determine the phenotypic variation. When the region containing the QTL is significantly reduced so that it includes few genes, those can be examined for polymorphisms. Knockout mice may provide additional evidence for the functionality of the gene, and, eventually, transgenic mice, in which the alternative phenotype is rescued, can provide ultimate proof that the gene responsible for the quantitative phenotype has indeed been identified. The details of this stage are beyond the scope of this chapter.

2. Methods

2.1. Evidence of Genetic Variation

When considering a genetic study, one must first inspect whether there is a significant genetic contribution to the relevant phenotype. A principal source of evidence that genes contribute to variation in a trait is found in studies showing, for example, significant behavioral variation, or distinct phenotypes, between genetically distinct inbred strains. The description of existing data on behavior genetics of rodents can be found elsewhere (e.g., **refs. *36*** and ***37***).

A comparison of several strains can be undertaken if no evidence is available regarding the phenotype of interest. Sampling strains with different genetic origins optimizes the chances of uncovering the genetic contribution to variation in a phenotype. Genetic comparisons of stocks of the laboratory mouse and rat show that there is ample diversity among existing laboratory stocks. Consequently, one may reasonably expect to find evidence of a genetic component if it exists (*see* **Note 1**).

2.2. QTL Mapping (Stages I and II)

Initial detection of a QTL involves genetic mapping in a two-generation cross (an intercross [F2] or a backcross [BC]. The process includes phenotyping

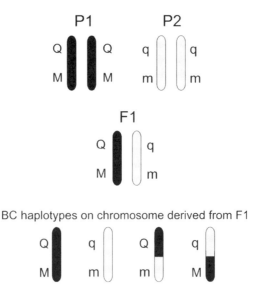

Fig. 1. QTL and marker segregation in a backcross design. Parents P1 and P2 differ at both QTL and marker alleles. Only the segregant chromosome is shown in the backcross generation.

the progeny of the cross of interest, followed by genotyping them for the markers and the use of linkage analysis to detect and map the QTL. This process is outlined briefly here and described in more detail in Chapter 7.

For simplicity we shall describe the general rationale for QTL detection in a BC population, where only two genotypes are present for each locus (*see* **Fig. 1**). It is assumed that parents from two inbred lines are crossed to produce an F1: parent 1 having MM and QQ genotypes at a marker and a linked QTL, respectively, and parent 2 having an mm and qq genotype at the same loci. All of the F1 offspring will have Mm and Qq genotypes. The segregating BC population is obtained by crossing the F1 to the recessive parental strain. The BC will always carry an m and q allele on one chromosome. Four possible haplotypes (M-Q, m-q, m-Q, and M-q) will segregate on the other chromosome, with expected frequencies of respectively $(1-r)/2$, $(1-r)/2$, $r/2$ and $r/2$, where r is the recombination fraction between the marker and the QTL. The simplest analysis takes the form of a t-test to determine whether the group of individuals with the M allele differ significantly in their trait value from the group of individuals with the m allele (see Chapter 7, Subheading 2.1.1.). Equivalently, if a particular marker allele is found to occur at a statistically higher frequency in high- (or low-) scoring individuals, it can be inferred that a nearby gene affects the trait. The above theoretical aspects of QTL detection have been presented by Soller et al. (*38*). This approach has subsequently been improved and refined, and the more complex likelihood methods allowing QTL localization are now routinely used (*see* Chapter 7, Subheading 2.). Interval mapping, based on the examination of a pair of markers and application of maximum likelihood techniques to test for significance, was introduced by Lander and Botstein (*39,40*), with subsequent variations (*41–45*). Attempts to improve the cost-effectiveness of the procedure led to the development of additional strategies (*see* **Note 2**). When looking at multiple correlated traits, power can be increased by controlling the residual variance (*46,47*). The sample size can be reduced by selective genotyping of the phenotypic extremes, which carry most of the statistical power for QTL detection (*40,48,49*). Consistent savings may be achieved by selective DNA pooling (*50*) of the phenotypic extremes, followed by allele frequency estimation in the pools. In addition, an alternative way to increase efficiency has been suggested through sequential sampling (*51*) and recurrent testing, until significance is reached. Finally, optimum marker spacing (*52*) improves the cost-effectiveness of an initial screen by appropriately choosing markers, usually two markers per chromosome.

2.3. Strategies for QTL Fine Mapping (Stage III)

Standard QTL mapping will usually locate genes to a relatively large chromosomal interval (10–50 cM). Fine mapping involves examination of individual QTLs, rather than the genomewide paradigm used for QTL detection. Typically, a QTL that has been previously detected and preferably confirmed is selected for further analysis. In order to define a restricted location for a QTL, greater accuracy and greater confidence are required. Chromosome partition, via recombination, was first introduced by *Drosophila* geneticists (*53–55*). With the advent of DNA-level polymorphisms, these methods were pioneered with great success by researchers using the tomato as the model organism (*22,24,56*). A number of adaptations to rodents have also been suggested (*57–59*). Various fine-mapping strategies are presented next, based on the recombination-defined-interval methodology and involving the thorough genetic analysis of a restricted interval.

2.3.1. Selective Phenotyping

This strategy may be especially attractive to neuroscientists who are involved in measurements of phenotypes such as electrophysiological recordings, which are arduous and time-consuming. A large F2 or BC population is produced and only individuals recombinant at an interval previously defined to contain a QTL are selected for phenotyping. This strategy is based on the rationale that once a gene is mapped to a given interval, only recombinant individuals within that interval contribute to further mapping accuracy. Genotyping is made possible by extracting DNA from tissues such as tail tips, thus allowing an early detection of the recombinants to be phenotyped.

2.3.2. Recombinant Progeny Testing

Individuals from BC or F2 populations carrying a distinguishable recombinant chromosome at the region of interest are crossed to one of the parental strains to determine the location of the QTL relative to the recombination point. A sample N_S of F2 animals is subsequently screened, according to the desired chromosomal interval reduction, for example from y to x cM (this is discussed in **Subheading 3.3.2.**).

2.3.3. Generation of Interval-Specific Congenic Strains (ISCS)

Similar to recombinant progeny testing, a sample N_S of BC or F2 individuals are genotyped to detect y/x recombinant individuals (where y is the original interval and x is the desired interval), with recombination equally distributed within the y-cM interval. These animals, however, are now backcrossed a number of times to one parental strain (the background strain) to eliminate alleles from the other (donor) parental strain at all other QTLs affecting the trait. Then, animals are intercrossed and homozygotes for the recombinant haplotype are selected to establish one interval-specific congenic strain (ISCS).

Selection at the DNA level is done with the aid of markers, reducing significantly the number of generations required with little additional genotyping (*57*). The resulting ISCSs are pure lines, each retaining a short (approx 1 cM) chromosomal fragment from the donor strain. Because all of the residual genetic variance has been eliminated through the intensive backcrossing process, they result in the approximation of the QTL to a monogenic trait. Phenotyping y/x selected ISCS will assign the QTL to the relevant fragment. As many individuals as required may be phenotyped from the same ISCS, thus allowing control of the environmental variance (*see* **Note 3**).

2.3.4. Recombinant Inbred Segregation Test

The recombinant inbred segregation test (RIST) takes advantage of the theoretical high mapping resolution present in recombinant inbred (RI) strains (*see* **Subheading 2.4.1.** and **Fig. 2**), applied to QTL mapping (*35*). To reduce the QTL-containing interval from y cM to x cM, y/x RI strains are selected with recombinations equally distributed within the y-cM interval. The RIST population (**Fig. 2**) is constructed by crossing the chosen RI, separately to each of the parent strains, P1 and P2, to produce either two distinct F2 (RIST-F2) or, if preferred, two distinct BC (RIST-BC) populations. The F2 or BC populations are phenotyped and genotyped with few markers. The $F2_l$ or BC_l population is genotyped with markers located in the region where P2 alleles

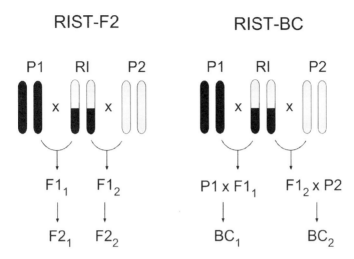

Fig. 2. Producing RIST populations. P1 and P2 are two inbred strains and were crossed to generate the RI strains. A selected RI strain with a recombinant haplotype in the region of interest is crossed with both parental strains to produce two separate F1 populations, F1₁ and F1₂. Subsequently, RIST-F2 and RIST-BC populations are obtained through intercross and backcross, respectively.

are present in the selected RI strain, and the $F2_2$ or BC_2 is genotyped with markers located in the region where P1 alleles are present in the selected RI strain. Because the QTL has been previously mapped in this region, it will necessarily segregate in one of the F2 or BC populations but not in the other. This will define whether the QTL is to one side or the other, relative to a recombination point in one RI strain. By overlapping regions by the use of several RI strains, the QTL can be accurately located.

2.4. Existing Mapping Resources

Although QTL detection is often effectively achieved on BC or F2 populations, this genetic scheme requires generating the appropriate population, a time-consuming process. An alternative to the BC or F2 scheme resides in using existing mapping populations. Although they may not be the theoretically optimum populations, they definitely have the advantage of being ready to use and may not require the lengthy generation procedure. In the following, we discuss the major types of resources available.

2.4.1. Recombinant inbred strains

The RI strains are one of the oldest resources available. They are established pure lines, originally proposed by Bailey (*60*) and developed as a major mapping resource by Taylor (*61*). Each strain was derived from an intercross of two genetically distinct strains, followed by inbreeding of the F2 progeny, to obtain a new pure line, with an approximately 1 : 1 ratio of the original breeds genetic material, and defined recombination points. RI strains have usually been typed on a large number of markers, such that in most events, no further genotyping will be required. Although there is no limitation to the trait being tested on existing strains, in most instances the size of the QTL effects will be unknown and, therefore, the efficiency of RI strains for this purpose will be difficult to estimate *a priori*. (*see* **note 4**). For a comprehensive list of existing mouse RI strains and the status to which they have been genotyped, refer to www.jax.org. The use of this resource is further discussed in **Subheading 3.4.1.**

2.4.2. Chromosome Substitution Strains

Chromosome substitution strains (CSS or consomics) result from introgressing individual chromosomes from a donor to a host strain, by recurrent backcrossing. They have been broadly used to examine the role of the Y chromosome in biobehavioral processes (*62,63*). More recently, in an attempt to develop a set of CSS to encompass the entire genome, Nadeau (*64*) has backcrossed individual A/J chromosomes to the C57BL/6J background by selection for appropriate microsatellite markers. Consomics can only locate the QTL to a specific chromosome. Therefore, they are excellent for QTL detection, but without additional crosses they have no use for fine mapping of QTLs.

2.4.3. Advanced intercross lines

Advanced intercross (AI) lines were proposed as a means of systematically increasing the density of recombination events to facilitate mapping (*65*). AI lines (**Fig. 3**) are produced by intercrossing two parental strains to produce a standard F2 generation. Starting with the F2, animals are semirandomly intercrossed to produce successive generations while systematically avoiding matings between relatives. A parental population of 50 males and 50 females is maintained in each generation to minimize inbreeding. Each generation accumulates recombination at a rate of $r_t=[1-(1-r)^{t-2}(1-2r)]/2$, where r_t is the proportion of recombinants at the tth generation and r is the initial proportion of recombination. When employed for the estimation of map location, AI lines improve accuracy by reducing the confidence interval (*see* **Subheading 3.2.2.**). More importantly, however, they constitute a highly effective tool for fine mapping.

2.4.4. Heterogeneous Stocks

In addition to bilineally derived AI stocks, stocks of mice and rats were derived by systematic crossing of many inbred strains and are being maintained on a semirandom basis for many generations. McClearn et al. (*66*) systematically intercrossed 8 inbred mouse strains to produce a heterogeneous stock (HS) that

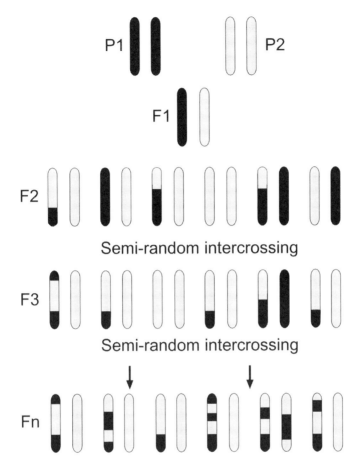

Fig. 3. Production of an advanced intercross line (AIL). Two parental strains (P1 and P2) are crossed to produce an F1, then intercrossed to produce a standard F2. Subsequently, each generation is semirandomly intercrossed within itself, from F3 to Fn (see text).

has now accumulated approximately 60 generations of intercrossing and a dense pattern of recombinations. A similar stock of rats has been developed by Dr. Carl Hansen at the National Institutes of Health. Like the mouse HS stock, it has been systematically intercrossed for many generations and can be expected to greatly facilitate fine mapping.

2.4.5. Recombinant congenic strains

Recombinant congenic strains (RCS) are derived by inbreeding strains after performing several independent backcrosses from a donor to a host strain (*67,68*). Existing RCS each carry from between 6.25% and 12.5% of donor genome alleles at random and sets of RCS strains are designed to sample 95% of the donor-strain genome. Following identification of phenotypic differences in the relevant trait between the two progenitor strains, RCS studies usually continue with a comparison of an RCS set with the host strain. Discovery of a significant difference between host and individual RCS indicate the existence of a QTL(s) residing on one or more of the donor chromosomal regions that have been fixed within that particular RCS strain. Because RCS are based on short chromosomal fragments from the donor strain, they may also provide some degree of usefulness for fine mapping.

2.4.6. Congenics

Congenic strains have been developed by repeated backcrossing from a donor to a host strain accompanied by selection for histocompatibility variants (*69,70*). Each congenic strain retains a single chromosomal segment from the donor strain. The length of the transferred segment varies with the number of backcross generations. At 10 generations, the segment is expected to be, on average, 20 cM in length (*71*). Some existing congenic strains have been partially defined by microsatellite polymorphism typing (*72*).

Bailey (*73,74*) calculated that the chromosomal inserts carried along with the selected variants in the C57BL/6By/Balbc/By bilineal congenic series would sweep approximately one-third of the genome and suggested that they had general applicability for mapping of a variety of traits, including behavior, and illustrated their use in a study of the mandible morphology (*75*).

3. Interpretation

3.1. Genetic Variation

Choosing strains for study on the basis of their polymorphism rate has the practical advantage of providing access to ample numbers of polymorphic markers. This can be particularly important at the fine-mapping stage, when the number of markers within a particular chromosomal region may be restricted. The polymorphic rates between *Mus castaneus*, *Mus spretus*, and the other mouse inbred strains are in excess of 90%, according to microsatellite typing by Dietrich et al. (*76*). This degree of diversity can also be exploited during the fine-mapping stage.

In the rat, typing of more than 5000 microsatellite polymorphisms in 48 inbred rat strains has been initiated by Jacob et al. (*77*) and further refined by Brown et al. (*78*). Polymorphism rates between pairs of strains can be accessed at http://waldo.wi.mit.edu/rat/public/. As shown there, polymorphism between strains is high, usually above 50%, reaching 82% in a few cases (e.g., SHRSP × BN/SSN. A few strains, however, show a poor polymorphism rate, as seen for BB(DP) × BB(DR), with only 18% polymorphism between the strains.

Although one cannot assume a one-to-one relationship between microsatellite polymorphism rates and variation in genes, judicious selection of strains of rats or mice using the interstrain polymorphism rate as criterion would likely provide a sample with an excellent degree of heterogeneity.

3.2. QTL Mapping (Stages I and II)

3.2.1. Power

Larger sample sizes and larger QTL effect increase power for detection as well as mapping accuracy. When considering F2 versus BC for QTL detection, it is important to define the precise purposes of the research. F2 will generally be more efficient for a primary estimation of the number of QTL segregating in the population, as well as their additive or dominance effects. A BC will be preferred, however, for an efficient detection of the major QTLs. The advantage of BC resides in the relatively higher gene effect than for an F2, as a result of the reduction in residual genetic variance (*79,80*). Genetic variance caused by gene interactions is also expected to be reduced, making the BC design even more powerful (*81*). The power variation between the alternative schemes is best summarized by the size of the mapping population in each case. For additive effects, an F2 requires about 30% less progeny than BC. For dominance effects, however, a BC requires about half of an F2 population.

For most practical cases, RI strains will be less powerful than BC or F2. If, however, a QTL explains a significant proportion of the genetic variation and the genetic variation itself is small compared to trait variation, RI strains can be considerably more efficient than BC or F2 (*82*).

3.2.2. Confidence Intervals

Following QTL detection, estimation of map location is carried out, usually on the same population, applying specific software for the interval mapping procedure or one of its variations. Interval mapping assigns a LOD score to the presence of the QTL at specific points across the genome. The point estimate for the QTL is the location with the highest LOD score value.

The most important parameter for evaluating QTL strategies in this stage is mapping accuracy. A number of methods have been suggested to estimate QTL mapping accuracy (*34,40,83,84*). In statistics, the concept of a 95% confidence interval (CI) for parameter estimates is used to describe the range of values, which has a 95% probability of containing the true value for that parameter. Lander and Botstein (*40*) suggested an equivalent approximation to the confidence interval in QTL mapping, defined by the points on either side of the QTL peak where the LOD score was one LOD score lower than at the peak (usually called the 1-LOD support interval). A 2-LOD score support interval was later found to be more appropriate in representing a 95% CI (*85*). The confidence interval of QTL map location can also be estimated using an empirical formula (*83*). The general expression for CI has the form $k/(Nd^2)$, where k is a constant that depends on the design and level of confidence, N is sample size, and d is the standardized gene effect. This equation was developed under an assumption of a dense genetic map, but it is also a close approximation to situations where marker spacing is up to half the CI itself. For QTL with additive effect, F2 will allow an increased mapping accuracy, whereas BC is preferred for dominance effects. Recombination is the main variable that affects stages I and II differently. For QTL detection, less recombination is desired to reduce the total amount of markers required for the genome scan, because markers will still be linked to the QTL even when they are at a considerable distance away. Conversely, for mapping accuracy, a greater density of recombination events improves mapping resolution by reducing the confidence interval; only markers that are closely linked to a QTL will detect an effect, and, therefore, a smaller interval will be defined. RI strains are produced by a large number of intercrosses, thus increasing the number of recombination events, leading to a reduction in the CI of up to fourfold.

3.3. Issues Regarding QTL Fine Mapping (Stage III)

In this process, the mapping interval is reduced to a minimum, in order to facilitate physical/molecular access to the chromosomal region to which the QTL is mapped. Reducing the mapping interval is essential for positional cloning of the gene of interest (stage IV) and is usually achieved through recombinant analysis. N individuals are analyzed for each recombinant haplotype, to determine the QTL allelic state (i.e., whether a specific recombinant haplotype retained an increasing/decreasing allele affecting the quantitative trait in question). Throughout this process, the smallest common region will eventually be determined by two recombinant haplotypes only. The QTL will be located between two recombination points, defined by the recombinant haplotypes. With an estimate of gene effect, two symmetrical hypotheses are tested, representing the two alternative states of the QTL alleles. The number of progeny that needs to be tested varies according to the chosen strategy, the QTL effect size, and its dominant state (*35*). These parameters, as well as the required target accuracy, availability of RI strains, time, and money constraints, will determine which fine-mapping strategy to use. In the following, we discuss several aspects of the various strategies.

3.3.1. Selective Phenotyping

Any number of recombinants phenotyped will reduce the width of the QTL-containing interval, and, subsequently, a smaller interval can be considered to search for new recombinants. For practical reasons, however, probably not more than two steps will be applied. At each stage of selective phenotyping, the total number of animals phenotyped is reduced by a factor of $1/2r(1-r)$ for an F2 population and by $1/r$ for a BC population (r being the proportion of recombination between the markers bracketing the interval in question). With selective phenotyping, savings are in phenotyping only, total number of animals produced being equal to that necessary with an F2 or a BC. This number increases rapidly as the CI decreases. Therefore, selective phenotyping is fast, but not very efficient. It will be most appropriate for mapping QTL with large effects, although the target resolution is rather low, not below approx 5 cM.

3.3.2. Recombinant Progeny Testing

Reducing the confidence interval from y cM to x cM will require y/x recombinant individuals, each with a recombination at one of the y/x intervals covering the initial y-cM interval. The number of F2 animals that need to be screened to detect these recombinants increases for shorter target intervals. Recombinant progeny testing requires only one additional generation compared to selective phenotyping (which usually requires two). It is also more efficient, especially for QTLs with a dominant effect, for a target interval as short as 1 cM.

3.3.3. Interval-Specific Congenic Strains

In this design, a series of strains, each containing a short fragment from the donor strain, is used; thus, the tested population is nonsegregating, as opposed to other types of mapping population. In such nonsegregating population, the QTL effect may be confused, through fixation of residual genetic loci or interaction effects (such as maternal effects), which are extraneous to the tested QTL. To avoid this risk, one can detect linkage on a small segregating population produced by crossing the ISCS to the background parental strains. Alternatively, ISCS can be applied on a single congenic strain, produced for the relevant region. ISCS require a significant number of generations to produce. Because of their genetic design, they cannot take advantage of dominant effects. They are, however, particularly suited for the analysis of QTLs with moderate or small effect, and they require a limited number of progeny, and very few genotyped samples, to achieve a short target interval of 1 cM.

3.3.4. Recombinant Inbred Segregation Test

The analysis of the two populations will locate the QTL above or below the recombination point in the segregating population (**Fig. 2**). The overlapping results of all selected RI strains will locate the QTL to the desired interval. For additive effects RIST-F2 is preferred, in which case, homozygotes at the marker locus will contribute most of the information. Thus, only homozygous individuals will be selected for phenotyping. When a dominant effect is considered, RIST-BC will be more efficient. Using the RIST strategy is both cost-

effective and fast: The phenotyping is drastically reduced and only two genera-
tions are required. Its application is limited only by the availability of appropriate
RI strains. It is expected, however, that for a target interval of 1 cM, appropriate
RI strains will be found for 50% of chromosomal regions, when a set of 25
RI strains is available.

3.4. Existing Mapping Resources in the Context of QTL Analysis
3.4.1. RI Strains

Recombinant inbred strains can be used for QTL detection, mapping, and
fine mapping through the RIST design. The greatest advantage of RI strains
is, indeed, for fine mapping. During their generation, a large amount of recombination has been established in a segregating population based on two original
genomes. Because recombination is the source of mapping accuracy, this ready-
made population is an efficient mapping tool. Although not optimal for QTL
detection, it should not be overlooked. When QTLs under study explain a
significant portion of the genetic variation and particularly when the entire
genetic variation is relatively low, RI strains present an excellent resource for
QTL detection. In such an instance, environmental variations can be controlled
by phenotyping several individuals from each RI strain.

3.4.2. Chromosome Substitution Strains

A CSS differs from its parental strain by one entire chromosome. Therefore,
a set of CSS, each with a different introgressed chromosome, represents an
excellent tool for QTL detection. Simply phenotyping few individuals from
each CSS will detect QTL(s) to specific chromosomes whenever a significant
phenotypic difference appears between the CSS and its parental strain. The
CSS itself does not provide any information as to the location of the gene; it
only detects its presence in a specific chromosome. Nevertheless, CSS are an
excellent starting point to further fine-map the gene to a small region through
the generation of specific congenics.

3.4.3. Advanced Intercross

The AI approach may be especially appropriate in the presence of a genetic
architecture characterized by many genes, each with a small effect size. The
presence of a QTL with large effect size may interfere with precise localization
of small-effect QTL(s) on other chromosomes, unless the position of the former
is defined with enough precision to permit appropriate statistical adjustment.
Use of a single generation in the AI approach also has the practical advantage
of saving time compared to the multiple-generation breeding required for the
various recombination-defined-interval approaches.

3.4.4. Heterogeneous Stock

The use of HS allows the simultaneous mapping of many QTLs at a high level of resolution (1 cM and less), for QTL with small effect sizes. Because mouse HS strains include alleles from commonly used inbred strains, they can be used to refine the localization of many QTLs involved in behavioral traits. The HS is similar to the AI with the difference that eight parental strains originated the cross and that it has been kept heterogeneous for a very large number of generations, and, therefore, it may allow increased mapping accuracy.

3.4.5. Recombinant Congenic Strains

The RCS present a reduction of variation as compared to the parental strain. A series of RCS will include the entire range of variation but scattered over a number of strains. In many instances, this is not an efficient mapping tool. When available, it can, however, be exploited for a phenotype study, where this scheme may uncover potential interaction between genes.

3.4.6. Congenics

Congenics are time-consuming to produce. However, once existent, they provide an important resource. An observed phenotypical difference between congenics and their parental background genome permits the localization of a QTL to a well-defined small interval. Additionally, because as many animals as required can be obtained from the same congenic strain, they allow for a thorough examination of the QTL-dependent phenotype.

3.5. Application to Human QTL Mapping

The main contribution of mouse QTL mapping results to human genetics is expected to be achieved through comparative genomics. Model organisms have long been recognized as an outstanding useful tool for the study of human complex traits and diseases. Their strength in genetic studies resides in the short generation time, the wealth of well-defined inbred lines, and the genetic schemes applicable for genetic dissection, as described in the present chapter. The crosses between inbred lines, along with powerful genetic analysis, allow the detection of much subtler effects for minor QTLs than is possible in outbred human populations.

With the parallel development of the Human Genome Project and model organism genetic mapping, we are reaching a stage where homologous chromosomal intervals can be precisely assigned, from species to species (*86*). This is particularly true for the mouse, where a very dense marker map is already available, including a YAC-based map with an average marker spacing of 224 kb on chromosome X (*87*). Comparative genomics allows the precise localization, on the human genome, of genes initially mapped in the mouse. This, in turn, may lead to mutational analysis of the gene in human populations.

Table 1
Software for QTL Analysis

Name	URL
Mapmaker/QTL 3.0	ftp://genome.wi.mit.edu/pub/mapmaker3
QTL Cartographer 1.12	http://statgen.ncsu.edu/qtlcart/cartographer.html
Map Manager QT b28	http://mcbio.med.buffalo.edu/mapmgr.html
QGene™ 2.30	qgene@clarityconnect.com
MapQTL™ 3.0	http://www.cpro.dlo.nl/cbw/
PLABQTL 1.0	http://www.unhohenheim.de/~ipspwww/soft.html
MQTL 0.98	ftp://gnome.agrenv.mcgill.ca/pub/genetics/software/MQTL/
Multimapper	http://www.RNI.Helsinki.FI/~mjs/
MultiQTL	http://www.multiqtl.com/
The QTL Café	http://web.bham.ac.uk/g.g.seaton/
Epistat	http://www.larklab.4biz.net/epistat.htm

Following positional cloning, assessment of the role of a particular gene in the studied complex trait may be strengthened by genetic manipulation, such as the generation of transgenic mice and knockout mice. These allow the realization of thorough functional analysis, a crucial step to the unraveling of physiological mechanisms.

4. Software

There exists a large variety of software, developed for the specific purpose of QTL mapping. An exhaustive list of the available software can be found at http://www.stat.wisc.edu/biosci/linkage.html. Manly and Olson (**88**) presented an excellent overview of existing software for QTL mapping and we encourage the reader to examine that work when choosing software. **Table 1** presents a list of some of the major programs and the websites where they can be downloaded. Additional software resources are given in Table 1 in Chapter 7.

5. Examples from the Literature

In this section, we briefly describe a sample of published studies that illustrate several experimental strategies in QTL analysis. We have focused to some extent on examples related to behavioral phenotypes, but also other complex phenotypes are presented where the experimental strategy may be of interest. This sample, obviously, does not include the entire work done on QTL analysis nor does it necessarily represent the most important studies.

5.1. Selective Genotyping

Flint et al. (**11**) used *selective genotyping* on an F2 population for the identification of QTLs affecting emotionality in mice. They took advantage of existing inbred lines, known to differ in their emotionality. Their first screening was based on one emotionality test (Open-Field Activity, OFA), and they further examined the detected QTLs for their possible effect on additional emotionality criteria. Out of the six initially detected QTLs, three were found to affect all emotionality tests and seem to account for all or the major part of the genetic component of the trait.

Gershenfeld and Paul (*89*) carried out a similar study for fearlike behavior QTLs and simultaneously measured two phenotypic criteria. From their F2 screening, they detected distinct QTLs for the different phenotypic criteria and were able to locate several QTLs, each with a moderate effect, explaining 2.3–8.4% of the phenotypic variance.

5.2. Backcross Populations

Melo et al. (*13*) exploited the advantages of BC populations to identify QTLs for sex-specific alcohol preference. They conducted a two-way backcross between B6, known as an alcohol-preferring strain, and DBA/J2, a recognized avoider strain. Selective genotyping of the phenotypic extremes led to the definition of five unlinked chromosomal regions involved in alcohol preference. These regions were further examined on the whole populations and this led to the assessment of one male-specific QTL and one female-specific QTL, affecting alcohol preference. Both QTLs have a strong effect, with 22.5% and 23% of the total genetic variance for male and female, respectively. It should be noted that a previous attempt to identify QTLs involved in alcohol preference had been made, using RI strains of the same origins, and failed to reach significance. This is expected because of the low power that RI strains provide for QTL detection.

5.3. Selective DNA Pooling

Collin et al. (*90*) took advantage of a modifier, known to enhance the susceptibility to germ-cell tumors, and applied the efficient *selective DNA pooling* strategy on a backcross population segregating for tumorigenesis factors. The pooling enabled a differential screening of unilateral versus bilateral tumors. The screening, using an average marker spacing of approx 9 cM, uncovered three candidate QTLs. The authors calculated that by using the DNA pooling approach they achieved a 7.2-fold reduction in genotyping.

5.4. Congenic Strains for Chromosomal Localization

Frankel et al. (*12*) constructed *congenic strains* for the study of epilepsy and were able to differentiate between the E12 locus and other QTLs. The use of congenics allowed for the chromosomal localization of E12 to chromosome 2, where a few functional candidate genes are known to reside.

5.5. Chromosome Substitution Strains

Matin et al. (*91*) produced a 129.MOLF-Chr19 *CSS* (chromosome 19 from the MOLF strain, substituted in the 129 strain). They used this *CSS* to investigate the tumorigenic effect of MOLF chromosome 19 on the 129 background, as detected in their previous study. This *CSS* was further intercrossed with the 129 parent, as well as with the MOLF parent. Both F2's were examined for tumor incidence, and a marked effect was found for the MOLF-Chr 19, on 129 background only. Segregation analysis of the 129 × CSS F2 also allowed for the localization of the tumorigenic effect to proximal chromosome 19.

5.6. Heterogeneous Stock

Talbot et al. (*92*), in search for a higher-resolution mapping for behavioral traits, used a *selective genotyping* approach on the *heterogeneous stock* (HS) of mice. Their study focused on QTLs previously identified by Flint et al. (*11*) and located on chromosome 1. With the *HS*, they could reduce the CI to 1.2 cM. Using the same population, they could also identify a QTL on chromosome 12, thus demonstrating the possibility of simultaneously mapping multiple QTL, using the heterogeneous stock.

5.7. Advanced Intercross

Iraqi et al. (*93*) described the construction of two trypanosomiasis susceptibility *AI lines*, issued from one resistant strain, crossed with two alternative sensitive strains. Genetic analysis of the segregating populations was performed by selective genotyping. Using this approach, they reduced the CI by 2.5- to 15-fold, for three resistance QTL that had previously been mapped, each to a 10- to 50-cM interval. Moreover, because of the high recombination level present in the AIL, one QTL on chromosome 1 could now been shown to consist of three independent loci. Another QTL was mapped to a 0.9-cM interval, a degree of resolution allowing positional cloning.

5.8. Congenic Strains for Fine Mapping

Encinas et al. (*94*) took advantage of *congenic strains* of mice, previously established for the analysis of diabetes on chromosome 3, to examine QTL effect on experimental autoimmune encephalomyelitis (EAE). Using this strategy, they were able to identify a 1.5-cM region, affecting EAE, and including the Iddm2 diabetes locus.

5.9. Transgenic mice

A recent study, by Symula et al. (*95*), described the use of YAC-transgenic mice to study factors altering an asthma QTL. Using a panel of transgenic mice, they were able to demonstrate a transgene-effected modulation of the mouse immune response.

6. Notes

1. Evidence of a genetic component. It is advisable, when probing genetic variation of a trait, to carry out a small-scale cross between phenotypically different strains and examine trait segregation in the F2. Alternatively, recombinant inbred lines may also be valuable for this purpose. When the genetic variation between the strains is demonstrated to occur and segregate, then proceed with genetic dissection of the trait.
2. Cost-effectiveness. Cost-effectiveness is controlled mainly in two different ways: (1) by limiting the genotyping cost (e.g., the number of genotyping test that are to be carried out and (2) by reducing the cost of establishing and maintaining a specialized mapping population (either by using an existing population or by reducing the generation × individual effective number).
3. Environmental variance. When phenotyping for a complex trait, it is necessary to keep in mind the possible environmental contribution to the phenotype. In this aspect, ISCS are of considerable advantage, as they represent established, genetically simplified, pure strains. Phenotyping a number of individuals for each genotype permits to minimize the error resulting from environmental variance.
4. Limitations of RI strains. The RI strains are of advantage for the localization and detection of QTLs with large effects. In most cases, however, the small number of RI strains available will not allow the required statistical power to be attained.

Acknowledgments

The authors thank Dr. Meira Sternfeld for critical reading of the manuscript. Ariel Darvasi was supported by the FIRST foundation of the Israel Academy of Sciences.

References

1. Gelderman, H. (1975) Investigations on inheritance of quantitative characters in animals by gene markers. I. Methods. *Theor. Appl. Genet.* **46,** 319–330.
2. Hu, S., Pattatucci, A. M., Patterson, C., Li, L., Fulker, D. W., Cherny, S. S., et al. (1995) Linkage between sexual orientation and chromosome Xq28 in males but not in females. *Nature Genet.* **11(3),** 248–256.
3. Satsangi, J., Parkes, M., Louis, E., Hashimoto, L., Kato, N., Welsh, K., et al. (1996) Two stage genome-wide search in inflammatory bowel disease provides evidence for susceptibility loci on chromosomes 3, 7 and 12. *Nature Genet.* **14(2),** 199–202.
4. Hanis, C. L., Boerwinkle, E., Chakraborty, R., Ellsworth, D. L., Concannon, P., Stirling, B., et al. (1996) A genome-wide search for human non-insulin-dependent (type 2) diabetes genes reveals a major susceptibility locus on chromosome 2 [see comments]. *Nature Genet.* **13(2),** 161–166.

5. Mahtani, M. M., Widen, E., Lehto, M., Thomas, J., McCarthy, M., Brayer, J., et al. (1996) Mapping of a gene for type 2 diabetes associated with an insulin secretion defect by a genome scan in Finnish families [see comments]. *Nature Genet.* **14(1),** 90–94.

6. Ginns, E. I., Ott, J., Egeland, J. A., Allen, C. R., Fann, C. S., Pauls, D. L., et al. (1996) A genome-wide search for chromosomal loci linked to bipolar affective disorder in the Old Order Amish. *Nature Genet.* **12(4),** 431–435.

7. Hugot, J. P., Laurent-Puig, P., Gower-Rousseau, C., Olson, J. M., Lee, J. C., Beaugerie, L., et al. (1996) Mapping of a susceptibility locus for Crohn's disease on chromosome 16 [see comments]. *Nature* **379(6568),** 821–823.

8. Sawcer, S., Jones, H. B., Feakes, R., Gray, J., Smaldon, N., Chataway, J., et al. (1996) A genome screen in multiple sclerosis reveals susceptibility loci on chromosome 6p21 and 17q22 [see comments]. *Nature Genet.* **13(4),** 464–468.

9. Ebers, G. C., Kukay, K., Bulman, D. E., Sadovnick, A. D., Rice, G., Anderson, C., et al. (1996) A full genome search in multiple sclerosis [see comments]. *Nature Genet.* **13(4),** 472–476.

10. Daniels, S. E., Bhattacharrya, S., James, A., Leaves, N. I., Young, A., Hill, M. R., et al. (1996) A genome-wide search for quantitative trait loci underlying asthma. *Nature* **383(6597),** 247–250.

11. Flint, J., Corley, R., DeFries, J. C., Fulker, D. W., Gray, J. A., Miller, S., et al. (1995) A simple genetic basis for a complex psychological trait in laboratory mice. *Science* **269(5229),** 1432–1435.

12. Frankel, W. N., Johnson, E. W., and Lutz, C. M. (1995) Congenic strains reveal effects of the epilepsy quantitative trait locus, El2, separate from other El loci. *Mammal Genome* **6(12,)** 839–843.

13. Melo, J. A., Shendure, J., Pociask, K., and Silver, L. M. (1996) Identification of sex-specific quantitative loci controlling alcohol preference in C57BL/ 6 mice [see comments]. *Nature Genet.* **13(2),** 147–153.

14. Berrettini, W. H., Ferraro, T. N., Alexander, R. C., Buchberg, A. M., and Vogel, W. H. (1994) Quantitative trait loci mapping of three loci controlling morphine preference using inbred mouse strains [see comments]. *Nature Genet.* **7(1),** 54–58.

15. Moen, C. J., Groot, P. C., Hart, A. A., Snoek, M., and Demant, P. (1996) Fine mapping of colon tumor susceptibility (Scc) genes in the mouse, different from the genes known to be somatically mutated in colon cancer. *Proc. Natl. Acad. Sci. USA* **93(3),** 1082–1086.

16. Manenti, G., Gariboldi, M., Elango, R., Fiorino, A., De Gregorio, L., Falvella, F. S., et al. (1996) Genetic mapping of a pulmonary adenoma resistance (Par1) in mouse. *Nature Genet.* **12(4),** 455–457.

17. Taylor, B. A. and Phillips, S. J. (1996) Detection of obesity QTLs on mouse chromosomes 1 and 7 by selective DNA pooling. *Genomics* **34(3),** 389–398.

18. Rubattu, S., Volpe, M., Kreutz, R., Ganten, U., Ganten, D., and Lindpaintner, K. (1996) Chromosomal mapping of quantitative trait loci contributing to stroke in a rat model of complex human disease [see comments]. *Nature Genet.* **13(4),** 429–434.

19. Stuber, C. W. (1995) Mapping and manipulating quantitative traits in maize. *Trends Genet.* **11(12)**, 477–481.

20. McCouch, S. R. and Doerge, R. W. (1995) QTL mapping in rice. *Trends Genet.* **11(12)**, 482–487.

21. Haley, C. S. (1995) Livestock QTLs—bringing home the bacon? *Trends Genet.* **11(12)**, 488–492.

22. Alpert, K. B. and Tanskley, S. D. (1996) High-resolution mapping and isolation of a yeast artificial chromosome contig containing fw2.2: a major fruit weight quantitative trait locus in tomato. *Proc. Natl. Acad. Sci. USA* **93,** 15,503–15,507.

23. Cormier, R. T., Bilger, A., Lillich, A. J., Halberg, R. B., Hong, K. H., Gould, K. A., et al. (2000) The Mom1AKR intestinal tumor resistance region consists of Pla2g2a and a locus distal to D4Mit64. *Oncogene* **19(28)**, 3182–3192.

24. Paterson, A. H., DeVerna, J. W., Lanini, B., and Tanksley, S. D. (1990) Fine mapping of quantitative trait loci using selected overlapping recombinant chromosomes, in an interspecies cross of tomato. *Genetics* **124(3)**, 735–742.

25. Rothschild, M., Jacobson, C., Vaske, D., Tuggle, C., Wang, L., Short, T., et al. (1996) The estrogen receptor locus is associated with a major gene influencing litter size in pigs. *Proc. Natl. Acad. Sci. USA* **93(1)**, 201–205.

26. Ebstein, R. P., Novick, O., Umansky, R., Priel, B., Osher, Y., Blaine, D., et al. (1996) Dopamine D4 receptor (D4DR) exon III polymorphism associated with the human personality trait of Novelty Seeking. *Nature Genet.* **12(1)**, 78–80.

27. Benjamin, J., Li, L., Patterson, C., Greenberg, B. D., Murphy, D. L., and Hamer, D. H. (1996) Population and familial association between the D4 dopamine receptor gene and measures of Novelty Seeking. *Nature Genet.* **12(1)**, 81–84.

28. Crabbe, J. C., Phillips, T. J., Feller, D. J., Hen, R., Wenger, C. D., Lessov, C. N., et al. (1996) Elevated alcohol consumption in null mutant mice lacking 5-HT1B serotonin receptors. *Nature Genet.* **14(1)**, 98–101.

29. Konig, M., Zimmer, A. M., Steiner, H., Holmes, P. V., Crawley, J. N., Brownstein, M. J., et al. (1996) Pain responses, anxiety and aggression in mice deficient in pre- proenkephalin. *Nature* **383(6600)**, 535–538.

30. Dietrich, W. F., Copeland, N. G., Gilbert, D. J., Miller, J. C., Jenkins, N. A., and Lander, E. S. (1995) Mapping the mouse genome: current status and future prospects. *Proc. Natl. Acad. Sci. USA* **92(24)**, 10,849–10,853.

31. Frankel, W. N. (1995) Taking stock of complex trait genetics in mice. *Trends Genet.* **11(12)**, 471–477.

32. Flint, J. and Corley, R. (1996) Do animal models have a place in the genetic analysis of quantitative human behavioural traits? *J. Mol. Med.* **74(9)**, 515–521.

33. Georges, M. (1997) QTL mapping to QTL cloning: mice to the rescue. *Genome Res.* **7(7)**, 663–665.

34. Darvasi, A., Weinreb, A., Minke, V., Weller, J. I., and Soller, M. (1993) Detecting marker-QTL linkage and estimating QTL gene effect and map location using a saturated genetic map. *Genetics* **134(3)**, 943–951.

35. Darvasi, A. (1998) Experimental strategies for the genetic dissection of complex traits in animal models. *Nature Genet.* **18(1)**, 19–24.

36. Blizard, D. A. and Darvasi, A. (1999) Experimental strategies for quantitative trait loci (QTL) analysis in laboratory animals, in *Handbook of Molecular–Genetic Techniques for Brain and Behavior Research* (Crusio, W. E. and Gerlai, R. T., eds.) Elsevier, Amsterdam, Vol. 13, pp. 82–99.

37. Crabbe, J. C., Phillips, T. J., Buck, K. J., Cunningham, C. L., and Belknap, J. K. (1999) Identifying genes for alcohol and drug sensitivity: recent progress and future directions. *Trends Neurosci.* **22(4)**, 173–179.

38. Soller, M., Genizi, A., and Brody, T. (1976) On the power of experimental designs for the detection of linkage between marker loci and quantitative loci in crosses between Inbred Lines. *Theor. Appl. Genet.* **47**, 35–39.

39. Lander, E. S. and Botstein, D. (1987) Homozygosity mapping: a way to map human recessive traits with the DNA of inbred children. *Science* **236(4808)**, 1567–1570.

40. Lander, E. S. and Botstein, D. (1989) Mapping mendelian factors underlying quantitative traits using RFLP linkage maps. *Genetics* **121(1)**, 185–199; erratum: **136(2)**, 705 (1994).

41. Jansen, R. C. and Stam, P. (1994) High resolution of quantitative traits into multiple loci via interval mapping. *Genetics* **136(4)**, 1447–1455.

42. Zeng, Z. B. (1994) Precision mapping of quantitative trait loci. *Genetics* **136(4)**, 1457–1468.

43. Haley, C. S. and Knott, S. A. (1992) A simple regression method for mapping quantitative loci in line crosses using flanking markers. *Heredity* **69**, 315–324.

44. Zeng, Z. B. (1993) Theoretical basis for separation of multiple linked gene effects in mapping quantitative trait loci. *Proc. Natl. Acad. Sci. USA* **90(23)**, 10,972–10,976.

45. Jansen, R. C. (1993) Interval mapping of multiple quantitative trait loci. *Genetics* **135(1)**, 205–211.

46. Korol, A. B., Ronin, Y. I., and Kirzhner, V. M. (1995) Interval mapping of quantitative trait loci employing correlated trait complexes. *Genetics* **140(3)**, 1137–1147.

47. Jiang, C. and Zeng, Z. B. (1995) Multiple trait analysis of genetic mapping for quantitative trait loci. *Genetics* **140(3)**, 1111–1127.

48. Lebowitz, R. J., Soller, M., and Beckmann, J. (1987) Trait-based analyses for the detection of linkage between marker loci and quantitative trait loci in crosses between inbred lines. *Theor. Appl. Genet.* **73**, 556–562.

49. Darvasi, A. and Soller, M. (1992) Selective genotyping for determination of linkage between a marker locus and a quantitative trait locus. *Theor. Appl. Genet.* **85**, 353–359.

50. Darvasi, A. and Soller, M. (1994) Selective DNA pooling for determination of linkage between a molecular marker and a quantitative locus. *Genetics* **138**, 1365–1373.

51. Motro, U. and Soller, M. (1993) Sequential sampling in determining linkage between marker loci and quantitative trait loci. *Theor. Appl. Genet.* **85**, 658–664.

52. Darvasi, A. and Soller, M. (1994) Optimum spacing of genetic markers for determining linkage between marker loci and quantitative trait loci. *Theor. Appl. Genet.* **89**, 351–357.

53. Breeze, E. L. and Mather, K. (1957) The organization of polygenic activity within chromosome in *Drosophila*. 1. Hair characters. *Heredity* **11,** 373–395.

54. Shrimpton, A. E. and Robertson, A. (1988) The isolation of factors controlling bristle score in *Drosophila melanogaster*. I. Allocation of third chromosome sterno-pleural bristle effects to chromosome sections. *Genetics* **118,** 437–443.

55. Davies, R. W. (1971) The genetic relationship of two quantitative characters in *D. melanogaster:* II. Location of the effects. *Genetics* **69,** 363–375.

56. Eshed, Y. and Zamir, D. (1995) An introgression line population of *Lycopersicon pennellii* in the cultivated tomato enables the identification and fine mapping of yield-associated QTL. *Genetics* **141(3),** 1147–1162.

57. Darvasi, A. (1997) Interval-specific congenic strains (ISCS): an experimental design for mapping a QTL into a 1-centimorgan interval. *Mammal Genome* **8(3),** 163–167.

58. Jacob, H. J., Lindpaintner, K., Lincoln, S. E., Kusumi, K., Bunker, R. K., Mao, Y. P., et al. (1991) Genetic mapping of a gene causing hypertension in the stroke-prone spontaneously hypertensive rat. *Cell* **67(1),** 213–224.

59. Rapp, J. P. and Deng, A. Y. (1995) Detection and positional cloning of blood pressure quantitative trait loci: is it possible? Identifying the genes for genetic hypertension. *Hypertension* **25(6),** 1121–1128.

60. Bailey, D. W. (1971) Recombinant-inbred strains: an aid to identify linkage and function of histocompatibility and other genes. *Transplantation* **11,** 325–327.

61. Taylor, B. A. (1978) Recombinant inbred strains: use in gene mapping, in *Origins of Inbred Mice* (Morse, H. C., III, ed), Academic, New York.

62. Hudgins, C. C., Steinberg, R. T., Klinman, D. M., Reeves, M. J., and Steinberg, A. D. (1985) Studies of consomic mice bearing the Y chromosome of the BXSB mouse. *J. Immunol.* **134(6),** 3849–3854.

63. Maxson, S. C. (1996) Searching for candidate genes with effects on an agonistic behavior, offense, in mice. *Behav. Genet.* **26(5),** 471–476.

64. Nadeau, J. H., Singer, J. B., Matin, A., and Lander, E. S. (2000) Analysing complex genetic traits with chromosome substitution strains. *Nature Genet.* **24(3),** 221–225; erratum: **25(1),** 125 (2000).

65. Darvasi, A. and Soller, M. (1995) Advanced intercross lines, an experimental population for fine genetic mapping. *Genetics* **141(3),** 1199–1207.

66. McClearn, G. M., Wilson, J. R., and Meredith, W. (1870) The use of isogenic and heterogenic mouse stock in behavioral research, in *Contributions to Behavior Genetic Analysis: The Mouse as Prototype.* (Lindzey, G. and Thiessen, D., eds.), Appleton Century Crofts, New York, pp. 3–22.

67. Demant, P. and Hart, A. A. (1986) Recombinant congenic strains—a new tool for analyzing genetic traits determined by more than one gene. *Immunogenetics* **24(6),** 416–422.

68. Fortin, A., Diez, E., Rochefort, D., Laroche, L., Malo, D., Rouleau, G. A., et al. (2001) Recombinant congenic strains derived from a/j and c57bl/6j: a tool for genetic dissection of complex traits. *Genomics* **74(1),** 21–35.

69. Snell, G. D. (1948) Methods for the study of histocompatibility genes. *J. Genet.* **49,** 87–103.

70. Klein, J. (1981) The histocompatibility-2 (H-2) complex, in *The Mouse in Biomedical Research* (Foster, H. L., Small, J. D., and Fox, J. G., eds.), Academic, New York

71. Flaherty, L. (1981) Congenic strains, in *The Mouse in Biomedical Research. Vol. 1: History, Genetics and Wild Mice* (Foster, H. L., Small, J. D., and Fox, J. G., eds.), Academic, New York.

72. Jiang, P. P., Hansen, T. H., Shreffler, D. C., and Miller, R. D. (1995) Mouse H2 congenic intervals: analysis and use for mapping. *Mammal. Genome* **6(9)**, 586–591.

73. Bailey, D. W. (1981) Recombinant inbred and bilineal congenic strains, in *The Mouse in Biomedical Research. Vol I: History, Genetics and Wild Mice* (Foster, H. L., Small, J. D., and Fox, J. G., eds.), Academic, New York, pp. 223–238.

74. Bailey, D. W. (1981) Strategic use od recombinant inbred and congenic strains in behavior genetics research, in *Genetic Research Strategies for Psychobiology and Psychiatry* (Gershon, E. S., Mattysse, S., Breakefield, X. O., and Ciaranello, R. D., eds.), Boxwood Press, Pacific Grove, CA, pp. 189–198.

75. Bailey, D. W. (1985) Genes that affect the shape of the murine mandible. Congenic strain analysis. *J. Heredity* **76(2)**, 107–114.

76. Dietrich, W., Katz, H., Lincoln, S. E., Shin, H. S., Friedman, J., Dracopoli, N. C., et al. (1992) A genetic map of the mouse suitable for typing intraspecific crosses. *Genetics* **131(2)**, 423–447.

77. Jacob, H. J., Brown, D. M., Bunker, R. K., Daly, M. J., Dzau, V. J., Goodman, A., et al. (1995) A genetic linkage map of the laboratory rat, Rattus norvegicus. *Nature Genet.* **9(1)**, 63–69.

78. Brown, D. M., Matise, T. C., Koike, G., Simon, J. S., Winer, E. S., Zangen, S., et al. (1998) An integrated genetic linkage map of the laboratory rat. *Mammal. Genome* **9(7)**, 521–530.

79. Lander, E. S. and Schork, N. J. (1994) Genetic dissection of complex traits. *Science* **265(5181)**, 2037–2048; erratum: **266(5184)**, 353 (1994).

80. Lander, E. and Kruglyak, L. (1995) Genetic dissection of complex traits: guidelines for interpreting and reporting linkage results [see comments]. *Nature Genet.* **11(3)**, 241–247.

81. Silver, L. M. (1995) *Mouse Genetics Concepts and Applications.* Oxford University Press, New York.

82. Belknap, J. K., Mitchell, S. R., O'Toole, L. A., Helms, M. L., and Crabbe, J. C. (1996) Type I and type II error rates for quantitative trait loci (QTL) mapping studies using recombinant inbred mouse strains. *Behav. Genet.* **26(2)**, 149–160.

83. Mangin, B., Goffinet, B., and Rebai, A. (1994) Constructing confidence intervals for QTL location. *Genetics* **138(4)**, 1301–1308.

84. Visscher, P. M., Thompson, R., and Haley, C. S. (1996) Confidence intervals in QTL mapping by bootstrapping. *Genetics* **143(2)**, 1013–1020.

85. Van Ooijen, J. W. (1992) Accuracy of mapping a quantitative trait locus in autogamous species. *Theor. Appl. Genet.* **84**, 803–811.

86. O'Brien, S. J., Menotti-Raymond, M., Murphy, W. J., Nash, W. G., Wienberg, J., Stanyon, R., et al. (1999) The promise of comparative genomics in mammals. *Science* **286(5439)**, 458–462, 479–481.

87. Nusbaum, C., Slonim, D. K., Harris, K. L., Birren, B. W., Steen, R. G., Stein, L. D., et al. (1999) A YAC-based physical map of the mouse genome. *Nature Genet.* **22(4)**, 388–393.

88. Manly, K. F. and Olson, J. M. (1999) Overview of QTL mapping software and introduction to map manager QT. *Mammal. Genome* **10(4)**, 327–334.

89. Gershenfeld, H. K. and Paul, S. M. (1997) Mapping quantitative trait loci for fear-like behaviors in mice. *Genomics* **46(1)**, 1–8.

90. Collin, G. B., Asada, Y., Varnum, D. S., and Nadeau, J. H. (1996) DNA pooling as a quick method for finding candidate linkages in multigenic trait analysis: an example involving susceptibility to germ cell tumors. *Mammal. Genome* **7(1)**, 68–70.

91. Matin, A., Collin, G. B., Asada, Y., Varnum, D., and Nadeau, J. H. (1999) Susceptibility to testicular germ-cell tumours in a 129.MOLF-Chr 19 chromosome substitution strain. *Nature Genet.* **23(2)**, 237–240.

92. Talbot, C. J., Nicod, A., Cherny, S. S., Fulker, D. W., Collins, A. C., and Flint, J. (1999) High-resolution mapping of quantitative trait loci in outbred mice. *Nature Genet.* **21(3)**, 305–308.

93. Iraqi, F., Clapcott, S. J., Kumari, P., Haley, C. S., Kemp, S. J., and Teale, A. J. (2000) Fine mapping of trypanosomiasis resistance loci in murine advanced intercross lines. *Mammal. Genome* **11(8)**, 645–648.

94. Encinas, J. A., Wicker, L. S., Peterson, L. B., Mukasa, A., Teuscher, C., Sobel, R., et al. (1999) QTL influencing autoimmune diabetes and encephalomyelitis map to a 0.15-cM region containing I12 [letter]. *Nature Genet.* **21(2)**, 158–160.

95. Symula, D. J., Frazer, K. A., Ueda, Y., Denefle, P., Stevens, M. E., Wang, Z. E., et al. (1999) Functional screening of an asthma QTL in YAC transgenic mice. *Nature Genet.* **23(2)**, 241–244.

9

Approaches to the Analysis of Complex Quantitative Phenotypes and Marker Map Construction Based on the Analysis of Rat Models of Hypertension

Dominique Gauguier and Nilesh Samani

1. Introduction

1.1. Essential Hypertension

Essential hypertension is among the best examples of inherited complex quantitative phenotypes. Although this syndrome is well characterized for multiple pathophysiological circuits that have led to the development of potent pharmacological agents influencing blood pressure (BP), it remains a major health issue in Westernized populations because of its high prevalence and the increased risk of end-organ complications, including stroke, coronary heart disease, heart failure, peripheral vascular disease, and renal failure. Both genetic factors and "environmental" factors such as diet, alcohol intake, and obesity are involved in the development of hypertension and its complications and contribute to its phenotypic heterogeneity. Investigating the genetic basis of BP control represents a paradigm to analyze gene–gene and gene–environment interactions. Although BP shows a continuous distribution in both human populations and experimental models, hypertension is arbitrarily defined by values above 140 mm Hg systolic and 90 mm Hg diastolic pressure. The utilization of quantitative values of the trait for statistical analysis of data derived from genetic studies represents a key strategy to overcome the arbitrary classification of hypertensive and normotensive individuals. This approach takes into account extreme values of the phenotypes, as well as quantitative values of the traits for *a priori* unaffected or undiagnosed individuals.

From: *Methods in Molecular Biology: vol. 195: Quantitative Trait Loci: Methods and Protocols.*
Edited by: N. J. Camp and A. Cox © Humana Press, Inc., Totowa, NJ

1.2. The Use of Rat Models

The quantitative trait locus (QTL) approach, which uses the continuous values of phenotypic variables in each individual of a population, is therefore particularly appropriate in genetic studies of BP control. Taking advantage of this strategy, genetic studies in rat models of spontaneous hypertension have played an important role in the identification of genetic loci that regulate BP. The rat is, by far, the leading model species in pharmacology and toxicology and provides the most relevant model for the accurate analysis of whole-organism, organ, and cellular phenotypes relevant to essential hypertension. Many of the noninvasive and invasive phenotyping techniques that are readily available in the rat are, at present, difficult or impossible to apply in other species, including the mouse. The rat is therefore the most relevant model organism for the dissection of blood pressure into distinct subphenotypes that participate in the pathophysiological process leading to hypertension through possible distinct molecular mechanisms and gene pathways. However, transgenic experiments in mice remain essential to investigating and validating the role of potential candidate genes on BP regulation.

The analysis of the genetic basis of complex phenotypes, is, in theory, simplified in inbred models. Studies of the genetic control of BP in spontaneously hypertensive rat strains (*see* **Subheading 2.1.**) have pioneered the QTL strategy in rats and opened a new field of investigation for other multifactorial disorders in rats, including type 1 and type 2 diabetes mellitus, atopy, arthritis, and behavioral traits. Most BP QTL studies have applied standard genetic strategies based on genetic and phenotypic analyses in a segregating population (F2 or first backcross), often supported by a comprehensive pathophysiological screening of the hybrids. The ultimate goal of genetic studies in experimental models remains the application to human health. Investigating BP QTLs in rat models represents one of the most demonstrative examples of an integrated scientific strategy applied to the identification of etiological pathways relevant to a human-complex disorder. This chapter synthesizes the individual components of QTL analysis based on results from numerous studies carried out with spontaneously hypertensive rat models and emphasizes the contribution of BP QTL results in models to our understanding of the etiology of human essential hypertension.

2. Methods

2.1. Susceptible and Resistant Rat Strains

In contrast to rodent models in which spontaneous obesity and diabetes are induced by naturally occurring single-gene mutations (*fa, db, ob, Agouti*), no monogenic rodent models of severe hypertension have been described. A pro-

Table 1.
Rat Strains Commonly Used for QTL Analysis of BP Phenotypes

Strains	Strain designation	Original outbred stock
High BP		
S	Dahl salt-sensitive	Sprague–Dawley
SHR	Spontaneously hypertensive	Wistar
SHRSP	SHR stroke prone	SHR
MHS	Milan hypertensive	Wistar
LH	Lyon hypertensive	Sprague–Dawley
GH	Genetically hypertensive	Wistar
SBH	DOCA salt-sensitive	Unknown
FHH	Fawn-hooded hypertensive	German brown × White Lashley
ISIAH	Inherited stress-induced hypertension	Wistar
PHR	Prague hypertensive	Wistar
Normal or low BP		
R	Dahl salt-resistant	Sprague–Dawley
WKY	Wistar Kyoto	Wistar
MNS	Milan normotensive	Wistar
LN	Lyon normotensive	Sprague–Dawley
LL	Lyon low blood pressure	Sprague–Dawley
SBN	DOCA salt-resistant	Unknown
FHL	Fawn-hooded low blood pressure	German brown × White Lashley
PNR	Prague normotensive	Wistar
Normotensive inbred rats		
unrelated to hypertensive strains		
BN	Brown Norway	
LEW	Lewis	
F344	Fisher	

cess of repeated selective breeding of increasingly hypertensive animals isolated from an outbred normotensive stock has been used to produce hypertensive lines. This procedure, based on the existence of naturally occurring alleles altering BP alleles in outbred animals, has been used to derive a wide range of inbred rat strains that have been specifically selected for high BP (**Table 1**). In most cases, the normotensive or low-BP strains have been concomitantly produced from the same outbred stock (**Table 1**). The main phenotypic and genetic characteristics of these strains have been recently reviewed (*1*). There is not much genetic diversity in commonly used hypertensive strains because most of them were developed from either Wistar and Sprague–Dawley outbred stocks, which share a common origin. This may limit the detection of susceptibility loci in experimental crosses. Other inbred rat strains such as the Brown Norway (BN), Fisher (F), and Lewis (LEW), which are often models for other disorders, are well characterized for the absence of BP alterations and appropriate for the generation of genetic crosses with hypertensive strains.

2.2. Design of the Experimental Cross

The critical stage of experimental genetic projects lies in the selection of the susceptible and resistant strains that will be used for the experimental cross. Two different empirical concepts have been used to choose the most appropriate cross. The first assumes that the analysis of hybrids derived from closely related strains that were isolated from the same outbred stock using the same selection criterion (i.e., SHR×WKY, SHRSP×WKY, LH×LN, S×R, MHS×MNS) would identify major genetic loci regulating BP. The second approach consists of the generation of hybrid cohorts from a hypertensive strain bred with a completely unrelated normotensive inbred strain (BN, F344, LEW), which allows the potential of contrasting alleles at additional BP QTLs. Each strategy has its advantages and drawbacks. Applying the first one will result in poor QTL mapping resolution of variables selected in the strain selection process, whereas the latter will provide a high coverage of the QTLs linked to traits that may not be relevant to the characteristics of the disease strain. Polymorphism rates between inbred rat strains could be a significant criterion to be considered for the choice of the experimental cross, as high mapping resolution is required in the long term for the characterization of speed congenic lines (*see* Chapter 8, **Subheading 2.3.3.**) derived for the QTL intervals.

Based on the obvious polygenic nature of high BP in hypertensive rats, intercrosses have been generally preferred to backcross breedings (which are better for oligogenic dominant traits). Highly significant QTLs have been identified with relatively small crosses (<200 animals). In most studies, only males have been considered for the genetic analysis to minimize the sex effect on BP. Analyzing male hybrids has often been prioritized because BP measurement procedures are easier in males and males develop evidence of high BP faster than females. However, genetic studies in crosses derived from SBH, GH, and SHRSP rats that included both males and females have shown sex specificity in the detection of BP QTLs, which may be relevant to the differential progression of hypertension in male and female rats. Reciprocal crosses could also be considered in order to test the respective effects of susceptible and resistant alleles and genetic background on BP control.

A panel of 31 recombinant inbred lines have been derived from BN and SHR rats (*2*) and are maintained at the Czech Academy of Sciences in Prague. Each line carries a different combination of homozygous chromosomal segments originated from the founding parental strains and potentially represents a mosaic of BP contrasting alleles from the original strains. The panel has been character-ized for a large number of genetic markers and provides useful resources of inbred animals that can be repeatedly tested for various phenotypes likely to play a role on BP regulation.

2.3. Phenotype Analysis

Indirect BP using the tail-cuff method and/or direct BP via a femoral or carotid cannula are the most common ways of measuring BP, although more sophisticated methods such as radiotelemetry have also been applied. On the one hand, BP measurement based on the tail-cuff method was the selection criterion used to derive all hypertensive rat strains and is therefore expected to be the most appropriate procedure. On the other hand, radiotelemetry allows a follow-up recording of BP for several weeks in individual animals, improves the accuracy of BP measures, and represents an efficient system to evaluate variations of BP during the light/dark cycles. In several studies, animals have been placed on a high-salt diet (2–8% NaCl) prior to BP measurement. Supple-mental dietary NaCl is required in crosses derived for the S strain. Variation in BP responses to changes in dietary intake of NaCl involves the interaction of multiple environment and genetic factors and creates an additional level of complexity in the interpretation of QTL results. The analysis of individual BP variables builds upon our knowledge of the multiple pathways involved in the pathophysiology of hypertension. Although systolic and diastolic BP are the major phenotypes measured in the hybrids, a number of subphenotypes that are directly relevant to BP, including mean arterial pressure, pulse pressure, circadian variation (telemetry), and heart rate, are also tested. BP-related pheno-types that may have their own additional genetic control have also been ana-lyzed, including cardiac mass and variables relevant to complications (renal failure and stroke). In most hypertensive strains, high BP is associated with effects on heart weight, as the heart hypertrophies in response to chronically increased BP. Similarly, stroke and renal damage occur in response to either spontaneous hypertension or high BP experimentally induced. It is, however, reasonable to hypothesize the existence of loci that influence these variables independent of BP.

2.4. Marker Resources for Genomewide Searches

More than 10,000 rat microsatellite markers have been produced over the past 5 yr and public databases have been implemented mainly on two sites (http://www.well.ox.ac.uk/rat_mapping_resources; http://rgd.mcw.edu/) to pro-vide the scientific community with all information required to efficiently carry out a genomewide search in almost any rat cross. These large collections of rat microsatellite markers have been characterized for allele variation between strains most commonly used in experimental crosses. The maximum polymorphism rate between two rat strains is unlikely to exceed 70% (*3*). An optimal panel of polymorphic microsatellite markers can be chosen from the repositories for a specific cross, assuming that the strains are derived from identical colonies to those used in the polymorphism assays. In this context, it should be noted that a very high level of allele variations was found among colonies of WKY and SHR strains (*3*), which were distributed to various laboratories and commercial suppliers before either strain was fully inbred.

An initial genomewide search is generally carried out with an average spacing of 10–15 cM between adjacent markers. The vast majority of rat microsatellite markers are integrated in dense linkage maps that allow the selection of a collection of markers evenly spaced for the genomewide search (http://www.well.ox.ac.uk/rat_mapping_resources; http://rgd.mcw.edu/). Markers are usually robust, and standardized touch-down PCR protocols (*3*) can be applied for high-throughput fluorescent genotyping. However, genotype analysis in hybrids derived from fully inbred strains is relatively simple and based on the detection of only two genotypes in a backcross and three genotypes in an intercross. Allele size differences of approx 10 bp or more between parental strains can be easily analyzed on a standard 4% agarose gel. With the increasing density of the rat linkage maps, a panel of such markers can be selected in public databases, thus substantially reducing the cost of genotype analysis as compared to fluorescent genotyping.

Several database systems are suitable for storing information on pedigree structure and both phenotype and genotype data, including Access, Discovery Manager, Sybase, and, more simply, File Maker Pro. Export files of the data are generally in text files appropriate for subsequent map construction and QTL analysis.

2.5. Map Construction

Prior to statistical analyses and QTL identification, genetic maps are constructed to confirm the appropriate genome coverage in the cross and identify possible typing errors and inconsistencies between the resulting maps and published data. JoinMap 2.0 (JM) is one of the most robust and user-friendly packages available for linkage analysis and genetic mapping (*4,5*). It was designed by Stam and Van Oijen (*5*), initially for the analysis of results from plant breeding, and can be applied to most experimental crosses in mammals. All files handled and produced by JM are ASCII text files. Each phase of the mapping analysis is summarized in **Table 2** and briefly described in the following subsections. An example is also given in Chapter 10, Subheading 5.1.

2.5.1. Creation of a Locus Genotype File ("loc-file")

Export files from the database system used to store data from a study may not comply to the format required for JM. For example, they may provide

Table 2.
Summary of the Main Steps Required for the Construction and Verification of Linkage Maps with the JoinMap Program

Step	Module	Input files	Output file
1. Formatting	jmdma	file.dat	file.loc
2. Linkage groups	jmgrp	file.loc	file.out
3. Grouping files	jmspl	file.loc and file.out	file1.loc, file2.loc, etc.
4. Recombination frequency analysis	jmrec	file1.loc, file2.loc, etc.	file1.pwd, file2.pwd, etc.
5. Linkage mapping	jmmap	file1.pwd, file2.pwd, etc.	file1.jmo, file2.jm,. etc.
6. Marker ordering	jmdma	file1.loc, file2.loc, etc. file1.map, file2.map, etc.	file1.loc, file2.loc, etc.
7. Unexpected double recombinants	jmchk	file1.loc, file2.loc, etc.	file1.chk, file2.chk, etc.
8. Distorted segregation	jmsla	file1.loc, file2.loc, , etc.	file1.sla, file2.sla, etc.

marker data in columns and individuals in rows and may use different genotype-coding systems. One of the roles of the **jmdma** utility program is to transform raw data into an appropriate format for the first stage of JM, using a translation file (**file.tra**) and a **file.dat** as input file.

The translation file (**file.tra**) (see following example) allows the transformation of genotype codes in the original datafile (0, 1, 2, 3 in an F2 cross for unknown, homozygote for each allele, and heterozygote, respectively) in a coding system that can be analyzed by JM (–, a, b, h):

```
1 - > a
2 - > b
0 - > -
3 - > h
```

Examples of a **file.dat**:

```
transpose skip=          Number of columns to be skipped (pedigree
                         type, individual number, phenotypes, etc)
translate=File.tra       File.tra
name=                    Name of the study
popt=                    Population type (f2, bc, . . .)
nloc=                    Number of loci
nind=                    Number of individuals
1                        column 1: Pedigree (to be skipped)
```

```
2                              column 2: Individuals (to be skipped)
3                              column 3: First phenotype (to be skipped)
D1Wox1                         column 4: First genetic marker
D1Wox2                         column 5
D1Wox3                         column 6
Etc...
f2    1    456    2    2    2    2    1    0    3    3    0...
f2    2    557    2    3    3    2    2    2    1    3    3...
f2    3    675    1    1    2    2    1    1    3    2    1...
f2    4    890    2    3    3    2    3    3    3    3    3...
f2    5    555    1    1    2    2    1    0    3    3    0...
Etc...
```

The output file is the **file.loc**, which will be used throughout the analysis with the following format:

```
; original file: LEIC1.dat
; no individuals removed
name = LEIC
popt = F2
nloc = 875
nind = 403
D1Wox1
  bbaba . . .
D1Wox2
  bhaha . . .
D1Wox3
  bhbhb . . .
```

2.5.2. Chromosome-Specific "loc" Files

The **jmgrp** module is used to assign markers to linkage groups, based on the calculation of log odds (LOD) scores of pairs of markers; that is, to determine those markers that are linked to each other that most often translates to those on the same chromosome. This module runs through several LOD thresholds in order to obtain the best grouping file. In our experience, using a LOD range between 3 and 6, with a step size of 1, generates linkage groups that are consistent with published maps, regardless of the number of markers analyzed (100 to >1500) and the size of the pedigree (100–400 hybrids). Greater LOD thresholds can be applied to analyze a possible marker clustering in a particular chromosomal region.

The input and output files are the **file.loc** and the **file.out**, respectively. A new **file.out** is created with results from the most appropriate LOD threshold. Ideally, for a genomewide search, the best LOD threshold will lead to a number of groups corresponding to the number of chromosomes, or greater.

The module **jmspl** will create a loc-file for each linkage group (e.g., file1.loc, file2.loc, etc). This module requires both the **file.loc** and the appropriate **file.out**.

2.5.3. Calculation of Recombination Frequencies

The **jmrec** module calculates estimates of recombination frequencies from the raw data in each of the chromosome-specific loc-files and produces LOD scores. The input file is a chromosome (linkage group)-specific **file.loc** and the output file (**file.pwd**) contains a list of pairwise recombination estimates. The parameters required for the **jmrec** module are a LOD threshold and recombination (REC) threshold. In the tutorial, the authors recommend values in the range 0.01–0.50 and 0.45–0.49 for LOD and REC thresholds, respectively. In our experience, thresholds of 0.01 (LOD) and 0.49 (REC) provide a reasonable choice for the analysis of large datasets.

An example of pwd-file is as follows:

```
; JoinMap JMREC output  Fri, 14 Feb 1997, 16:01
; data taken from LEIC1.loc
; LOD-threshold:  0.0100
; REC-threshold:  0.4900

name = LEIC1

   D1Wox1      D1Wox2      0.1083      13.6677
   D1Wox1      D1Wox3      0.1299      13.8006
   D1Wox1      D1Wox4      0.1202      13.2372
   D1Wox1      D1Wox5      0.1885       8.2965
Etc...
```

The recombination frequency between pairs of markers in the pwd-file should be between 0 and 0.5. If an estimate exceeds a value of 0.5, a "SUSPECT" warning is issued and genotypes should be double-checked prior to linkage mapping analysis. The module **jmrec** can be applied for calculations of recombination frequencies even when the genotype of the parental strains is unknown or missing. In this case, suspect estimates may be the result of an inverted genotype phase between linked markers that can be easily corrected in the loc-file.

It must be noted that when data from reciprocal crosses are analyzed, a loc-file must be created for each population and the module **jmrec** must be independently applied to each loc-file in order to account for different recombinant frequencies in the two crosses. As a result, two independent pwd-files are produced that are merged for subsequent mapping. For the construction of an integrated map from different crosses, the analysis is performed with population specific pwd-files

2.5.4. Constructing the Chromosomal Maps

A linkage map is produced by the module **jmmap**, which uses the pairwise list of recombination estimates stored in the **file.pwd** created for each chromosome/ linkage group. The module **jmmap** requires the creation of a **file.rsp** (response file) containing the chosen criteria for the analysis. The response file refers to the corresponding pwd (input) and jmo (output) files as follows:

```
pwd= LEIC
jmo= LEIC
fix=
map=Kosambi
lod=0.001
rec=0.499
jum=4
tri=6
rip=3
top=0
int=n
opd=n
```

For the construction of the first map, it is reasonable to analyze the data without specifying a fixed marker order (fix). Two mapping functions (Haldane and Kosambi) can be used. LOD and REC thresholds of 0.001 and 0.499, respectively, enable the use of all information in the pwd-file. The three mapping parameters correspond to the following:

1. "Jumps in goodness to fit" (jum) which evaluate changes in the map (chi square) when a new marker is analyzed. It should be in the range 3.0–5.0.
2. Triplet (tri) which is used by JoinMap to calculate LOD of the three possible orders within a triplet before map construction starts. Threshold value should be above 5.0.
3. Ripple (rip), which corresponds to a local search through permutations for improvements in the order of three adjacent markers.

The three parameters correspond to the number of top linkages to output for each locus (top), the output of intermediate results (int: yes or no), and the output of ordered pairwise data (opt: yes or no), respectively.

The maps are produced in three rounds of marker–marker linkage analysis, the last one being the least stringent and including all markers. It is recommended to exclude from the dataset any marker mapped at the last round and creating either a large gap in the chromosome or a substantial expansion in the chromosomal extremities when compared to the maps derived in rounds 1 and 2. The resulting maps and the statistics related to their construction are in a **file.jmo**. Markers excluded after rounds 1 and 2 that are likely to be problematic for mapping are reported as "removed <marker>," followed by the reason of removal (jump, conflict, or negative distance). For each of the three cycles, a map is constructed (in two orientations) reporting the cumulative map position (cM). Following error checks and remapping, a **file.map** containing the most appropriate map is created. The module **jmdma** can be used again here to organize markers in the loc-file in the same order as in the map-file. This is particularly useful for the final error checking step. The specifications for the module **jmdma** at this stage are as follows:

```
Data file?                file.loc
Map file for sorting?     file.map
Output file?              file.loc
```

The final loc-file overwrites the initial one.

2.5.5. Maker Error Checking

The last stages of the analysis consist of the identification of improbable genotypes originating from suspect double recombinants between closely linked markers, and distortion in the genotype ratio for each markers locus using the **jmchk** and **jmsla** modules, respectively.

The **jmchk** module analyses the three locus genotypes that are not considered with the **jmmap** module, which is based on pairwise recombination frequencies. The input file is a **file.loc** and the output file is a **file.chk**, which is organized as follows. Individuals, problematic genotypes, and flanking markers are reported as well as a statistical estimation of the magnitude of the problem.

```
ind   previous locus    locus                  next locus        log (1/p)
---   ----------------   --------------------   ---------------   ---------------
25    b: D1Wox31         h: D1Wox32             b: D1Wox75        3.092 *
50    a: D1Wox31         b: D1Wox32             a: D1Wox75        6.786 ****
31    h: D1Wox32         b: D1Wox75             h: D1Wox78        2.672
log(1/p) values: *>3; **>4; ***>5; ****>6; *****>7
```

Because markers in the loc-file are in the same order as in the map, problematic genotypes can be easily identified and double checked:

```
original file:          file.loc
; map file for sorting:   file.map
; no individuals removed
name = LEIC
popt = F2
nloc = 149
nind = 403
; linkage group  1 (bottom-up):
D1Wox31
```

```
    hhhha hhhhb hbhab aaahb abhbb hab-b hbbbb hhhhb babhh babba...
D1Wox32
    hhhha hhhhb hbhab aaahb abhbh habab hbbbb hhhhb babhh babbb...
D1Wox75
    hhhha hhhab hbhab aaahb hbhbb aabab bbbbb hahhb aabhh babba...
D1Wox78
    hbaha hhhab hhhah ahahb hbhbb aabab hbbbb hahhh aabha babba...
```

The **jmsla** module analyzes the genotype frequency distribution and provides statistics (chi square) to estimate distorted segregations. The input file is the loc-file.

```
JoinMap Single Locus Analysis 2.0/a
locus genotype file:    file.loc
population name:        Leic
population type:        F2
number of loci:         149
number of individuals: 403
significance levels:   *:0.1   **:0.05   ***:0.01   ****:0.005   *****:0.001
******:0.0005   *******:0.0001
frequency distributions per locus   (149 loci):
             a     h     b     c     d     -     X2    (df) :signif.[classes]
   ---- ---- ---- ---- ---- ----    ------------------------------------
1: D1Wox31  86    156   105   0     0     56    0.47  (2):            [a:h:b]
2: D1Wox32  101   162   83    0     0     57    0.76  (2):            [a:h:b]
3: D1Wox75  83    190   113   0     0     17    2.01  (2):            [a:h:b]
4: D1Wox78  90    123   151   0     0     39    12.51 (2):    ****    [a:h:b]
```

2.6. QTL Analysis and Fine Mapping

Genetic linkage analysis of BP data generated in crosses has received much attention by statistical geneticists. The analysis is expected to prove the existence of QTLs, give statistical support to their map position, detect possible interactions between QTLs, evaluate different inheritance modes and identify the allele contributing to the disease phenotype. Several different techniques have been developed that are based on the utilization of maximum likelihood techniques to calculate LOD scores at many selected positions in an interval between markers and plotted versus map location. These techniques are reviewed in Chapter 7, Subheadings **2.2.** and **2.3.** Although optimized for experimental crosses and broadly used for most of the QTL mapping projects, applying these programs requires statistical expertise.

For example, all phenotypes in the cross must be analysed for Normal distribution and possible correlation prior to linkage analysis, because most of the test statistics are either based on the Normal distribution or on distributions that are related to and can be derived from Normal. The property of the Normal distribution is that 68% of all its observations fall within a range of ±1 standard deviation from the mean, and a range of ±2 standard deviations includes 95% of the values. Obviously, the shape of the sampling distribution becomes Normal as the sample size increases and Normal distribution is usually obtained for most BP phenotypes. Validation of Normality and evidence of correlation between traits can be easily tested with standard statistical softwares, including, for example, SPSS 9.0.

2.6.1. Preparation of JM files for MAPMAKER/QTL

The most popular and readily available programs for QTL analysis are Map Manager QT for Macintosh computers and MAP-MAKER/QTL, JoinMap/QTL, and MultiQTL for PC and other platforms. The majority of BP QTLs in rats have been identified using the program MAP-MAKER/QTL. Mapping files constructed with JoinMap can be entered in MAP-MAKER/QTL using the module **prepare chr.raw** of MAPMAKER/EXP 3.0. MAPMAKER/EXP requires the creation of two files. The first is a raw data file similar to the loc-file of JoinMap and containing the phenotype data in addition to the genotypes. The header of the raw data file (**file.raw**) should include information on the cross used (F2 backcross or F2 intercross) and the total numbers of individuals, markers, and phenotypes as follows:

```
Data type f2 backcross
403     149     17
*D1Wox1 b b a b a ...
*D1Wox2 b h a h a ...
*D1Wox3 b h b h b ...
*Phenx  456  557  675  890  555 ...
```

The second file that is required (file.prep) reports the correspondence between marker order in the genetic map and in the raw data file (this order is actually identical in the map [file.map] and in the final JoinMap loc-file [file.loc] when loci are sorted by map position, as described earlier using **jmdma**). Distances from the centromere in the JoinMap files must be converted in interval size between adjacent markers:

```
print name on
make chromosome chr1
seq  1  2  3  4
anchor chr1
seq  1=3.5  2=3.6  3=5.7  4=2.1
framework chr1
save data
```

Four files are generated by the module prepare chr.raw of MAPMAKER/EXP 3.0 (file.dat, file.maps. file.traits, file.xmaps) that can be subsequently processed by MAPMAKER/QTL, as described in Chapter 7, Subheading 5.3.

Following initial linkage analysis, fine mapping is required in order to confirm the existence of the QTLs, identify the peak of linkage, and define the genetic size of the QTLs. The observation of several peaks within the same QTL after linkage map saturation and complete genotyping of the progeny set could indicate the existence of several independent QTLs. Some approaches to fine mapping are discussed in Chapter 8.

3. Interpretation

3.1. Phenotypic Analysis

The accurate measurement of BP or related phenotypes (see above) is, of course, crucial to the genetic analysis. However, even when BP measurement procedures are standardized, alterations in experimental conditions, such as age of hybrids and diet composition (including salt intake), may affect the detection and significance of QTLs. Alterations may be subtle and even unrecognized but can significantly affect results. With regard to phenotyping, the panel of recombinant inbred strains (Chapter 8, Subheading 2.4.1.) derived by Pravenec and colleagues (*2*), which is already genetically characterized, provides a powerful system to carry out comprehensive and serial screening of multiple phenotypes and study their possible genetic control. Although phenotype analysis in this panel would only reflect the expression of SHR alleles on a BN genetic background (or vice versa), a similar thorough screening in a classical F2 or backcross population would require a genomewide search for several series of hybrids.

3.2. QTL Mapping

Our knowledge of BP QTLs in rats is based on data from approximately 25 different crosses that were able to identify more than 60 QTLs throughout the rat genome. Results from genomewide searches in these crosses have recently been reviewed (*1,6*). Although it is impossible to assess if an appropriate significance criterion was applied in each of the studies, they provide a comprehensive overview of the complex genetic basis of BP regulation. As expected, the allele of the hypertensive strain at the QTLs is usually associated with high BP. However, at some QTLs, alleles that originate from the hypertensive strain have an opposite effect and actually lower BP! The likely reason for this is the random fixing of a "hypotensive" allele at the locus during the initial selection of the hypertensive strain. This important observation serves to emphasize the complex way in which a quantitative variable such as BP is actually determined in an individual. Once initial evidence of linkage have been detected, additional markers can be chosen in public databases for subsequent fine mapping of the QTLs. The identification of the peak of linkage and the definition of 1-LOD and 2-LOD confidence intervals are particularly important for the subsequent derivation of congenic lines for the QTLs. Determinants of statistical resolution of a QTL include the strength of its genetic effect, the number of animals studied, and the number of markers analyzed, although, in most of the studies, increasing marker density beyond a resolution of one marker every 5–10 cM does not significantly improve the QTL position. As a consequence, BP QTLs based on classical F2 and backcross populations are localized in fairly large chromosomal regions (>30 cM), which makes the isolation of the underlying gene(s) impossible through classical positional cloning methodologies.

3.3. Significance of the QTLs

As a rough estimation, a LOD of 3 or higher is generally considered as statistically significant. However, factors such as the size of the genome, the assumed genetic model for the effect, and the experimental cross (backcross or intercross) influence the LOD plot. Lander and Kruglyak (7) calculated values for LOD scores under various conditions to determine threshold for suggestive significance and significance in specific inheritance models and in a given cross. Under various models of inheritance (additive, recessive, dominant), suggestive linkage corresponds to a LOD score of 1.9–2.0 ($p<3.4 \times 10^{-3}$ and $p<2.4 \times 10^{-3}$) in a backcross and an intercross, respectively, whereas significant linkage corresponds to a LOD score of 3.3–3.4 ($p<1.0 \times 10^{-4}$ and $p<7.2 \times 10^{-5}$, respectively. Suggestive linkage is defined as "a statistical evidence that would be expected to occur one time at random in a genome scan." Significant and highly significant linkages are supported by statistical evidence expected to occur 0.05 and 0.001 times in a genome scan, respectively. However, when subphenotypes are analyzed, it may be worth considering a QTL supported by suggestive LODs when it colocalizes with a strongly significant QTL already identified in the same cross for another phenotype. This somewhat reflects the fourth class of linkage ("confirmed linkage") proposed by Lander and Kruglyak. Confirmed linkage applies to a significant QTL that is replicated in a further study, for which a nominal *p*-value of 0.01 should be required. However, as described later in this chapter, although BP QTLs identified in different hypertensive rat strains tend to aggregate in the same chromosomal regions, further analysis in congenic lines demonstrates that the genes involved are likely to be strain-specific. The criterion of confirmed linkage should therefore be applied to data from identical crosses, or at least from crosses derived from the same hypertensive strain.

3.4. QTL Replication and QTL Clustering

The genetic background of a normotensive strain appears to strongly influence the replication of QTLs in different crosses. The most comprehensive analysis of BP QTLs that supports this observation has been performed by Rapp who derived crosses from the same colony of hypertensive rats (S) bred with five different normotensive strains (R, LEW, MNS, WKY, BN) (*1*). Results from QTL analysis demonstrated that although some QTLs can be replicated in different crosses, the majority of them are unique to a pair of strains (*1*). Genetic studies performed in backcrosses F1 (S×R)×R and F1 (S×R)×S and in the intercross F2(S×R) have demonstrated the importance of the genetic background and allele dosage in the detection of linkage. In these crosses, the higher the proportion of S alleles in the genetic background, the more significant the linkage to BP (*1*).

Blood pressure QTLs in rat are spread along the genome, but evidence of linkage with BP has been consistently found on rat chromosomes 1, 2, 10, and 13. For example, evidence of linkage between BP and a region of rat chromosome 13 containing the Renin gene has been detected in five different crosses (SHR×WKY, SHR×LEW, SHR×BB, S×R and LH×LN) and in the SHR×BN recombinant inbred panel (*6*). In the first approximation, this clustering of QTLs linked to the same trait in a similar region of the genome suggests that hypertensive strains may share alleles, significantly influencing BP at the same locus and possibly in the same gene. However, subsequent analysis of congenic lines demonstrated that this QTL is likely to be either a composite locus containing multiple alleles increasing or decreasing BP, with an overall net effect significantly increasing BP in the hypertensive strain, or strongly influenced by permissive alleles elsewhere in the genome (*8*). A similar clustering of QTLs linked to BP and related phenotypes was identified in rat chromosome 1 in S, SHRSP, and SHR strains (*1*). Subsequent analysis of congenic lines for these loci ruled out the possibility of variants in a single gene affecting BP (*9,10*).

3.5. How Many BP QTLs in a BP QTL?

At the stage of QTL mapping in an experimental cross, the interpretation of results from linkage analysis in terms of the number of loci detected in the same chromosomal region is difficult and results can be misleading. A single broad peak is generally observed spanning a large chromosomal interval. Refining a QTL map may lead to the identification of either "ghost" peaks or multiple significant peaks (see Chapter 7, Subheading 2.3.). Although they may be the result of the presence of several alleles on the same chromosome independently affecting BP, they may also indicate genotyping errors and incomplete typing of the progeny set. The existence of multiple linked QTLs can only be confirmed by dissecting the locus in a series of congenic lines that carry overlapping regions of the QTL. For example, chromosome 1 harbors strongly significant BP QTLs identified in the S, SHR, and SHRSP strains. Linkage analysis initially identified several peaks in a S×LEW cross and the existence of several independent BP QTLs was suggested (*11*). Recent results from the screening of congenic lines independently derived from the S and SHR strains for this region showed that the initial QTL defined in an experimental cross contains at least three QTLs in the S rat and two in the SHR (*9,10*). Obviously, the observation of several gene loci at the same QTL able to significantly increase BP raises the possibility that two closely linked QTLs may also cancel each other out and may remain undetected in a cross if the alleles at the two loci have opposite effects on BP.

3.6. Gene–Gene and Gene–Environment Interactions

Additive effects are assumed as a first approximation for the statistical analysis of QTLs. However, numerous examples of interactions between alleles at QTLs (epistasis) have been reported. For example, evidence of a strong interaction between BP QTLs on chromosomes 2 and 10 was observed in an F2(S×MNS) population and was subsequently confirmed in congenic lines carrying both QTLs introgressed into a S genetic background (*12*). Time-dependent detection of linkage, which may be relevant for ecogenetic factors and/or epistatic effects between QTLs, has been observed on chromosome 13 in a SHR×WKY cross (*13*). The identification of BP QTLs specifically in hybrid populations treated with a high-salt diet may also indicate the influence of ecogenetic factors. Results from QTL analysis in a classical F2 or backross population can only suggest such effects and data from other experimental systems are required to confirm the hypothesis.

3.7. Intermediate Phenotypes

Mapping QTLs for BP-related phenotypes such as cardiac hypertrophy, stroke, or renal failure has led to the successful identification of susceptibility loci for these traits that, however, do not cosegregate with BP in the cross. These results raised the hypothesis that intermediate phenotypes have their own genetic control independent of BP, although most of these regions were previously characterized for BP QTLs in other crosses and/or hypertensive strains. For example, stroke phenotypes in the SHRSP rat were investigated in two intercrosses (SHRSP×SHR and SHRSP×WKY) and gave fundamentally different results. In the SHRSP×SHR cross, stroke latency appears to be a polygenic trait controlled by three chromosomal regions that are not linked to BP in the cross but have been previously described for BP QTLs in other hypertensive strains (*14*). Using a different phenotype based on brain infarct size following occlusion of the middle cerebral artery, which would reflect stroke sensitivity, a single strongly significant QTL was identified (LOD=16.6) on chromosome 5 and accounts for 67% of the total variance in the cross (*15*). Thus, based on a different cross and different experimental conditions to determine stroke phenotype, different QTL location and effects can be identified. Although these phenotypes may underly different mechanisms, the analysis of congenic lines derived for these loci represents the most efficient system to confirm the existence of these QTLs and their BP-independent genetic control.

3.8. Beyond QTL Mapping

Quantitative trait loci mapping is only a preliminary stage in the genetic analysis of BP control. Further investigations are required to prove the existence of the QTLs and, most importantly, to test their relevance to human essential hypertension. The construction of congenic strains where segments of chromosomes harboring a QTL are introgressed into a permissive background (usually the reciprocal strain used in the intercross), by marker-selected breeding ("speed congenics"), currently provides the most reliable way of progressing from mapping of a QTL to identification of the susceptibility gene (*16*). With recent improvements in the number of genetic markers available for the rat and the construction of dense genetic maps, this strategy can be applied to rat congenic lines (*17*). The strategy usually involves an initial transfer of a large chromosomal regional (at least the 2-LOD confidence interval) to ensure that the QTL is "captured" in the congenic strain, and the subsequent development of congenic substrains by further rounds of backcrossing to narrow the interval containing the QTL. Often multiple substrains containing overlapping introgressed segments are developed and, by comparing the BP in each substrain with that of the parental strain (which should be different if the QTL is still present in the substrain), the smallest interval containing the QTL is defined. Although the strategy is generally robust, difficulties of interpretation can arise if there are multiple QTLs in the targeted chromosomal interval, some with opposing effects harbored within the original segment (see above). However, the ultimate expectation is that the interval can be narrowed to a segment of approx 1 cM. Although subcentimorgan narrowing can be attempted (depending on the availability of polymorphic markers and an accurate genetic map), the process becomes more cumbersome because of the need to type increasingly larger numbers of animals to find suitable recombinants.

At this stage, identifying high-BP candidate genes located in QTLs refined by congenic analyses can occur in various ways. Candidates can be identified in rat gene maps constructed for the QTLs as well as in maps for the homologous chromosomal intervals in the human and mouse genomes (*18,19*). An alternative approach that is being increasingly utilized is to identify a likely tissue or organ (e.g., kidney) through which the QTL may manifest its effect and comparison gene-expression profiles in such a tissue between the congenic and parental strain. Any differentially expressed gene that also maps to the congenic interval would be a strong candidate. An advantage of the approach is that other differentially expressed genes, even if they do not map to the region, may play important downstream roles and allow pathophysiologic pathways to be defined. Finally, progress in sequencing of the rat genome may provide information on other potential candidates. In addition, improved comparative genome analysis between rat and human can be applied to the identification of short chromosomal intervals that can be analyzed for evidence of linkage and association with hypertension in appropriate family collections. Evidence of linkage between hypertension and human chromosome 17, in a region showing synteny conservation with rat chromosome 10 BP QTLs, is a clear demonstration of the potential application of rat BP QTL analysis to human essential hypertension (*20*).

3.9. Conclusions

The identification of BP QTLs in rat models is a tedious process involving sound phenotypic analysis and valid statistical support for the analysis of phenotypes and genotypes. At best, linkage analysis in a classical cross will identify QTLs spanning 20 to 30 cM regions, even when supported by high LOD-score values and dense maps. Data already obtained in congenic lines generally confirm QTL mapping data, although, for reasons discussed here, they do not prove that the phenotypic effect observed in congenic actually accounts for the effect detected in the cross. The emergence of new resources for genetic studies in the rat, including genomic libraries (*21,22*), gene maps (*18,19*), radiation hybrid maps (*18*), EST sequences (*23*), and rat genomic sequencing data, combined with modern high-throughput expression-profiling technologies will assist disease gene isolation in hypertensive rat models.

Multiple analyses of BP QTLs in experimental rat crosses have demonstrated the complexity of the genetic control of BP even in inbred models that are expected to facilitate the identification of susceptibility genes for human-complex disorders. Both resources for genomewide searches in rat crosses and statistical programs applied to QTL mapping in experimental crosses have progressed to increase the speed and efficiency of QTL detection and analysis. Consequently, the limiting step in quantitative genetics in high-BP rat models remains the extensive and accurate phenotype screening of large cohorts of hybrids. It is anticipated that BP QTL maps, which seem already thoroughly characterized in the rat, will progress in the future with the use of numerous and precise BP subphenotypes and related phenotypes based on the application of extensive physiological, biochemical, and histological analyses. Others panels of hybrid animals, such as advanced intercross lines (AIL; Chapter 8,

Subheading 2.4.3.) (*24*) and heterogeneous mouse stocks (Chapter 8, Subheading 2.4.4.) (*25*) may also provide additional information on BP QTL mapping in the future. Overall, QTL mapping studies in the rat will contribute to improving our knowledge of BP homeostasis and should provide new insights in the definition of novel disease pathways for drug development.

4. Software

4.1. SPSS

Many of the basic statistical analyses can be performed in standard statistical software packages, such as SPSS. SPSS 9.0 is available from http://www.spss.com/.

4.2. JoinMap 2.0

JoinMap™ version 2.0 was created in 1995 by Stam and Van Oijen (*5*). It is a registered trademark software which can be obtained from Johan W. Van Oijen (CPRO-DLO, P.O. Box 16, 6700 AA Wageningen, the Netherlands, e-mail: mapping@CPRO.DLO.NL). It operates on almost all computer systems, including PC/MSDOS, VAX/OpenVMS, Alpha/OpenVMS, SUN/SunOS, and Apple Macintosh. The software package comes with a licence file (joinmap.lic) that must not be altered, as the integrity of the file is verified by each JoinMap module. Instructions for the installation of the software in each platform are described in the tutorial. The analysis of data derived from other experimental crosses than F2 cross and first backcross as well as genotype data from codominant markers are described in the tutorial.

4.3. MAPMAKER/QTL

See Chapter 7, Table 1, for information on this program.

5. Worked Example

5.1. Experimental Cross and Phenotypes

The example chosen to illustrate the various aspects of QTL analysis described in this chapter is based on results from a SHR×WKY F2 cross that was derived by Samani (*13*). A total of 233 male hybrids were generated and indirect BP was measured in 12-, 16-, and 20-wk-old hybrids by tail plethysmography. Direct BP was measured in a subset of 193 hybrids at 25 wks of age, and systolic BP, diastolic BP, and heart rate were determined. At the end of the experiment, heart weight and ventricular mass were determined. Prior to genetic analysis, phenotypes measured in the hybrids were checked for Normal distribution using the SPSS software (**Table 3**). Phenotypes that failed to pass the Normal distribution test (RV, SBP2M, DBP2M, and PPMAP)

Table 3.
**Physiological Variables Measured in the SHR×WKY Cross, Test of
Normality for the Phenotypes, and Analysis of Correlations Between
Phenotypes**

	Phenotypes	Test of Normality (Kolmogorov–Smirnov)			Significant correlations ($p<0.001$)
		Statistic	df	Significance	
BPS16	Indirect BP (16 wk-old)	0.054	84	0.200	BPS18, 20, DBP/SBP, V, LV, MAP, PP
BPS18	Indirect BP (18 wk-old)	0.048	84	0.200	BPS16, 20, DBP/SBP, V, LV, MAP
BPS20	Indirect BP (20 wk-old)	0.073	84	0.200	BPS16, 18, DBP/SBP, V, LV, MAP
BW	Body weight	0.065	84	0.200	V, LV, RV
V	Total ventricular weight	0.055	84	0.200	BPS16, 18, BW, LV, RV, HR
LV	Left ventricular weight	0.045	84	0.200	BPS16, 18, 20, BW, V, RV, HR
RV	Right ventricular weight	0.154	84	**0.000**	BW, V, LV, HR
SBP	Direct systolic BP	0.092	84	**0.073**	BPS16, 18, 20, DBP, PP, MAP
DBP	Direct diastolic BP	0.099	84	**0.040**	BPS16, 18, 20, SBP, MAP, PPMAP
MAP	Mean arterial BP	0.080	84	0.200	BPS16, 18, 20, DBP/SBP, PP, PPMAP
HR	Mean heart rate	0.064	84	0.200	BW, V, LV, RV
PP	Pulse pressure	0.082	84	0.200	BPS16, SBP, MAP, PPMAP
PPMAP	Pulse pressure/mean blood pressure	0.109	84	**0.016**	DBP, PP, MAP

were adjusted prior to linkage analysis. Correlation tests between phenotypes
were carried out using the SPSS software (**Table 3**).

5.2. Genetic Mapping

A collection of markers showing allele variations between the colonies of
SHR and WKY used to derive the intercross were selected for the genomewide
search. Based on microsatellite markers, the overall polymorphism rate between
these strains was 50%. Genotypes of the hybrids were determined for a total
of 195 markers evenly spaced in the 20 rat autosomes (average spacing 8 cM

with no gap greater than 10 cM). Genetic maps were constructed using the JoinMap software and unlikely double recombinants were verified.

5.3. QTL Analysis

Linkage analysis between genetic markers and phenotypes was carried out with the MAPMAKER/QTL package. Among the BP QTLs identified in this intercross, loci mapped to chromosomes 1 and 13 illustrate the careful analysis that is required in interpreting results from genetic linkage analysis.

Chromosome 13 was the primary target of linkage analysis in the SHR×WKY cross because conflicting results from linkage analysis between BP and a region containing the Renin gene were obtained in various crosses (*1,6,8*). Surprisingly, in the SHR×WKY cross, strong evidence of genetic linkage between BP and a 50 cM region of rat chromosome 13 (maximum LOD score of 5.75) was found to be maximal in 20-wk-old animals and disappeared in 25-wk-old hybrids (**Fig. 1**). The existence of linkage with other loci in 12- to 25-wk-old animals ruled out the possibility of a bias in phenotype measurements. These observations emphasize the difficult interpretation of negative results (absence of genetic linkage in a cross or absence of significant phenotypic effects in congenics derived for a QTL), which may be the consequence of an age-dependent expression of the phenotype, as well as other factors, including cross or gender-specific effects. More sophisticated hypotheses involving epistatic and ecogenetic factors may also explain these controversial results.

A major QTL spanning 40 cM of rat chromosome 1 strongly influences blood pressure regulation in the SHR×WKY cross (maximum LOD>7 for marker D1Mit2 and D1Wox19) (**Fig. 2**). In first approximation, the localization of the QTL supports BP QTL mapping data obtained in other crosses and/or strains (*1,6*). A series of reciprocal congenic lines (WKY alleles at the locus introgressed onto a SHR genetic background and SHR alleles at the QTL onto a WKY background) were subsequently derived. Results from BP analysis in the congenics confirmed the existence of a gene or a group of linked genes controlling BP regardless of major influences from resistant/susceptible alleles in the genetic background. However, analysis of congenic sublines designed to further dissect the QTL in a region containing the SA gene demonstrated that the original QTL contains at least two genes independently regulating BP (*10*) (**Fig. 2**). This complex situation is consistent with results obtained by Rapp in congenic derived from the S rat, in which the original QTL mapped to chromosome 1 in an intercross can be dissected in at least three regions independently controlling BP (S1a, S1b, and S2) (*9*) (**Fig. 2**). By comparing the localization of the QTLs in the different series of congenics, it appears that intervals S2 and SHR1 and SHR2 contain hypertensive alleles are specific to the S and SHR strains, respectively. On the other hand, intervals S1a and S1b

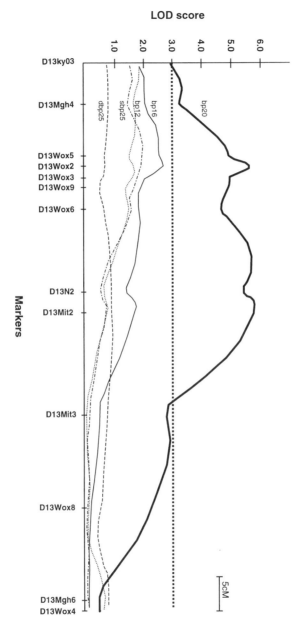

Fig. 1. BP QTL maps of rat chromosome 13 in the SHR×WKY intercross. Linkage analysis was performed using BP phenotypes measured in 12- (bp12), 16- (bp16), 20- (bp20), and 25 (sbp25 and dbp25)-wk-old hybrids. The horizontal dotted line indicates the threshold of significant linkage as calculated by Lander and Kruglyak (**7**) for an F2 cross.

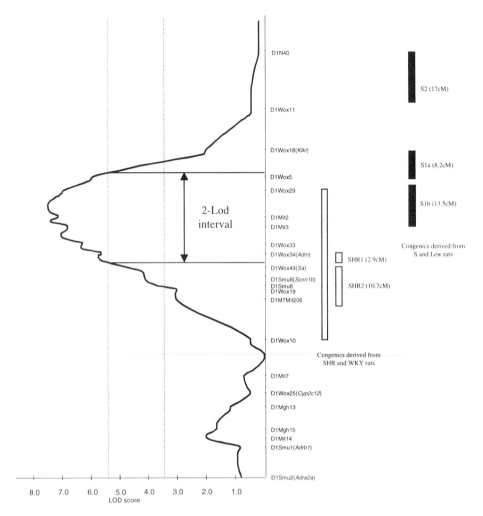

Fig. 2. BP QTL map of rat chromosome 1 in the SHR×WKY intercross and subsequent refinement of the QTL maps in reciprocal congenic lines derived from the SHR and WKY rats (congenic intervals SHR1 and SHR2). The horizontal dotted line indicates the threshold of significant linkage as calculated by Lander and Kruglyak (*7*) for an F2 cross. Intervals S1a, S1b and S2 refer to the approximate position of the chromosome 1 BP QTLs determined in congenic lines of the S rat (*9*).

correspond to regions of significant linkage in the SHR×WKY cross and the effect of a common gene on BP in the two strains cannot be excluded. A cluster of QTLs for BP-related phenotypes, including mean arterial pressure, ventricular mass, stroke, and renal failure have been localized in rat chromosome 1 within the region of significant linkage, with BP identified in the SHR and S rats. The genetic dissection of these QTLs and the extensive characterization of BP variables controlled by genes at these loci should provide important insights in the mechanisms involved in the development of hypertension and associated complications. Results from chromosome 1 BP QTL maps demonstrate that, even when a QTL is accurately mapped in a classical cross and supported by highly significant LOD scores, the susceptibility locus in unlikely to uncover the effect of a single gene in congenic lines. They also demonstrate that, in addition to possible influences of resistant and/or susceptible alleles throughout the genome on the detection of the original QTL, strains derived from different outbred stocks (e.g., SHR and S) are likely to carry different combinations of susceptibility alleles in similar chromosomal regions.

6. Note

1. Data repositories for rat genetic/genomic resources
   a. http://www.well.ox.ac.uk/rat_mapping_resources/. The Wellcome Trust Centre for Human Genetics, Oxford, UK. Microsatellite markers; linkage maps; radiation hybrid maps; physical mapping data; polymorphism information between strains; gene maps and comparative genome analysis based on linkage and/or radiation hybrid maps.
   b. http://ratmap.gen.gu.se/. Göteborg University, Sweden. Repository of gene, locus, and QTL maps. Comparative genome analysis.
   c. http://rgd.mcw.edu/. Medical College of Wisconsin, Madison, WI. Microsatellite markers; linkage maps; radiation hybrid maps; physical mapping data; polymorphism information between strains; EST mapping data.
   d. http://ratest.uiowa.edu/. University of Iowa, Ames, IA. EST sequencing and mapping.
   e. http://ratmap.ims.u-tokyo.ac.jp/. The Otsuka GEN Research Institute, Tokushima, Japan. Microsatellite markers; radiation hybrid maps.

Acknowledgments

Dominique Gauguier holds a Wellcome Trust Senior fellowship in basic biomedical science. We thank Dr. Gina Kearsey for her help with the analysis of QTL data. Work in the SHR is supported by the EURHYPGEN II concerted action of the European Community.

References

1. Rapp, J. P. (2000) Genetic analysis of inherited hypertension in the rat. *Physiol. Rev.* **80**, 135–172.
2. Pravenec, M., Klir, P., Kren, V., Zicha, J., and Kunes, J. (1989) An analysis of spontaneous hypertension in spontaneously hypertensive rats by means of new recombinant inbred strains. *J. Hypertens.* **7**, 217–222.

3. Bihoreau, M. T., Gauguier, D., Kato, N., Hyne, G., Lindpaintner, K., Rapp, J. P., et al. (1997) A linkage map of the rat genome derived from three F2 crosses. *Genome Res.* **7,** 434–440.

4. Stam, P. (1995) Construction of integrated genetic linkage maps by means of a computer package: JoinMap. *Plant J.* **5,** 739–744.

5. Stam, P. and Van Ooijen, J. W. (1995) *JoinMap ™ version 2.0: Software for the calculation of genetic linkage maps.* Centre for Plant Breeding and Reproduction Research, Wageningen, The Netherlands.

6. Stoll, M. and Jacob, H. J. (1999) Improved strategies for the mapping of quantitative trait loci in the rat model, in *Molecular Genetics of Hypertension* (Dominiczak, A. F., Connell, J. M. C., and Soubrier, F., eds.), Bios Scientific, Oxford, pp. 31–52.

7. Lander, E. S. and Kruglyak, L. (1995) Genetic dissection of complex traits: guidelines for interpreting and reporting linkage results. *Nature Genet.* **11,** 241–247.

8. St Lezin, E. M., Pravenec, M., Wong, A. L., Liu, W., Wang, N., Lu, S., et al. (1996) Effects of renin gene transfer on blood pressure and renin gene expression in a congenic strain of Dahl salt-resistant rats. *J. Clin. Invest.* **97,** 522–527.

9. Saad, Y., Garrett, M. R., and Rapp, J. (2001) Multiple blood pressure QTL on rat chromosome 1 defined by Dahl rat congenic strains. *Physiol. Genomics* **4,** 201–214.

10. Frantz, S., Clemitson, J., Bihoreau, M. T., Gauguier, D., and Samani, N. J. (2001) Genetic dissection of region around the Sa gene on rat chromosome 1: Evidence for multiple loci affecting blood pressure. *Hypertension,* **38,** 216–221.

11. Garrett, M. R., Dene, H., Walder, R., Zhang, Q. Y., Cicila, G. T., Assadnia, S., et al. (1998) Genome scan and congenic strains for blood pressure QTL using Dahl salt-sensitive rats. *Genome Res.* **8,** 711–723.

12. Rapp, J. P., Garrett, M. R., and Deng, A. Y. (1995) Construction of a double congenic strain to prove an epistatic interaction on blood pressure between rat chromosomes 2 and 10. *J. Clin. Invest.* **101,** 1591–1595.

13. Samani, N. J., Gauguier, D., Vincent, M., Kaiser, M. A., Bihoreau, M. T., Lodwick, D., et al. (1996) Analysis of quantitative trait loci for blood pressure on rat chromosomes 2 and 13: age-related differences in effect. *Hypertension* **28,** 1118–1122.

14. Rubattu, S., Volpe, M., Kreutz, R., Ganten, U., Ganten, D., and Lindpaintner, K. (1996) Chromosomal mapping of quantitative trait loci contributing to stroke in a rat model of complex human disease. *Nature Genet.* **13,** 429–434.

15. Jeffs, B., Clark, J. S., Anderson, N. H., Gratton, J., Brosnan, M. J., Gauguier, D., et al. (1997) Sensitivity to cerebral ischaemic insult in a rat model of stroke is determined by a single genetic locus. *Nature Genet.* **16,** 364–367.

16. Markel, P., Shu, P., Ebeling, C., Carlson, G. A., Nagle, D. L., Smutko, J. S., et al. (1997) Theoretical and empirical issues for marker-assisted breeding of congenic mouse strains. *Nature Genet.* **17,** 280–284.

17. Jeffs, B., Negrin, C. D., Graham, D., Clark, J. S., Anderson, N. H., Gauguier, D., et al. (2000) Applicability of a "speed" congenic strategy to dissect blood pressure quantitative trait loci on rat chromosome 2. *Hypertension* **35,** 179–187.

18. Watanabe, T. K., Bihoreau, M. T., McCarthy, L. C., Kiguwa, S. L., Hishigaki, H.,

Tsuji, A., et al. (1999) A radiation hybrid map of the rat genome containing 5,255 markers. *Nature Genet.* **22,** 27–36.

19. Kaisaki, P. J., Rouard, M., Danoy, P. A. C., Wallis, R. H., Collins, S. C., Rice, M., et al. (2000) Detailed comparative gene map of rat chromosome 1 with mouse and human genomes and physical mapping of an evolutionary chromosomal breakpoint. *Genomics* **64,** 32–43.

20. Julier, C., Delepine, M., Keavney, B., Terwilliger, J., Davis, S., Weeks, D. E., et al. (1997) Genetic susceptibility for human familial hypertension in a region of homology with blood pressure linkage on rat chromosome 10. *Hum. Mol. Genet.* **6,** 2077–2085.

21. Cai, L., Schalkwyk, L. C., Stehli, A. S., Zee, R. Y. L., Haaf, T., Georges, M., et al. (1997) Construction and characterization of a 10-genome equivalent yeast artificial chromosome library for the laboratory rat, *Rattus norvegicus. Genomics* **39,** 385–392.

22. Woon, P. Y., Osoegawa, K., Kaisaki, P., Zhao, B., Catanese, J., Gauguier, D., et al. (1998) Construction and characterization of a 10-fold genome equivalent rat P1-derived artificial chromosome library. *Genomics* **50,** 306–316.

23. Scheetz, T. E., Raymond, M. R., Nishimura, D. Y., McClain, A., Roberts, C., Birkett, C., et al. (2001) Generation of a high-density rat EST map. *Genome Res.* **11,** 497–502.

24. Darvasi, A. and Soller, M. (1995) Advanced intercross lines, an experimental population for fine genetic mapping. *Genetics* **141,** 1199–1207.

25. Talbot, C. J., Nicod, A., Cherny, S. S., Fulker, D. W., Collins, A. C., and Flint, J. (1999) High-resolution mapping of quantitative trait loci in outbred mice. *Nature Genet.* **21,** 305–308.

10

A Case Study of QTL Analysis in a Mouse Model of Asthma

Youming Zhang and William Cookson

1. Introduction

1.1. Background

Asthma is the most common childhood disease (*1*). It is characterized by inflammation of the small airways of the lung that produces intermittent narrowing of the respiratory bronchioles, airflow limitation, and the symptoms of wheezing, chest tightness, and breathlessness. The most common form is allergic asthma, also known as atopic asthma. The atopic state is distinguished by the strength of the immunoglobulin E (IgE) response to commonly inhaled proteins, known as allergens.

Asthma is a complex genetic disorder with a high population prevalence compared with other, Mendelian, pulmonary disorders such as cystic fibrosis. The complex inheritance of asthma suggests oligogenic inheritance and genetic heterogeneity (*2*). Asthma is also described as "multifactorial" because it is determined by the interaction between major and minor genes and involves important nongenetic factors such as the environment. Genes that influence atopy and asthma can be detected most simply by testing for associations with particular polymorphisms of candidate genes in samples of affected and unaffected individuals. The candidate approach is limited by the number of known genes with roles in the pathophysiology of atopy and asthma. A second approach to gene identification, known as "positional cloning," relies on the localization of disease genes to a particular chromosomal segment by genetic linkage. Genome-wide screens using linkage analysis in humans have identified several loci with potential linkage to asthma or asthma-associated traits, such as the total serum IgE concentration, allergen skin test responses, eosinophil

From: *Methods in Molecular Biology: vol. 195: Quantitative Trait Loci: Methods and Protocols.*
Edited by: N. J. Camp and A. Cox © Humana Press, Inc., Totowa, NJ

count in blood, and bronchial hyperresponsiveness (BHR) (*3–6*). The direct candidate approach and genome screens have revealed potential roles for various genes (for both asthma and atopy) in a number of regions; most notably in the 11q13, 5q31–33, 6p31–33, 12q14.3–q24.1, 13q14, and 14q11.2–13 regions in humans (*7*). Bronchial hyperresponsiveness of the airways to a wide range of different stimuli is an important feature of asthma. These stimuli include allergens, smoking, air pollution, and infections. The degree of sensitivity of the airway to various stimuli can be quantified by measuring the concentration of a nonspecific bronchoconstrictor, usually histamine or methacoline, necessary to cause a 20% fall in the FEV1 (forced expiratory volume in 1 s). This is termed the provocative concentration that causes a 20% fall (Pc20). BHR may also be represented as the provocative dose of spasmogen that produces a 20% fall in FEV1 (PD20) or as the slope between the initial FEV1 and the FEV1 following the last dose of spasmogen.

Bronchial hyperresponsiveness is clearly associated with airway inflammation and there is increasing evidence that in asthma, BHR may be the result of thickening of the bronchial wall. The presence of BHR is suggestive of ongoing airway inflammation and may be an independent predictor of the development of overt clinical asthma (*8*). In the general population, there is a normal distribution in the dose-response slope to bronchoconstrictors. This is generally regarded as suggestive of a polygenic pattern of inheritance, although a single gene with variable penetrance could also be consistent with a normally distributed phenotype.

1.2. The Use of Animal Models

The use of animal models of disease has proved useful in the study of the biochemistry, physiology, and pharmacology of asthma. A large degree of syntenic homology exists between mouse and human chromosomes (*9*). Mice can reproduce the features of human diseases spontaneously and large numbers of offspring can be used for genetic studies. Inbred strains provide a homogenous genetic background in which to study disease phenotypes. Environmental effects can be controlled or reduced by maintaining all experimental mice in the same living conditions.

Bronchial hyperresponsiveness is one of the most studied quantitative traits underlying asthma. Continuous variation in the expression of the trait can be the result of both genetic and nongenetic factors. Nongenetic factors can be either environmental or random variation. In mice, it is relatively straightforward to separate genetic from nongenetic contributions through the analysis and comparison of animals within and between inbred strains. If individual members of an inbred strain are maintained under identical environmental conditions, then the existing variation is likely to be the result of chance alone.

A major advance in the genetics of complex traits was the development of statistical methods that take account of the fact that multiple genes make different quantitative contributions to the phenotype. Quantitative trait locus (QTL) mapping has now become commonplace and has accelerated the analysis of polygenic susceptibility to various diseases (*10*). The development of comprehensive chromosomal maps of microsatellites and SNPs has made it possible to carry out mapping studies for quantitative traits such as BHR.

Bronchial hyperresponsiveness is the most often studied phenotype in mouse models of asthma. A/J mice are consistently hyperresponsive to cholinergic challenge and have been extensively studied. One segregation and linkage analysis indicated that a major locus on chromosome 6 acting additively with a polygenic effect segregates with airway press–time index (APTI) (the measure of BHR used in this study) in the progeny of hyperresponsive A/J and hyporesponsive C3H/HeJ mice (*11*). The chromosome region contains the candidate gene interleukin-5 (IL-5) receptor. A genome screen of the progeny of a cross between the A/J strain and C57BL/6J mice found that BHR failed to segregate as a Mendelian trait (*12*). However, the results showed significant linkage at two loci, Bhr1 (log odds [LOD] = 3.0) and Bhr2 (LOD = 3.7) on chromosomes 2 and 15, respectively. A third locus, Bhr3 (LOD = 2.83), mapped to chromosome 17. In a BN × LEW rat cross, a region on rat chromosome 10 containing the candidate genes IL-4 and IL-13 has been found to show linkage with serum IgE levels (*13*). The results of these studies are summarized in **Table 1.**

1.3. Strategy Used for This Study

BP2 mice, "Bon Producteurs 2," are derived from Biozzi mice. Biozzi mice have been produced by repeated assortative mating from a population of outbred albino mice. Biozzi mice have two extreme phenotypes: one is a high-antibody production line and the other is a low-antibody production line (*14,15*). Several quantitative trait loci contributing to extreme phenotypes of the selected high (H) and low (L) antibody-responder lines of mice have been mapped to mouse chromosomes 6, 8, 12, and 17 (*16,17*).

BP2 higher-responder mice were bred by bidirectional selection for antibody responsiveness (agglutinin titres) to sheep erythrocytes. They have been shown to be homozygous for that character in F14–F17 generations (*18,19*). BP2 mice have subsequently been shown to provide a good model of human asthma, following presensitization and inhalation of ovalbumin (OA) (*20*).

In our studies, we have crossed BP2 mice with BALB/c mice. The BP2 strain differs from BALB/c in at least four ways: (1) The first and essential difference is that BP2 mice display BHR following antigenic challenges; (2) BP2 mice show very high levels of serum IgE, which doubles after immunization, whereas the BALB/c mice have a considerably lower amount, which, as

Table 1
Linkage Results for Asthma-Associated Quantitative Traits in Rodent Genome Screens

Animal	Breeding	No. of animals	No. of markers	Quantitative traits	Results	Ref.
Mouse	(C3H/HeJ × A/J)F1 × A/J	196	94	APTI (BHR)	Chromosome 6 (LOD = 3.1)	11
Mouse	(C57BL/6J × A/J)F1 × C57BL/6J	321	157	ED_{200} (R_L) (BHR)	Chromosome 2 (LOD = 3.0) Chromosome 15 (LOD = 3.7) Chromosome 17 (LOD = 2.83)	12
Rat	(LEW × BN)F1 × F1	186	8 (chromosome 10)	IgE	Chromosome 10 ($p = 0.0002$)	13

expected, also augments upon immunization; (3) BP2 mice undergo an intense anaphylactic bronchoconstriction when challenged with iv OA, whereas the BALB/c mice are unresponsive; (4) eosinophils may be identified in the bronchiolar epithelium of BP2 mice after challenge, but are absent in BALB/c mice (**21**). Our mapping strategy was based on an intercross between BP2 and BALB/ c. The use of intercross breeding need not assume any genetic model of BHR and, thus, an intercross has two main advantages over a backcross. First, it can be used to map loci defined by recessive deleterious mutations, which cannot be detected in a backcross. The second advantage is a consequence of the occurrence of informative meiotic events in both parents. This will lead to twice as much recombination information per animal compared to the backcross. However, the data obtained from intercross breeding are more complex and more difficult to analyze because of the impossibility of determining which allele at each heterozygous F2 locus came from which parent (**22**).

2. Methods

2.1. Mouse Breeding and Crossing Strategies

Bronchial responsiveness (BHR: expressed as ΔP_{enh}, defined in **Subheading 2.2**) was measured in 18 BP2 mice, 18 BALB/c mice, 27 F1s (generated by BALB/c × BP2), and 10 F1s (generated by BP2 × BALB/c). Female BP2 and male BP2 had no significant difference in the trait ΔP_{enh} (data not shown). Two hundred nineteen F2 animals were used in the genome screen and were generated from a BALB/c (M) × BP2 (F) intercross. All of the mice were provided by the Centre d'Elevage R. Janvier (Le Genest Saint-Isle, France). The F2 generation contained 110 males and 109 females. Two male mice died during the allergen challenge and were excluded from the study. The mice were 6 wk old at the beginning of experiment.

2.2. Mouse Immunization and Provocation Procedure

The mice were immunized subscutaneously with 0.4 mL immunization solution (containing 100 µg OA) when they were 6 wk old (day 1). On day 8, the mice were immunized again with 0.4 mL immunization solution. On d 15 and 16, the mice were twice challenged intranasally under light ether anesthesia with 50 µL provocation solution (containing 10µg OA). On d 17, mouse bronchial responsiveness to methacholine was evaluated in a plethysmographic chamber to analyze their respiratory waveforms. After a few minutes for stabilization (during which at least five values had been obtained), an aerosol of methacholine was delivered for 20 s. The airway resistance was expressed as P_{enh} (enhanced pause) calculated as follows:

$$P_{enh} = 0.67[(0.4T_r/T_e) - 1] (P_{ef}/P_{if}) \tag{1}$$

Table 2
Statistics for $\sqrt{\Delta P_{enh}}$ (Square Root Transformed) in Nonsegregating and Segregating Generation

$\sqrt{\Delta P_{enh}}$	BALB/c	BP2	BALB/c × BP2	BP2 × BALB/c	F2
Mean	0.941	1.783	1.186	1.134	1.372
Variance	0.046	0.173	0.074	0.073	0.159
SE	0.051	0.098	0.052	0.085	0.027
N	18	18	27	10	217

where T_e is the expiratory time, T_r is the relaxation time, P_{ef} is the peak expiratory flow, and P_{if} is the peak inspiratory flow.

To calculate the ΔP_{enh} (difference between the basal and maximal value; the basal value was measured in the stabilization period and the maximum value was measured after methacholine administration), an average of five maximal values was used. A higher ΔP_{enh} means that the airway resistance is higher and so the mouse has a higher airway reactivity. A square root transformation was applied to the ΔP_{enh} to normalize the data. The results of ΔP_{enh} measurements in nonsegregating and segregating generations are listed in **Table 2.**

2.3. Mouse DNA Extraction and Genotype Generation

Mouse DNA was extracted from tails using a salting-out method (**23**). Forward primers for most polymerase chain reactions (PCRs) were labeled with either 6-FAM, HEX, or TAMRA fluorescent dyes (Oswel DNA, Edinburgh; Pekin-Elmer, UK). The PCR of mouse microsatellite loci was performed in 25-mL reactions containing (1) 50 ng genomic DNA, (2) 67 mM Tris-HCl, pH 8.8, 16.6 mM $(NH_4)SO_2$, 0.1% Tween-20 (Bioline, UK), (3) 0.2 mM each of dATP, dTTP, dCTP, and dGTP, (4) 62.5 ng of each primer used, and (5) 0.3 U of BIOTAQ polymerase (Bioline, UK) overlaid with 50 μL mineral oil. Reactions were performed in Hybaid Omnigene™ thermocyclers by use of 32 successive cycles, each cycle consisting of (1) 60 s at 94°C, followed by (2) 60 s at 45–60°C, and then (3) 30 s at 72°C. TaqGold can be used instead of BIOTAQ, in which case PCR was begun at 94°C for 8 min (hot start).

In order to reduce the cost of experiments we used [F]dNTP instead of fluorescent primers to differentiate between BALB/c and BP2 alleles. Like other nucleotides, [F]dNTPs can be incorporated into both strands of a PCR amplification at random dC and dT sites and extended by DNA polymerase. The [F]dNTPs consist of either a 2′-deoxyuridine 5′-triphosphate (dUTP) or a 2′-deoxycytidine 5′-triphosphate (dCTP) coupled to one of the following rhodamine dyes: [R110], [R6G], and [TAMRA]. [F]dNTPs PCR was only used to test marker polymorphism between BLAB/c and BP2. Markers were organized into different sets according to the sizes of the products of the PCR and labeled primers. PCR products from the sets were pooled before electrophoresis and analyzed on an ABI 373 automated sequencer. An internal lane size standard was used in each run for calculation of the size of allele peaks using Genescan™ software and calling of alleles using Genotyper™.

The whole mouse genome is estimated to be 1360.9 cM in length. The rate of polymorphism in microsatellites between two lab strains usually approximates 50% (*24*). We tested 507 microsatellites covering the entire mouse genome in order to find markers that were polymorphic between BALB/c and BP2 strains. A total of 245 markers (48%) showed a difference of allelic sizes between two strains (**Table 3**). These markers covered 1260.3 cM of the mouse genome (calculated from our F2 data).

2.4. First Stage of Genome Screen

2.4.1. Genotype Checking and Generation of the Marker Map Using JoinMap

A total of 122 polymorphic markers were used for the first stage of the whole-genome screen. These markers covered the whole genome at approximately 10 to 15 cM intervals. After the generation of the phenotype and genotype data, the genotype data were checked and the marker map generated using the program JoinMap. This process is illustrated in the worked example (**Subheading 5.1.**) and also discussed in Chapter 9, Subheading 2.5.

2.4.2. QTL Mapping Using MAPMAKER/QTL

MAPMAKER/QTL was used to test for additive and dominance effects for each marker; this is also illustrated in the worked example (**Subheading 5.2**) and this software is discussed in relation to other available softwares in Chapter 7. The positive linkage results are listed in **Table 4** (*p* values less than 0.05 and their likelihood ratio statistics (LRSs) and corresponding LOD scores are shown).

2.5. Saturation Mapping

Several potential loci that influenced the asthma-associated quantitative traits were located from the first stage of the genome screen. High-resolution mapping to narrow down the map interval was then carried out by selecting and typing additional microsatellite markers across 20 cM of the regions of interest. A total of 58 new polymorphic markers were used in saturation mapping around loci, showing linkages to ΔP_{enh} on chromosome 9, 10, 11, and 17. After all

Table 3
Marker Polymorphism Rates Between BALB/c and BP2 Strains

Chromosome	Markers tested	Polymorphic markers	Percentage	Markers used in genome screen	Length (cM)
1	40	22	55	17	92.3
2	35	18	51	13	105.2
3	26	9	35	7	58.6
4	16	13	81	7	71
5	17	9	53	7	77.3
6	11	9	82	6	72.7
7	20	12	60	6	63.5
8	27	13	48	9	64
9	50	18	36	13	67.7
10	49	20	41	13	62.1
11	51	28	55	24	74.4
12	14	8	57	6	55.6
13	18	8	44	5	53.8
14	23	8	35	5	37.7
15	11	6	55	5	53.9
16	17	7	41	5	53.3
17	44	20	45	17	51.3
18	11	7	64	6	55.3
19	13	5	38	5	52.1
x	14	5	36	4	38.5
Total	507	245	48	180	1260.3

genotypes were obtained, the data were analyzed for linkage. The positive linkage results to BHR from the genome screen, and the human chromosomal regions of syntenic homology are shown in **Table 5.**

2.5.1. Permutation Tests Using Map Manager QT

The permutation test is a method of establishing the significance of the LRSs generated by the interval mapping procedures. The permutation test was needed to provide genome-wide thresholds for suggestive, significant, and highly significant evidence for linkage in this study. The trait values are randomly permuted among the progeny, destroying any relationship between the trait values and the genotypes of the marker loci. The regression models are fitted for the permuted data and the LRS is recorded. This procedure is repeated hundreds or thousands of times, giving a distribution of statistical values that we would be expected if no QTL was linked to any of the marker loci. The critical values

Table 4
Results of the First Stage of Genome Screening of Quantitative Trait
$\sqrt{\Delta P_{enh}}$

Loci	Position (cM)	p Value	LRSs	LOD
D3Mit82	48.6	0.02	7.4	1.60
D4Mit59	71	0.03	6.9	1.50
D7Mit14	63.5	0.03	6.5	1.41
D9Nds6	14.7	0.04	6.1	1.32
D9Mit48	22.9	0.002	11.8	2.56
D10Nds1	0	0.004	11.4	2.47
D10Mit2	5.4	0.04	6.1	1.32
D10Mit91	36.2	0.01	8.8	1.91
D10Mit70	48.5	0.0006	14.8	3.21
D10Mit14	57.3	0.0003	16.2	3.51
D11Mit131	27.7	0.03	6.6	1.43
D11Nds1	39.9	0.0001	16.8	3.65
D11Nds5	57.6	0.0003	15.8	3.42
D17Mit60	5.3	0.031	6.9	1.50
D17Mit34	9.7	0.007	9.7	2.10

were calculated by this test using whole genome markers sets. One thousand permutations were calculated by the Map Manager QTb21 program. The results of the permutation tests are listed in **Table 6.** The threshold values of the permutation test, which was labeled suggestive, significant, and highly significant, correspond to the genomewide probabilities proposed by Lander and Kruglyak (**27**).

3. Interpretation

3.1. Phenotype Data from the Cross

The BP2 and BALB/c strains had overlapping but significantly different distributions of ΔP_{enh} (**Table 2**). The mean ΔP_{enh} in the F1 mice was significantly lower than the average of that of the two parents, indicating overall partial dominance for low ΔP_{enh}. The F2 mean was not significantly different from the average of the two parents.

3.2. Potential QTL

Potential QTL effects that controlled ΔP_{enh} were found on chromosomes 9 (LOD score 2.5), 10 (LOD score 3.8), 11 (LOD score 3.65), and 17 (LOD score 2.1); see **Table 5.** According to published criteria for interpreting the

Table 5
QTL Mapping Results of $\sqrt{\Delta P_{\text{enh}}}$ and the Human Chromosome Syntenic Homology

Chromosome	QTL position	±	m	a	d	d/a	LOD	LRS	%var_exp	Regions of human syntenic homology/candidate genes
9	18	10	1.300	-0.105	0.022	-0.210	2.5	11.5	5.2	Chromosome 11q23: IL10R
10	44	7	1.380	-0.220	0.116	-0.530	3.8	17.5	8.3	Chromosome 12q22–q24
11	52	7	1.372	0.146	0.097	0.664	3.65	16.8	7.5	Chromosome 17: inos, eotaxin
17	10	4	1.370	0	-0.155	11.9	2.1	9.7	4.4	Chromosome 6: MHC, TNF

Note: m, mean; *a*, additive effect; *d*, dominance ratio; LOD, LOD score; LRS, likelihood ratio statistics; %var_exp, percentage explained. The trait was square root transformed before analysis. The QTL positions, *m*, *a*, *d*, and *d/a* were given by the Marker Regression Program (**25,26**).

Table 6
Results of the Permutation Test

Trait	Suggestive LRS (LOD)	Significant LRS (LOD)	Highly significant LRS (LOD)
$\sqrt{\Delta P_{\text{erh}}}$	10.3 (2.23)	16.5 (3.58)	22.8 (4.95)

Note: Suggestive LRS corresponded to the 37th percentiles of genomewide probabilities. Significant LRS corresponded to the 95th percentiles of genome-wide probabilities. Highly significant corresponded to the 99.9th percentiles of genomewide probabilities (*37*).

significance of linkages in genomewide searches (**27**) and our permutation test results (**Table 6**), the chromosome 9 and 17 signals would be classified as "suggestive" and linkages to chromosome 10 and chromosome 11 as "significant." Together, the loci explained 25.4% of the phenotypic variance of ΔP_{enh} in the F2 mice (**Table 5**).

ΔP_{enh} was decreased by the BP2 allele on chromosomes 9 and 10, and increased by that allele on chromosome 11. Interpretation of the QTL effect on chromosome 17 was not straightforward, although the LOD score for this QTL was only 2.1. The additive effect (*a*) of the QTL on chromosome 17 was close to zero, and the dominance effect (*d*) was relatively large, leading to a dominance ratio (*d/a*) more than 10 (*see* **Table 5**). Such a situation may arise from two closely linked QTLs, with similar additive effects in opposite directions, but each showing dominance in the same direction. In other words, if a_1 and a_2 are the additive effects of loci 1 and 2 and d_1 and d_2 are the dominance effects, $a_1 + a_2$ is small (since a_1 and a_2 are similar in magnitude but opposite in sign), but $d_1 + d_2$ is large (because both are positive). Therefore, the results suggested that the QTL effect on chromosome 17 comprised more than one QTL. The region contains the major histocompatibility complex (MHC), which holds many genes that may influence immunologically mediated traits.

3.3. Relevance to Studies of Human Disease

Several of the potential linkages may be relevant to human loci linked to asthma-associated traits. The chromosome 10 ΔP_{enh} QTL shows syntenic homology with human chromosome 12q21.1–12q24.22. This region has previously been shown to be linked to human asthma-associated traits in several studies (**28,29**). It contains the important candidate gene interferon-γ. The chromosome 11 ΔP_{enh} QTL shows syntenic homology to human chromosome 17, which has been implicated in previous human linkage studies of asthma

(*5*). The region contains a cluster of chemokine genes that are involved in many inflammatory pathways. One of these, eotaxin, is a chemokine that acts as a potent inducer of eosinophil migration (*30*). The region also contains the important candidate inducible nitric oxide synthase (iNOS). The suggestive linkage of ΔP_{enh} to mouse chromosome 17 supports the previous study of De Sanctis et al. (**12**), who showed the region to be linked to spontaneous bronchial responsiveness in an AJ × C57/B6 cross. This region contains the MHC and tumor necrosis factor (TNF) genes, which may have diverse effects on antigen recognition and the promotion of airway inflammation. The MHC and TNF genes have also been implicated in gold salt-induced IgE nephropathy in a BN × LEW rat cross (**13**). In humans, class II human leukocyte antigen (HLA) genes are known to restrict the ability to react to particular allergens (*31,32*), and polymorphisms within TNF genes have been associated with asthma independently of class II effects (*33*). The suggestion that two or more loci are acting within this QTL in our murine model is, therefore, consistent with the observations in humans.

Although the BP2 mouse does show many features that typify human asthma, the induction of florid changes by intraperitoneal injection and inhalation of OA does not match the events that produce human disease. It should not be assumed, therefore, that either the pathophysiological or genetic mechanisms producing changes in airway histology or responsiveness are the same in mice and human. Nevertheless, the presence of loci that are potentially shared between our murine model and human families segregating asthma suggests that underlying genetic factors may also be shared to some extent. The sharing of loci between different mouse models of BHR may also aid in the dissection of the complex genetics underlying asthma.

4. Software

4.1. JoinMap

The JoinMap program is a software package program for linkage analysis and genetic mapping that was written by Piet Stam and Johan W. van Ooijien. The program can be run on UNIX-based workstations or VAX under the VMS operating system. They can be contacted either by e-mail (mapping@ CPRO.DLO.NL), fax (+313 174 16513), or mail: (CPRO-DLO, POBox 16, 6700 AA Wageningen, the Netherlands).

4.2. MAPMAKER/QTL

MAPMAKER/QTL is a pedigree-based program written by Dr. Eric Lander and his colleagues for constructing linkage maps from raw genotyping and phenotyping data recovered from large numbers of loci. The program uses a highly efficient algorithm for "likelihood of linkage" computations. It can be run on UNIX-based workstations or VAX minicomputers running under the VMS operating system. The program and a manual are available from the author for licensing to academic researchers. MAPMAKER/QTL can be used of the analysis of quantitative traits. For further information, contact Dr. Eric Lander, Whitehead Institute, 9 Cambridge Center, Cambridge, MA 02142, USA. The website is http://www-genome.wi.mit.edu/genome_software/genome_software_index.html.

4.3. Map Manager QT

The Map Manager QT program was written by Dr. Kenneth F. Manly and is made available without charge from the author. Dr. Manley can be contacted at his E-mail address (Kmanly@mchio.med.buffalo.edu) or at Roswell Park Cancer Institute, Buffalo, New York 14263, USA.

5. Worked Example

5.1. Generation of the Marker Map Using JoinMap

The JoinMap program (*34*) was used to check the genotypes and generate the linkage map. This process is outlined in more detail in Chapter 9, Subheading 2.5. The relevant files for the example described in this chapter, using the data from chromosome 10, are shown here.

5.1.1. Phenotypic Data Preparation

All values of the trait ΔP_{enh} are listed in **Table 7.** Missing values are indicated by a "–".

5.1.2. Preparation of loc.file

When the genotype data of the 219 F2 mice were generated by the Genotyper program (*see* **Subheading 2.3**), homozygosity for the BP2 allele was defined as "a," homozygosity for the BALB/c allele as "b," and heterozygosity for the BP2 allele and BALB/c allele as "h."

Unread genotypes were recorded as "–." The genotype data of the first four markers of chromosome 10 are listed in the correct format in **Table 8,** "chr10.loc." See Chapter 9, subheadings 2.5.1.–2.5.3. for how to generate this chromosome-specific file.loc file from other data formats. The order of markers used was according to published results (*24*).

5.1.3. Estimating Recombination and Constructing a Linkage Map Using JMREC and JMMAP

This is one of the core tasks in which the JoinMap program is used. The JoinMap recombination estimation module (JMREC) calculates estimates of

Table 7
The Phenotype $\sqrt{\Delta P_{enh}}$ Data of 219 F2 Mice

Penh

3.752	2.908	1.258	2.986	1.246	3.268	1.854	2.244	—	1.794
5.826	1.730	1.770	2.172	1.566	3.884	2.272	2.096	4.864	3.804
2.936	2.596	3.684	1.056	2.056	1.050	1.504	1.814	1.632	1.188
2.686	3.850	0.180	4.022	1.470	1.548	2.064	3.230	1.976	3.059
1.148	3.020	6.326	1.268	3.028	3.698	3.844	2.016	0.874	2.224
1.616	0.416	3.746	1.644	7.256	0.896	1.402	2.582	1.568	2.676
2.490	2.460	1.302	3.442	1.384	1.152	1.848	1.644	0.706	2.240
0.966	1.250	0.702	0.524	1.918	3.984	2.266	1.296	1.042	1.792
1.612	1.154	1.410	1.958	4.994	4.484	3.330	1.220	2.670	—
0.968	2.620	1.938	0.740	0.816	0.174	2.644	3.490	0.422	7.268
1.650	1.420	2.858	1.394	0.890	1.596	2.020	2.024	2.252	1.452
3.192	3.620	2.104	3.740	1.388	1.560	1.678	2.586	0.392	1.268
2.434	1.082	2.020	0.822	1.926	3.886	4.146	1.182	3.183	0.636
2.456	0.920	1.156	1.980	1.594	1.524	1.139	0.946	0.936	1.462
2.202	1.904	0.542	1.444	1.78	1.314	0.998	1.154	1.476	1.396
2.396	1.616	1.078	1.090	1.596	0.222	1.832	0.498	0.692	3.854
2.816	2.900	1.884	1.968	2.730	1.098	2.084	1.546	0.150	1.032
2.326	2.030	0.790	2.254	1.65	1.196	2.418	1.340	1.652	3.328
1.774	0.906	3.962	1.272	1.928	0.824	2.744	2.664	2.052	3.998
1.350	0.408	1.602	2.350	1.63	1.616	1.705	1.182	3.270	2.386
1.514	1.266	2.318	4.090	2.382	2.326	2.144	1.960	1.794	1.980
0.540	0.766	1.638	2.952	1.602	0.328	2.520	2.278	3.296	

recombination frequency from the raw data in a locus genotype file (e.g., chr10.loc; **Table 8**). The parameters used by JMREC are listed in **Table 9**. The output of JMREC is a simple list of pairwise recombination estimates, together with their marker–marker LOD scores: a so-called pairwise data file (pwd-file). The JoinMap map construction module (JMMAP) produces a linkage map from the pwd-file. Part of the pwd-file is shown in **Table 10**.

5.1.4. Checking the Genotypes in the Raw Data

The JoinMap genotype checking module (JMCHK) provides the opportunity to verify, after a map is calculated, whether the population contains very improbable genotypes such as those originating from double recombinations. It calculates for all loci and for all individuals the probability of obtaining the present genotype, conditional on each genotype at the two flanking loci and on their recombination frequency. It takes the chr10.loc file as input, and outputs a chr10.chk file (shown in **Table 11**). We considered problematic

Table 8
Loc.file of Genotypes of Mouse Markers on Chromosome 10

```
Chr10.loc
name = chromosome 10
popt = F2
nloc = 13
nind = 219
d10nds1
   aahha hahhh hhhha hhhba hhhha hhhhb ahbhh haahh ahaba bhahb
   hbhba hhhba abbab bbhhh bhhba bahb- bahba haaha hhhba abhbb
   hhbhb babha ahaba hhaba hhahh hbbah ahhah hbbhb hhah- hbbab
   bahbh bahhb aaahb bahhh aabhb hhhba hbahh ahhbh bbahh ha-h-
   abbah hbhbh b-hhh bhbh
d10mit2
   aahha hahhh hbhha hhhba hhhha hhhhb abbhh hhhhh ababa bhhhb
   hhhbh hhhba abhab bbhhh bhhba baabh ba-bh haaha hhhba abhbb
   hhbhb babba ababa hhaba hhahh hbbhh hhbah hbbhb hhaha hbbah
   bahbh bahhb ahahb hahhh ahbhb bhhba abaah ahhbh bbahh haahh
   abbah hbhbh baahh bhhh
d10mit36
   hahhh babhh hbahh hhhbh hhhha hhhhb hbhhh hbhhh abhbh hhhhb
   ahhbh hhhba abhbb bbhhb bhhbh bhabh ha-bh hahhh bhhba abahb
   h-bhh habbh hhaba bhbbh hhahb hbbhh hhhah bbhhh hhaha hhhah
   bahbh hhaab ahahb habhh hbhhh bbhba ahaah ahbbb bbaah hhaah
   abhhh hbbbh baahh bahh
d10mit113
   hhaah babab hbahh hhhhh hhhha hhhah hbhhh abhab abbbh hhhhb
   ahhhh hhahh abhbb bbhab bhhbh bhabh haabh hahhh bbhba abahb
   hhhhh habbh hhaba hhbhh hhahb hbahh hhhah bbahh hhaha hhhah
   bahba hhaab ahahb habhb hbhaa hbbba ahhhh abhhb bhaah hhaab
   abhhh hbbbh bhahh babh
```

Note: a: homozygotes of BP2 allele; h = heterozygotes; b: homozygotes of BALB/c allele.

genotypes to be those having a threshold of greater than 3 for the test statistic $\log_{10}(1/p)$. Problematic genotypes can be checked in original genotype results and subsequently removed from any further analyses if still problematic after the check.

5.1.5. Checking the Distribution of the Genotype Frequencies of Loci

The JoinMap single-locus analysis module (JMSLA) determines the frequency distribution of the numbers of informative loci and performs a chi-

Table 9
JMREC Parameters for Chromosome 10

Response file	y.rsp
Data taken from	chr10.pwd
LOD threshold for mapping	0.0010
REC threshold for mapping	0.4990
Jump threshold	4.0000
Triplet threshold	10.0000
Mapping function	KOSAMBI
Ripple value	3
No. of genes	13
No. of pairs	78
No. of linkage groups	1 (based on LOD = 1.0 and REC = 0.45)

square goodness-of-fit test for the expected segregation ratios. Genotypes of "a," "h," and "b" in the F2 should be present in roughly the ratio of 1:2:1, so if the marker segregation ratio was distorted in distribution, the genotypes were rechecked. This module takes as input the chr10.loc file and outputs chr10.sla. The results for the chromosome 10 loci are shown in **Table 12.** In this table, "c" refers to the genotype either homozygote "b" or heterozygote "h," "d" refers to the genotype either homozygote "a" or heterozygote "h."

5.1.6. Constructing the final marker map

Having corrected genotypes when necessary in the ".loc" file, the map was constructed anew (as in **Subheading 5.1.2.**) and tested again for distorted segregation ratios and unexplained double-recombination events. These cycles of checking and mapping were repeated until problematical genotypes and markers were either corrected or eliminated from the analysis. The final order of markers and pairwise recombination frequencies were verified against existing maps. Linear map distances were established using the Kosambi mapping function. The final chromosome 10 linkage map is shown in **Table 13.**

5.2. Application of the MAPMAKER/QTL Program

The MAPMAKER/QTL program was used to check the phenotype distribution and carry out linkage analysis (*35*). The use of this program is described in more detail in Chapter 7, Subheading 5.3.1. Before running MAPMAKER/QTL, a raw data file should be set up to include all of the genotype and phenotype data from each linkage group, which will usually correspond to data from one chromosome. For our data, the phenotypes are given in **Table 7** and the genotypes in **Table 8.** These data are included in the chr10.raw file (*see*

Table 10
Part of the pwd-file of Chromosome 10 (chr10.ptd)

```
; data taken from chr10.loc
; LOD-threshold:  0.0010
; REC-threshold:  0.4990
name = chromosome10
d10nds1 d10mit2      0.0529    62.2508
d10nds1 d10mit36     0.2106    18.5558
d10nds1 d10mit113    0.2987     7.4102
d10nds1 d10mit91     0.3303     4.4882
d10nds1 d10mit134    0.4145     0.5860
d10nds1 d10mit70     0.4098     0.6844
d10nds1 d10mit150    0.4146     0.7132
d10nds1 d10mit267    0.4854     0.1338
d10nds1 d10mit14     0.4801     0.1661
d10nds1 d10mit25     0.4848     0.1902
d10nds1 d10mit145    0.4949     0.1202
d10nds1 d10mit103    0.4942     0.3946
d10mit2 d10mit36     0.1497    30.0925
d10mit2 d10mit113    0.2480    12.5741
d10mit2 d10mit91     0.2818     7.9436
d10mit2 d10mit134    0.3787     1.0825
d10mit2 d10mit70     0.3754     1.2361
d10mit2 d10mit150    0.3828     1.0562
d10mit2 d10mit267    0.4619     0.0121
d10mit2 d10mit14     0.4516     0.0553
d10mit2 d10mit25     0.4604     0.0299
d10mit2 d10mit145    0.4699     0.0143
d10mit2 d10mit103    0.4607     0.1408
```

Table 14 for example). A chr10.prep file is set up using the mapping information obtained from JoinMap (data shown in **Table 13**). The example of the output generated from running MAPMAKER/QTL for the chromosome 10 data is given in **Table 15.** In this table, POS indicates positions relative to the flanking markers. On the right-hand side, the distance between the neighboring markers are shown in cM. WEIGHT is the additive effect which can have direction, DOM is the dominance deviation, and LOG-LIKE is the LOD score. In this table, there is evidence of a QTL between markers 5 and 13. The "show peak" command reveals that the peak of linkage for this QTL was detected between markers 8 and 9, exactly 5 cM from marker 8. The command "sequence [8–9: try]" instructs the program to perform the scan four times, once with each of

Table 11
Checking Results of Chromosome 10 Genotypes (chr10.chk)

```
JoinMap genotype Checking module 2.0/a
locus genotype file:        chr10.loc
population name:            chromosome10
population type:            F2
number of individuals:      219
number of loci:             13
map file:                   chr10.map
number of linkage groups:   1
analysing linkage groups:   1
list of genotype data with log(1/p) values > 2.0:
```

(log(1/p) is minus the 10-log of the probability of a genotype, conditional
   on the genotype of the neighboring loci and conditional on the map)

log(1/p) values: * > 3 ** > 4 *** > 5 **** > 6 ***** > 7

ind	previous locus	locus	next locus	log(1/p)
linkage group nr. 1 ((bottom up)):				
9	h: d10mit36	a: d10mit113	h: d10mit91	2.032
174	h: d10mit36	a: d10mit113	h: d10mit91	2.032
178	h: di0mit36	b: di0mit113	h: d10mit91	2.032
161	h: d10mit145	b: d10mit103	-	2.227

top 5% (=1) loci with high average (over n cases) log(1/p):

locus	log(1/p)	n
d10nds1	0.165	214

top 5% (=11) individuals (ind) with high average (over n cases) log(1/p):

ind	log(1/p)	n
161	0.268	12
174	0.257	13
178	0.235	13
9	0.235	13
70	0.234	13
133	0.232	13
176	0.227	11
162	0.206	13
55	0.206	13
213	0.198	13
28	0.185	13

Table 12
Checking Results of the Frequency Distribution of Chromosome 10 Loci (chr10.sla)

```
JoinMap Single Locus Analysis 2.0/a
locus genotype file:   chr10.loc
population name:       chromosome10
population type:       F2
number of loci:         13
number of individuals: 219
significance levels:  *:0.1  **:0.05  ***:0.01  ****:0.005  *****:0.001
******:0.0005  *******:0.0001
frequency distributions per locus  (13 loci):
```

	a	h	b	c	d	-	X2	(df):signif.	[classes]
1:d10nds1	55	100	59	0	0	5	1.07	(2):	[a:h:b]
2:d10mit2	53	105	60	0	0	1	0.74	(2):	[a:h:b]
3:d10mit36	41	118	58	0	0	2	4.33	(2):	[a:h:b]
4:d10mit113	50	114	55	0	0	0	0.60	(2):	[a:h:b]
5:d10mit91	49	116	50	0	0	4	1.35	(2):	[a:h:b]
6:d10mit70	50	119	48	0	0	2	2.07	(2):	[a:h:b]
7:d10mit134	51	119	47	0	0	2	2.18	(2):	[a:h:b]
8:d10mit150	52	118	49	0	0	0	1.40	(2):	[a:h:b]
9:d10mit267	49	119	51	0	0	0	1.68	(2):	[a:h:b]
10:d10mit14	47	119	51	0	0	2	2.18	(2):	[a:h:b]
11:d10mit25	48	119	52	0	0	0	1.79	(2):	[a:h:b]
12:d10mit145	46	120	52	0	0	1	2:55	(2):	[a:h:b]
13:d10mit103	42	115	52	0	0	10	3:07	(2):	[a:h:b]

```
frequency distribution of numbers of informative plants
in pairwise combinations of loci  (78 pairs):

informative  freq
-----------  ----
    0 -    9     0
   10 -   19     0
   20 -   29     0
   30 -   39     0
   40 -   49     0
   50 -   59     0
   60 -   69     0
   70 -   79     0
   80 -   89     0
   90 -   99     0
  100 -  109     0
  110 -  119     0
  120 -  129     0
  130 -  139     0
  140 -  149     0
  150 -  159     0
  160 -  169     0
  170 -  179     0
  180 -  189     0
  190 -  199     0
  200 -  209    12
  210 -  219    66
```

Table 13
Linkage Map of Chromosome 10 (cM) (chr10.map)

d10nds1	0.0
d10mit2	5.4
d10mit36	21.9
d10mit113	30.8
d10mit91	36.2
d10mit70	48.5
d10mit134	48.5
d10mit150	50.2
d10mit267	57.3
d10mit14	57.3
d10mit25	58.8
d10mit145	61.5
d10mit103	62.1

Table 14
Part of the chr10.raw File (chr10.raw)

```
data type f2 intercross
219 13 6
*d10nds1
  aahha hahhh hhhha hhhba hhhha hhhhb ahbhh haahh ahaba bhahb
  hhhba hhhba abbab bbhhh bhhba bahb- bahba haaha hhhba abhbb
  hhbhb babha ahaba hhaba hhahh hbbah ahhah hbbhb hhah- hbbab
  bahhh bahhb aaahb bahhh aabhb hhhba hbahh ahhbh bbahh ha-h-
  abbah hhhhh b-hhh bhhb
*d10mit2
  aahha hahhh hbhha hhhba hhhha hhhhb abbhh hhhhh ababa hhhhb
  hbhbh hhhba abhab bbhhh bhhba baabh ba-bh haaha hhhba abhbb
  hhbhb babba ahaba hhaba hhahh hbbhh hhbah hbbhb hhaha hbbah
  bahbh bahhb ahahb hahhh ahbhb bhhba abaah ahhbh bbahh haahh
  abbah hbhbh baahh bhhh
*d10mit36
  hahhh babhh hbahh hhhbh hhhha hhhhb hbhhh hbhhh abhbh hhhhb
  ahhbh hhhba ahhhb bbhhb bhhbh bhabh ha-bh hahhh bhhba abahb
  h-bhh habbh hhaba bhbbh hhahb hbbhh hhhah bbhhh hhaha hhhah
  bahbh hhaab ahahb habhh hbhhh bbhba ahaah ahbbb bbaah hhaah
  abhhh hbbbh baahh bahh
....
*Penh
3.752 2.908 1.258 2.986 1.246 3.268 1.854 2.244 - 1.794 5.826...
```

Table 15
MAPMAKER/QTL Outfile of Chromosome 10 Analyses

```
************************************************************************
*                                                                    *
*                          MAPMAKER/QTL                              *
*                          (version 1.1b)                            *
*                                                                    *
************************************************************************

'photo' is on: file is 'chn10.out'
3> sequence [all]
The sequence is now '[all]'
4> trait 4
The current trait is now: 4 (sgrphen)
5> scan 1 2 0.125
QTL maps for trait 4 (sgrphen):
Sequence: [all]
LOD threshold: 2.00    Scale: 0.12 per '*'
NO fixed-QTLs.
Scanned QTL genetics are free.

POS    WEIGHT    DOM     %VAR   LOG-LIKE |
-------------------------------------------| 1-2 5.6 cM
0.0    -0.114    0.019   4.4%    2.139   | **
1.0    -0.109    0.029   4.2%    1.947   |
2.0    -0.103    0.041   3.8%    1.763   |
3.0    -0.094    0.055   3.5%    1.599   |
4.0    -0.085    0.068   3.2%    1.465   |
5.0    -0.074    0.079   2.9%    1.362   |
-------------------------------------------| 2-3 17.8 cM
0.0    -0.068    0.084   2.7%    1.310   |
1.0    -0.065    0.086   2.7%    1.210   |
2.0    -0.061    0.088   2.6%    1.109   |
3.0    -0.056    0.090   2.4%    1.007   |
4.0    -0.051    0.092   2.3%    0.906   |
5.0    -0.046    0.092   2.1%    0.807   |
6.0    -0.040    0.092   2.0%    0.710   |
7.0    -0.034    0.091   1.8%    0.617   |
8.0    -0.028    0.089   1.6%    0.529   |
9.0    -0.021    0.085   1.4%    0.447   |
10.0   -0.014    0.081   1.1%    0.374   |
11.0   -0.007    0.076   1.0%    0.312   |
12.0    0.000    0.071   0.8%    0.262   |
13.0    0.007    0.065   0.7%    0.225   |
14.0    0.013    0.058   0.5%    0.203   |
15.0    0.020    0.052   0.5%    0.196   |
16.0    0.026    0.046   0.5%    0.202   |
17.0    0.032    0.041   0.5%    0.220   |
```

continued

Table 15.
Continued

POS	WEIGHT	DOM	%VAR	LOG-LIKE	
					3-4 9.9 cM
0.0	0.036	0.037	0.5%	0.244	
1.0	0.041	0.035	0.6%	0.279	
2.0	0.046	0.033	0.7%	0.321	
3.0	0.051	0.030	0.8%	0.370	
4.0	0.056	0.027	1.0%	0.427	
5.0	0.061	0.023	1.1%	0.489	
6.0	0.065	0.020	1.3%	0.555	
7.0	0.069	0.017	1.4%	0.624	
8.0	0.071	0.015	1.5%	0.693	
9.0	0.074	0.013	1.6%	0.760	
					4-5 5.7 cM
0.0	0.075	0.012	1.7%	0.818	
1.0	0.085	0.018	2.2%	1.005	
2.0	0.093	0.024	2.7%	1.203	
3.0	0.100	0.028	3.1%	1.402	
4.0	0.106	0.032	3.5%	1.596	
5.0	0.110	0.035	3.8%	1.781	
					5-6 13.4 cM
0.0	0.112	0.037	4.0%	1.904	
1.0	0.118	0.041	4.4%	2.038	*
2.0	0.123	0.045	4.8%	2.174	**
3.0	0.128	0.049	5.2%	2.310	***
4.0	0.132	0.054	5.6%	2.444	****
5.0	0.135	0.059	6.0%	2.574	*****
6.0	0.137	0.065	6.3%	2.700	******
7.0	0.139	0.070	6.5%	2.820	*******
8.0	0.140	0.076	6.8%	2.934	********
9.0	0.140	0.081	6.9%	3.039	*********
10.0	0.140	0.086	7.0%	3.136	**********
11.0	0.139	0.090	7.1%	3.223	**********
12.0	0.138	0.094	7.1%	3.300	***********
13.0	0.136	0.096	7.0%	3.365	***********
					6-7 0.0 cM
0.0	0.135	0.097	6.9%	3.387	************
					7-8 1.6 cM
0.0	0.135	0.097	6.9%	3.387	************
1.0	0.141	0.083	7.0%	3.382	************
					8-9 7.4 cM
0.0	0.140	0.077	6.8%	3.336	**********
1.0	0.145	0.086	7.4%	3.491	************
2.0	0.148	0.093	7.8%	3.624	*************
3.0	0.150	0.098	8.2%	3.729	**************
4.0	0.151	0.103	8.3%	3.802	***************
5.0	0.151	0.107	8.4%	3.840	***************
6.0	0.149	0.108	8.3%	3.837	***************
7.0	0.146	0.107	7.9%	3.782	***************

continued

Table 15.
Continued

```
POS      WEIGHT   DOM     %VAR    LOG-LIKE |
---------------------------------------| 9-10 0.0 cM
0.0      0.143    0.105   7.6%    3.742  | **************
---------------------------------------| 10-11 1.4 cM
0.0      0.143    0.105   7.6%    3.741  | **************
1.0      0.140    0.092   7.0%    3.261  | ***********
---------------------------------------| 11-12 2.6 cM
0.0      0.134    0.076   6.0%    2.920  | ********
1.0      0.133    0.080   6.0%    2.887  | ********
2.0      0.131    0.084   5.9%    2.846  | *******
---------------------------------------| 12-13 0.5 cM
0.0      0.129    0.086   5.8%    2.816  | *******
---------------------------------------|
```

Results have been stored as scan number 1.
6> show peak
LOD score peaks for scan 1.1 of trait 4 (sgrphen).
Sequence: [all]
No fixed-QTLs.
Scanned QTL genetics are free.

Peak Threshold: 2.00 Falloff: −2.00
```
================================================================
```
QTL-Map for peak 1:
Confidence Interval: Left Boundary= 5-6 + 0.0
                       Right Boundary= 12-13 (off end)
```
INTERVAL    LENGTH   QTL-POS   GENETICS    WEIGHT   DOMINANCE
8-9          7.4      5.0       free        0.1509   0.1065
```
chi∧2= 17.685 (2 D.F.)   log-likelihood= 3.84
mean= 1.163   sigma∧2= 0.145   variance−explained= 8.4 %
```
================================================================
```
7> sequence [8-9:try]
The sequence is now '[8-9:try]'
8> map
```
================================================================
```
QTL map for trait 4 (sgrphen):
```
INTERVAL    LENGTH   QTL-POS   GENETICS    WEIGHT   DOMINANCE
8-9          7.4      4.7       free        0.1512   0.1058
```
chi∧2= 17.655 (2 D.F.)   log-likelihood= 3.83
mean= 1.163   sigma∧2= 0.145   variance−explained= 8.4 %
```
================================================================
```
QTL map for trait 4 (sgrphen):
```
INTERVAL    LENGTH   QTL-POS   GENETICS    WEIGHT   DOMINANCE
8-9          7.4      5.0       dominant    0.1359   0.1359
```
chi∧2= 17.258 (2 D.F.)   log-likelihood= 3.75
mean= 1.162   sigma∧2= 0.145   variance−explained= 8.2 %
```
================================================================
```

continued

Table 15.
Continued

```
QTL map for trait 4 (sgrphen):
INTERVAL   LENGTH   QTL-POS   GENETICS    WEIGHT   DOMINANCE
8-9          7.4      3.6      recessive   0.0660   -0.0660
chi^2= 3.939   (2  D.F.)        log-likelihood= 0.86
mean= 1.341   sigma^2= 0.155    variance-explained= 2.0 %
============================================================
QTL map for trait 4 (sgrphen):
INTERVAL   LENGTH   QTL-POS   GENETICS    WEIGHT   DOMINANCE
8-9          7.4      3.7      additive    0.1513   0.0000
chi^2= 14.042 (2 D.F.)         log-likelihood= 3.05
mean= 1.220   sigma^2= 0.148    variance-explained= 6.7%
============================================================
9>q
save data before quitting? (yes) y
Now saving chn10.qtls...
Now saving chn10.traits...
...goodbye...
```

four genetic models; free, additive, dominant, and recessive. The free model fits separate regression coefficients for additive and dominance components, allowing these coefficients to have any values. The additive model fits a single coefficient for the additive component, forcing the dominant component to be 0. The dominant model fits a single coefficient that is used for both additive and dominant components. The recessive model fits a single coefficient that is used for both additive and dominance components, but with an opposite sign for each. The results of these four analyses are shown in the lower part of **Table 15** and indicate that the QTL on mouse chromosome 10 controlling BHR is a dominant effect.

6. Notes

1. Comparison of MAPMAKER/QTL and Map Manager QT. Both MAPMAKER/QTL and Map Manager can carry out data transformation, QTL detection, and genetic model analysis. MAPMAKER/QTL can give more details of the QTL's localization, but the Map Manager program can provide the strain distribution patterns obtained from each chromosome (data not shown), and like the MAPMAKER/QTL program, it can rapidly determine likely map positions relative to other loci in the database and can also give linkage results in LRS format. (The LRS can be converted to the conventional base-10 LOD score by dividing it by 4.61 [twice the natural logarithm of 10]). In addition, MapManager QT can be used to perform the permutation test. Map Manager QT is only available for the Macintosh platform, whereas MAPMAKER/QTL is available for other platforms.

Acknowledgments

The study was supported by the Wellcome Trust. We are grateful to Professor B. Boris Vargaftig and Jean Lefort in Pasteur Institute for phenotypic studies, to Dr. Virginia Kearsey for statistical advice, and to Dr. Denise Mouton for sharing her expertise with the Biozzi BP2 mice.

References

1. Strachan, D. P., Anderson, H. R., Limb, E. S., O'Neill, A., and Wells, N. (1994) A national survey of asthma prevalence, severity, and treatment in Great Britain. *Arch. Dis. Child.* **70,** 174–178.
2. Cookson, W. (1999) The alliance of genes and environment in asthma and allergy. *Nature* **402 (6760 Suppl.),** B5–B11.
3. Cookson, W. O. C. M., Sharp, P. A., Faux, J. A., and Hopkin, J. M. (1989) Linkage between immunoglobin E responses underlying asthma and rhinitis and chromosome 11q. *Lancet* **i,** 1292–1295.
4. Daniels, S. E., Bhattacharyya, S., James A., Leaves, N. I., Young, A., Hill, M. R., et al. (1996) A genome-wide search for quantitative trait loci underlying asthma. *Nature* **383,** 247–250.
5. CSGA (The Collaborative Study on the Genetics of Asthma) (1997) A genome-wide seat for asthma susceptibility loci in ethnically diverse populations. *Nature Genet.* **46,** 159–162.
6. Ober, C., Cox, N. J., Abney, M., Di Rienzo, A., Lander, E. S., Changyaleket, B., et al. (1998) Genome-wide search for asthma susceptibility loci in a founder population. *Hum. Mol. Genet.* **7,** 1391–1398.
7. Holgate, S. T. (1997) Asthma genetics: waiting to exhale. *Nature Genet.* **15,** 227–229.
8. Anto, J. M. (1998) Methods to assess and quantify BHR (bronchial hyperresponsiveness) in epidemiological studies. *Clin. Exp. Allergy* **28(S1),** 13–14.
9. DeBry, R. W. and Seldin, M. F. (1996) Human/mouse homology relationships. *Genomics* **33,** 337–351.
10. Paterson, A. H., Lander, E. S., Hewitt, J. D., Peterson, S., Lincoln, S. E., and Tanksley, S. D. (1998) Resolution of quantitative traits into Mendelian factors by using a complete linkage map of restriction fragment length polymorphisms. *Nature* **335,** 721–726.
11. Ewart, S. L., Mitzner, W., DiSilvestre, D. A., Meyers, D. A., and Levitt, R. C. (1996) Airway hyperresponsiveness to acetylcholine: segregation analysis and evidence for linkage to murine chromosome 6. *Am. J. Respir. Cell Mol. Biol.* **14,** 487–495.
12. De Sanctis, G. T., Merchant, M., Beier, D. R., Dredge, R. D., Grobholz, J. K., Martin, T. R., et al. (1995) Quantitative locus analysis of airway hyperresponsiveness in allergic airway hyperresponsiveness in A/J and C57BL/6J mice. *Nature Genet.* **11,** 150–154.
13. Kermarrec, N., Dubay, C., De Gouyon, B., Blanpied, C., Gauguier, D., Gillespie,

K., et al. (1996) Serum IgE concentration and other immune manifestations of treatment with gold salts are linked to the MHC and IL4 regions in the rat. *Genomics* **31**, 111–114.

14. Biozzi G., Stiffel, C., Mouton, D., Bouthillier, Y., and Decreusefond, C. (1972) Cytodynamic of the immune response in two lines of mice enetically selected for "high" or "low" antibody synthesis. *J. Exp. Med.* **135**, 1071–1094.

15. Biozzi, G., Mouton, D., Heumann, A. M., Bouthillier, Y., Stiffel, C., and Mevel, J. C. (1979) Genetic analysis of antibody responsiveness to sheep erythrocytes in crosses between lines of mice selected for high or low antibody synthesis. *Immunology* **36**, 427–438.

16. Puel, A., Mevel, J. C., Bouthillier, Y., Decreusefond, C., Fridman, W. H., Feingold, N., et al. (1998) Identification of two quantitative trait loci involved in antibody production on mouse. *Immunogenetics* **47**, 326–331.

17. Puel, A., Groot, P. C., Lathrop, M. G., Demant, P., and Mouton, D. (1995) Mapping of genes controlling quantitative antibody production in Biozzi mice. *J. Immunol.* **154**, 5799–5809.

18. Mouton, D., Siqueira, M., Sant'Anna, O. A., Bouthillier, Y., Ibanez, O., Ferreira, V. C., et al. (1988) Genetic regulation of multispecific antibody response: improvement of "high" and "low" characters. *Eur. J. Immunol.* **18**, 41–49.

19. Frangoulis, B., Mouton, D., Sant'Anna, O. A., Vidard, L., and Pla, M. (1990) H-2 typing of mice genetically selected for high and low antibody production. *Immunogenetics* **31**, 389–392.

20. Eum, S. Y., Haile, S., Lefort, J., Huerre, M., and Vargaftig, B. B. (1995) Eosinophil recruitment into the respiratory epithelium following antigenic challenge in hyper-IgE mice is accompanied by interleukin 5-dependent bronchial hyperresponsiveness. *Proc. Natl. Acad. Sci. USA* **92**, 12,290–12,294.

21. Vargaftig, B. B. Modifications of experimental bronchopulmonary hyperresponsiveness. *Am. J. Respir. Crit. Care Med.* **156**, s97–s102.

22. Silver, L. M. (ed.) (1995) *Mouse Genetics.* Oxford University Press, Oxford.

23. Miller, S. A., Dykes, D. D., and Polesky, H. F. (1988) A simple salting out procedure for extracting DNA from human nucleated cells. *Nucleic Acids Res.* **16**, 1215.

24. Dietrich, W. F., Miller, J., Steen, R., Merchant, M. A., Damron, Boles, D., et al. (1996) A comprehensive genetic map of the mouse genome. *Nature* **380**, 149–152.

25. Kearsey, M. J. and Hyne, V. (1994) QTL analysis: a simple "marker regression" approach. *Theor. Appl. Genet.* **89**, 698–702.

26. Kearsey, M. J. and Pooni, H. S. (1996) *The Genetical Analysis of Quantitative Traits.* Chapman & Hall, London.

27. Lander, E. and Kruglyak, L. (1995) Genetic dissection of complex traits: guidelines for interpreting and reporting linkage results. *Nature Genet.* **11**, 241–247.

28. Barnes, K. C., Neely, J. D., Duffy, D. L., Friedhoff, L. R., Breazeale, D. R., Schou, C., et al. (1996) Linkage of asthma and total serum IgE concentration to markers on chromosome 12q: evidence from Afro-Carribean and Caucasian. *Genomics* **37**, 41–50.

29. Nickel, R., Wahn, U., Hizawa, N., Maestri, N., Duffy, D. L., Barnes, K. C., et al. (1997) Evidence for linkage of chromosome 12q15–q24.1 markers to high total serum IgE concentrations in children of the German multicenter allergy study. *Genomics* **46,** 159–162.

30. Humbles, A. A., Conroy, D. M., Marleau, S., Rankin, S. M., Palframan, R. T., Proudfoot, A. E., et al. (1997) Kinetics of eotaxin generation and its relationship to eosinophil accumulation in allergic airways disease: analysis in a guinea pig model *in vivo. J. Exp. Med.* **186,** 601–612.

31. Levine, B. B., Stember, R. H., and Fotino, M. (1972) Ragweed hayfever: genetic control and linkage to HLA haplotypes. *Science* **178,** 1201–1203.

32. Young R. P., Dekker, J. W., Wordsworth, B. P., Schou, C., Pile, K. D., Matthiesen, F., et al. (1994) HLA-DR and HLA-DP genotypes and immunoglobulin E responses to common major allergens. *Clin Exp. Allergy* **24,** 431–439.

33. Moffatt, M. F. and Cookson, W. O. C. M. (1997) Tumour necrosis factor haplotypes and asthma. *Hum. Mol. Genet.* **6,** 551–554.

34. Stam, P. (1995) Construction of integrated genetic linkage maps by means of a computer package: Joinmap. *Plant J.* **5,** 739–774.

35. Lincoln, S., Daly, M., and Lander, E. (1992). Mapping genes controlling quantitative traits with Mapmaker/QTL 1.1. Whitehead Institute Technical report. 2nd ed.

36. Manly, K. F. (1993) A Macintosh program for storage and analysis of experimental genetic mapping data. *Mammal. Genome* **4,** 303–313.

37. Manly, K. F. (1998) User's Manual for Map Manager Classic and Map Manager QT. http://mcbio.med.buffalo.edu/MMM/MMM.html.

38. Manly, K. F. and Olson, J. M. (1999) Overview of QTL mapping software and introduction to Map Manager QT. *Mammal. Genome* **10,** 327–334.

III

MAPPING QUANTITATIVE TRAIT LOCI IN AGRICULTURAL SETTINGS

11

QTL Analysis in Plants

Shizhong Xu

1. Introduction

Quantitative traits are defined as traits that have a continuous phenotypic distribution (*1,2*). Variances of these traits are often controlled by the segregation of many loci, called quantitative trait loci (QTL). Therefore, quantitative traits are often synonymously called polygenic traits. Another characteristic of quantitative traits is that environmental variates can play a large role in determining the phenotypic variance. The polygenic nature and the ability of being modified by the environment make the study of genetic basis for quantitative traits more difficult than that for monogenic traits. Traditional methods of quantitative genetics that use only the phenotypic and pedigree information cannot separate the effects of individual loci but examine the collective effect of all QTL. With the rapid development of molecular technology, a large number of molecular markers (DNA variants) can be generated with ease. Most molecular markers are functionally neutral, but they normally obey the laws of Mendelian inheritance. Therefore, the relative positions of the markers along the genome (called the marker map) can be reconstructed using observed recombinant events. The joint segregating patterns of markers, in conjunction with phenotypic and pedigree information, provides additional information about the genetic basis of quantitative traits, including the number and chromosomal locations of QTL, the mode of gene action, and sizes (effects) of individual QTL. A complete description of the properties of QTL is called the genetic architecture. The study of the genetic architecture of quantitative traits using molecular markers is called QTL mapping.

Plants are ideal organisms for QTL analysis. Many plant species are self-compatible, which enables the generation of inbred lines quickly by recurrent

From: *Methods in Molecular Biology: vol. 195: Quantitative Trait Loci: Methods and Protocols.*
Edited by: N. J. Camp and A. Cox © Humana Press, Inc., Totowa, NJ

selfing. Crosses between inbred lines can be used for QTL analysis. For mapping purposes, inbred line crosses have the fewest complications. The progeny from such crosses display maximum disequilibrium. Using F_1 parents, a variety of populations, such as backcross (BC) and F_2, can be generated for mapping. We can control the mating designs with arbitrary complexity (e.g., diallel crosses) to maximize the interactions between founder alleles (3). We can deliberately choose fewer founders and increase family sizes so that each founder allele or allelic combination is well represented in the progeny. We can even take advantage of cloning and vegetative reproduction to obtain repeated measurements for each genotype. These unique properties possessed by plants provide a unique opportunity to detect additional QTL effects (e.g., dominance and epistatic effects), in addition to additive effects. In contrast, human geneticists cannot enjoy these luxuries as we plant people do.

There are numerous statistical methods and programs available for QTL mapping. The simplest and quickest one is the least square (LS) method (4,5). However, regression mapping is an *ad hoc* approach because it fails to take into account the heterogeneity of the residual variance (6). The iteratively reweighted least square (IRWLS) method (7,8) has corrected this defect in LS mapping but still ignores the mixture distribution of the residual error. Maximum likelihood (ML) mapping, developed by Lander and Botstein (9) and improved by Jansen (10), Zeng (11), and others, fully takes into consideration the mixture distribution of the residual error and thus is optimal. However, ML is computationally more intensive than LS and IRWLS. Therefore, LS and IRWLS are still commonly used in QTL mapping. Recently, Bayesian methodology has become popular because of the availability of simulation-based Markov chain Monte Carlo (MCMC) algorithms. Bayesian mapping was initiated by Hoeschele and VanRaden (12,13) and subsequently developed by Satagopan et al. (14) and Sillanpää and Arjas (15,16). Recently, Yi and Xu (17,18) extended the Bayesian methodology to map QTL for complicated binary traits. Bayesian mapping allows the use of prior knowledge of QTL parameters. Because Bayesian mapping provides a posterior distribution of QTL parameters, one automatically obtains the posterior variances and credibility intervals for the estimated QTL parameters. One of the major hurdles of ML mapping is finding the number of QTL. This involves a change in the dimensionality of the model. The recently developed reversible jump MCMC algorithm (19,20) allows the number of QTL to change in a convenient and objective way. This has revolutionized QTL mapping studies. Previous works of Bayesian mapping are primarily focused on simple line crosses. The work presented in this study intends to develop a Bayesian mapping for complicated mating designs involving multiple lines, as commonly seen in commercial stocks of plant breeding.

2. Methods

2.1. Data Preparation

Data required for QTL mapping include (1) phenotypic values of all individuals in the mapping population, (2) pedigree relationships among the individuals, and (3) marker genotypes.

2.1.1. Distributional Requirements

Because the Bayesian method is highly model dependent, we must make an assumption about the probability distribution of the phenotypic values. The Normal distribution is usually assumed, but other types of distribution can also be used. If the distribution severely deviates from Normality, one should perform a transformation to make it Normal before data analysis. For example, if the phenotypic value y is measured in ratio, the angular $y' = \sin^{-1}\sqrt{y}$ transformation is recommended (*21*). If the phenotypic distribution shows a scale effect (i.e., the standard deviation proportional to the mean), a logarithm transformation is desirable. Note that by Normal distribution we mean that the phenotypic distribution conditional on the genotypic value (i.e., the distribution of the residual error) is Normal. The usual way of diagnosing Normality by looking at the frequency histogram of phenotypic values is not valid because that distribution is actually the distribution of the sum of the genetic effect and residual error. If the trait is controlled by a few QTL with large effects, we expect the phenotypic distribution to deviate from Normality. Therefore, a skewed and multimode phenotypic distribution does not justify the transformation. Some characters have a binary or categorical phenotypic distribution but with a polygenic genetic background (i.e., disease resistant/susceptible). The phenotypic measurements of such discrete characters may be coded as numerals. Instead of transforming the phenotypic values to make them Normal, we should choose Bernoulli or multinomial distribution (*22–24*).

2.1.2. Pedigree Structure

Knowledge of pedigree relationships is essential in QTL mapping because without a family structure, it is not possible to construct any sort of genetic model (*25*). A line cross (e.g., backcross [BC]) is a simple pedigree because all of the progeny in the BC family are full sibs, resulting from the mating of a homozygous parent with its hybrid offspring. For multiple line crosses, the relationships of individuals become complicated. A special format is required to input the pedigree data. First, individuals are classified into founders and nonfounders. A founder in a pedigree is defined as an individual whose parents are not identified. A nonfounder is an individual whose both parents are identified and included in the pedigree. To identify the pedigree relationships, three

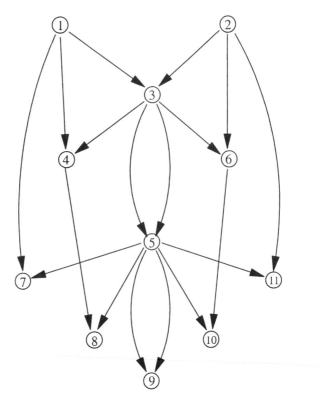

Fig. 1. A path diagram illustrating a complex pedigree with 11 individuals.

identifications (IDs) are required for each individual: the ID of the individual itself, the ID of its father, and the ID of its mother. The ID numbers of the parents for a founder should be treated as missing values (__; *see* **Table 1**). In many software packages, the records of individuals are assumed to be entered into the data sheet in a chronological order. In other words, the parents must be entered into the data sheet before their children or, equivalently, that the ID number of a parent must be smaller than those of its children (*see* **Note 1**).

Let us use the small pedigree shown as a path diagram in **Fig. 1** as an example to illustrate the required format of data entry. Individuals 1 and 2 are the founders of the pedigree. The cross of 1 and 2 produces 3, a hybrid. This hybrid individual is then crossed back to each founder and produces two BC-like individuals, 4 and 6. In the meantime, 3 is selfed to generate 5, an F_2-like individual. The relationships among the remaining plants in the pedigree are similarly traced by the path diagram (**Fig. 1**). We assume that the plant is hermaphroditic, so that an individual can serve as both male and female. Records of the 11 plants are entered into the data sheet in a chronological way as shown

Table 1
Format for Data Input, Example for the Small Pedigree Shown in Fig. 1

Individual ID	Father ID	Mother ID	Phenotype	Marker 1		Marker 2		Marker 3	
				P[a]	M[a]	P	M	P	M
1	—	—	y_1	1	1	2	1	1	2
2	—	—	y_2	2	3	3	3	1	3
3	1	2	y_3	1	2	2	3	2	1
4	1	3	y_4	1	1	1	2	1	1
5	3	3	y_5	2	2	2	3	1	2
6	2	3	y_6	3	1	3	3	3	1
7	1	5	y_7	1	2	1	2	1	2
8	4	5	y_8	1	2	1	2	1	1
9	5	5	y_9	2	2	2	2	2	2
10	5	6	y_{10}	2	3	3	3	1	3
11	2	5	y_{11}	2	2	2	3	3	2

[a]P and M stand for paternal and maternal alleles, respectively. However, if this is not known, the alleles can be entered arbitrarily.

in **Table 1.** The first three columns of Table 1 store the ID of individual plant, the father ID, and the mother ID, respectively. The phenotypic values are entered in the fourth column. The last three columns store the genotypes of three markers.

2.1.3. Marker Data

The third source of data is the array of marker genotypes for all individuals in the pedigree. In contrast to the traditional way of coding genotypic data in plants, we code the genotype by recording the two allelic forms. In the traditional coding system, the three genotypes in a F_2 family, A_1A_1, A_1A_2, and A_2A_2, may be coded as 0, 1, and 2, respectively. In the current system, we assign a unique number to each allele, such as allele A_1 is assigned value 2. Therefore, the three genotypes can now be coded as four allele-pairings: (1 1), (1 2), (2 1), and (2 2). The first number in each genotype represents the paternal allele and the second represents the maternal allele. When the genotype is unordered (phase unknown), the two alleles can be arbitrarily assigned. A missing allele should be assigned a special numerical value, such as 0 or 9.

2.1.4. The Marker Map

In addition to marker genotypes, we assume that the marker map is given or inferred using an existing mapping program [e.g., MAPMAKER (*26*) and JOINMAP (*27*)].

2.2. Linear Model

2.2.1. Single QTL Model

Let $n/2$ be the number of founders in the mapping population so that the total number of founder alleles at any locus is n. In plants, a founder can be an inbred line, which only carries one allelic form. If all the $n/2$ founders are inbred, the total number of different alleles is $n/2$. Let us use a single QTL as an example to demonstrate the derivation of the linear model. Multiple QTL will be discussed later. Define $\mathbf{a} = \{a_k\}_{n \times 1}$ as a vector for the n allelic values (i.e., the value that each allele contributes to the quantitative trait) and $\mathbf{d} = \{d_{kl}\}_{n \times n}$ as a symmetric matrix for the interaction (dominance) effects between each pairs of alleles. Let N be the total number of individuals in the mapping population, including the founders, the parents, and all progeny. If plant j happens to carry copies of founder alleles k and l, then the phenotypic value of j can be described by

$$y_j = b + a_k + a_l + d_{kl} + \varepsilon_j \tag{1}$$

where y_j is the phenotypic value, b is the overall population mean, and ε_j is the environmental error assumed $N(0, \sigma^2)$ distribution. We can replace b by $\mathbf{x}_j\mathbf{b}$ if there are classifiable environmental effects (covariates) that we wish to separate from the genetic effects. If the phenotypic value y_j is measured as a plot mean of r replicates of the same plant (genotype), the residual error variance should be σ^2/r. In plant QTL mapping, N (the total number of individuals) is usually much larger than n (number of founder alleles) so that each founder allele and allelic combination can be replicated many times in the descendants. A good mating design should be well balanced so that each allele and allelic combination is equally represented in the descendents. From this point of view, a cross-classified mating design is more efficient than a nested hierarchical mating design. The diallel cross is a cross-classified mating design in which k inbred lines served as male parents are crossed with the same k lines served as female parents. The number of matings is $k \times k$, which makes up a square matrix. The diagonal elements represent pure breeding and the off-diagonal elements represent cross-breeding. If one is not interested in cytoplasmic effects, only half of the off-diagonals are needed. Such a diallel design is called the half-diallel. If each male parent is mated with several female parents and each female parent is only mated with one male parent, the design is called half-sib design. The half-sib design is a typical nested hierarchical mating design.

The sum of the two allelic values for an individual is called the additive effect or the breeding value. Note that the allelic and dominance effects of all individuals in the mapping population can be traced back to the corresponding effects defined in the founders. Therefore, QTL analysis amounts to estimating and testing these effects in the founders, not the effects of descendents in the mapping population.

Unlike in a usual linear model where an observation can be unambiguously identified to a particular treatment combination, in QTL mapping we do not observe which founder alleles are actually carried by any particular plant at the QTL; instead, we use observed marker information to infer the allelic inheritance of the QTL. Therefore, a probability statement must be assigned to the design matrix of the QTL model. Let us define $i_j^p = 1, \ldots, n$ as the allelic identifier for the paternal allele of individual j and i_j^m as that for the maternal allele. For example, if the paternal allele of j is a copy of the first founder allele and the maternal allele of j is a copy of the fourth founder allele, then $i_j^p = 1$ and $i_j^m = 4$. Using the founder allele identifiers, we can rewrite the linear model using a pseudocode notation:

$$y_j = b + a(i_j^p) + a(i_j^m) + d(i_j^m) + \varepsilon_j \tag{2}$$

Here we have adopted the pseudocode notation of $a(i_j^p)$ to represent element i_j^p of the allelic value vector $\mathbf{a}$ instead of using the awkward expression $a_{i_j^p}$. Note that matrices $\mathbf{a}$ and $\mathbf{d}$ are parameters of the model.

2.2.2. Multiple QTL Model

For a multiple QTL model, the notation becomes complicated, but the basic principle of the linear model remains identical. Assume that the number of QTL is q. We now extend vector $\mathbf{a}$ into a matrix, $\mathbf{A} = \{(a_{ki}\}_{n \times q}$, so that the ith column vector of $\mathbf{A}$ stores the additive values for the ith QTL. Similarly, we extend matrix $\mathbf{d}$ into a three-dimensional matrix, $\mathbf{D} = \{d_{kli}\}_{n \times n \times q}$, so that the third dimension defines the loci. Again, let us use i_j^p and i_j^m as the founder allelic identifiers for individual j at the ith QTL. This time, the letter i in symbol i_j^p is a variable, the value of which varies depending on the locus. This leads to a rather unusual notation for a variable. For example, the allelic identifiers for the second QTL would be 2_j^p and 2_j^m. If the paternal allele of the second QTL for individual j is a copy of the third founder allele, then $2_j^p = 3$. Although 2 is a constant, with both a superscript and a subscript, 2_j^p becomes a symbol for a variable. Using this notation, the multiple QTL model is written

$$y_j = b + \sum_{i=1}^{q} \{a(i_j^p, i) + a(i_j^m, i) + d(i_j^p, i_j^m, i)\} + \varepsilon_j \tag{3}$$

With this notation, epistatic effects can be easily incorporated into the model. Let us take a two-QTL model, for example, to demonstrate the formulation. Define $\mathbf{H} = \{h_{kl}\}_{n \times n}$ as an epistatic effect matrix, where h_{kl} is the interaction effect between the kth founder allele at locus 1 and the lth founder allele at locus 2. In contrast to the dominance effect, d_{kl}, which is the interaction between the two alleles within a locus, the epistatic effect is the interaction effect between two alleles, one from each locus. Therefore, dominance and epistasis are also called allelic and nonallelic interactions, respectively (*1*). Hence, the two-locus epistatic model would be represented as follows:

$$
\begin{aligned}
y_j = b &+ a(1_j^p, 1) + a(1_j^m, 1) + d(1_j^p, 1_j^m, 1) \\
&+ a(2_j^p, 2) + a(2_j^m, 2) + d(2_j^p, 2_j^m, 2) \\
&+ h(1_j^p, 2_j^p) + h(1_j^p, 2_j^m) + h(1_j^m, 2_j^p) + h(1_j^m, 2_j^m) + \varepsilon_j
\end{aligned}
\tag{4}
$$

The epistatic effect matrix $\mathbf{H}$ only contains the interaction effects between a pair of alleles, called the additive-by-additive effects. There are many other types of epistatic effects, including additive-by-dominance, dominance-by-additive, and dominance-by-dominance effects (*28*). These higher-order interactions are difficult to represent and, thus, are not dealt with in this chapter. For a total of q QTLs, the total number of possible nonallelic interaction matrices (additive-by-additive) is $q(q - 1)/2$. Therefore, we need a third subscript for matrix $\mathbf{H}$ to define which two loci are interacting. The general expression of the linear model for q QTL is

$$
y_j = b + g_j + \varepsilon_j
\tag{5}
$$

where

$$
g_j = \sum_{i=1}^{q} \left\{ a(i_j^p, i) + a(i_j^m, i) + d(i_j^p, i_j^m, i) \right\}
\tag{6}
$$

$$
+ \sum_{i=1}^{q-1} \sum_{r=i+1}^{q} \left\{ h(i_j^p, r_j^p, t) + h(i_j^p, r_j^m, t) + h(i_j^m, r_j^p, t) + h(i_j^m, r_j^m, t) \right\}
$$

is the genetic value and $t = 1, \ldots, q(q - 1)/2$ indexes the pairs of loci that are interacting and is a function of i and r. If needed, epistatic effects involving three or more loci can be added into the model. However, it is prudent to limit what is included in the model to avoid severe overparameterization.

2.3. Tracing the Allelic Origins

Each of the two (paternal and maternal) alleles carried by j at locus i can, in principle, be traced back to its origin in the founders using the founder-allele identifiers, i_j^p and i_j^m. However, the precise segregations of these allele identifiers are not directly observed, and there may be many generations away between j and the founders; thus, it becomes difficult to directly sample i_j^p and i_j^m. Instead, we must sample possible allelic identifier configurations for our calculations by adopting a dynamic programming approach to generate samples for the allele identifiers, for example, via Markov chain methods. Allelic identifiers for individuals must be generated in a chronological order (i.e., parents must be generated before their children). We begin by arbitrarily assigning the alleles to the founders using the integers from 1 to n. By convention, we assign the paternal allele followed by the maternal allele for each founder. For example, the allele identifiers for individual k, who is the fth founder, will be $i_k^p = 2f - 1$ and $i_k^m = 2f$, for $f = 1, \ldots, n/2$. If individual j is not a founder, we know that its parents must be already generated. In this case, the designation of alleles is more complicated and depends on two factors. First, the allelic identifiers of the parents for j and, second, on the observed genotypic markers for individual j for the flanking markers to the proposed QTL. The dependence of allelic identifiers for j on the allelic identifiers of the parents can be expressed as follows. Define i_p^p and i_p^m as the founder-allele identifiers for the father of j, and i_m^p and i_m^m as the identifiers for the mother of j. Given the allele identifiers of the parents, the identifiers for j can be easily represented using the following recursive equations:

$$i_j^p = z_j^p i_p^p + (1 - z_j^p) i_p^m \tag{7}$$

and

$$i_j^m = z_j^m i_m^p + (1 - z_j^m) i_m^m \tag{8}$$

where $z_j^p = 1$ if the paternal allele of the father has been passed to j and $z_j^p = 0$ otherwise, regardless of the allelic form, and z_j^m is similarly defined, but for the paternal allele of the mother (**29**). If we assume the ordered genotypes of the father and mother are A_1A_2 and A_3A_4, respectively, then each child can take one of the four following genotypes: $A_1A_3, A_1A_4, A_2A_3, A_2A_4$. If a child is A_2A_3, we know that the maternal allele of the father and the paternal allele of the mother have been passed to the child; thus, $z_j^p = 0$ and $z_j^m = 1$.

By structuring the problem in this way, we have turned the problem of identifying the founder alleles into that of finding the allelic transmission from parents to the progeny, a much simpler problem. The distribution of z_j^p or z_j^m is Bernoulli with a probability depending on the genotypes of markers and their distances from the locus in question. The distributions of z_j^p and z_j^m conditional on marker information, however, are not independent, making it difficult to derive the joint distribution. Therefore, we need another variable U_j to indicate one of the four possible genotypes for a progeny. Define $U_j = k$ for $k = 1, \ldots,$ 4 if individual j takes the kth-ordered genotype. The values of z_j^p and z_j^m are solely determined by U_j with the following relationships: $z_j^p = I_{(U_j=1)} + I_{(U_j=2)}$ and $z_j^m = I_{(U_j=1)} + I_{(U_j=3)}$, where $I_{(U_j=k)} = 1$ for $U_j = k$ and $I_{(U_j=k)} = 0$ for $U_j \neq k$. Without marker information, we have $\Pr(U_j = k) = 1/4$ for $k = 1, \ldots, 4$. However, this marginal distribution is not useful for QTL mapping, because what we need here is the conditional distribution given the observed marker data. Next, we incorporate the observed genotypic data from flanking markers. Let us consider two markers, one in each side of the QTL. Define M_{1j} and M_{2j} as the genotypes for the left and right flanking markers, respectively. In other words, the values of M_{1j} and M_{2j} are defined in the same way as U_j, except that they are for the marker genotypes. We assume that both markers are fully informative so that the values of M_{1j} and M_{2j} are observed data (*see* **Note 2**). The joint distribution of the three loci, $\{M_{1j}, U_j, M_{2j}\}$, is determined by the relative positions of the loci along the chromosome. Let λ_i be the position of the ith QTL measured in Morgans from the left end of the chromosome. The positions of the two markers are assumed known and thus suppressed from the following derivation. Under the Haldane (**30**) map function, the joint distribution of $\{M_{1j}, U_j, M_{2j}\}$, can be described exploiting a property of Markov chains:

$$\Pr(M_{1j}, U_j, M_{2j} \mid \lambda_i) = \Pr(M_{1j}) \Pr(U_j \mid M_{1j}, \lambda_i) \Pr(M_{2j} \mid U_j, \lambda_i) \qquad (9)$$

where $\Pr(M_{1j} = k) = 1/4$ for $k = 1, \ldots, 4$ and $\Pr(U_j \mid M_{1j}, \lambda_i)$ is the transition probability from the left marker to the QTL and $\Pr(M_{2j} \mid U_j, \lambda_1)$ is the transition probability from the QTL to the right marker. These transition probabilities are obtained from the following transition matrix:

$$\mathbf{T} = \begin{bmatrix} (1-c)^2 & c(1-c) & c(1-c) & c^2 \\ c(1-c) & (1-c)^2 & c^2 & c(1-c) \\ c(1-c) & c^2 & (1-c)^2 & c(1-c) \\ c^2 & c(1-c) & c(1-c) & (1-c)^2 \end{bmatrix}$$

where c is the recombination fraction between the two loci in question. For instance, if $U_j = 1$ and $M_{1j} = 3$, then $\Pr(U_j = 1 \mid M_{1j} = 3, \lambda_i) = T(3,1) = c(1 - c)$, where c is the recombination fraction between the left marker and the QTL. In general, $\Pr(U_j = t \mid M_{1j} = s, \lambda_i) = T(s, t)$. From the joint distribution, we can calculate the conditional distribution,

$$\Pr(U_j \mid M_{1j}, M_{2j}, \lambda_i) = \frac{\Pr(M_{1j}, U_j, M_{2j} \mid \lambda_i)}{\Pr(M_{1j}, M_{2j})} \qquad (10)$$

where $\Pr(M_{1j}, M_{2j}) = \Pr(M_{1j})\Pr(M_{2j} \mid M_{1j})$. The above conditional distribution will be used in modeling the posterior distribution of U_j and thus the posterior distribution of z_j^p and z_j^m, which, in turn, determine the founder allele identifiers, i_j^p and i_j^m. These founder allele identifiers are the keys to our Bayesian analysis of QTL.

2.4. Bayesian Mapping

2.4.1. Background

In Bayesian analysis parameters such as the QTL locations, the additive and dominance effects are treated as unknown variables with prior distributions. The purpose of Bayesian analysis is to combine the prior distribution with the observed data to obtain a posterior distribution for the unknown parameters. It should be noted that the prior distributions are not actual distributions of the parameters, rather that the parameters themselves are fixed, and it is our belief of the parameter values that varies. Therefore, the prior distribution is actually the distribution of our subjective belief. Similarly, the posterior distribution of parameters is the updated distribution of our belief after incorporation of data information. Note that the parameters that define the prior distributions are referred to as hyperparameters to avoid confusion.

The observed data include phenotypic values, $\mathbf{y} = \{y_j\}_{N\times1}$, and observed marker genotype information. However, because it is cumbersome to derive the MCMC algorithm if marker genotypes are explicitly expressed as data, we have suppressed marker information from the likelihood for simplicity. Here, we will assume full information for all markers, with the function of markers only being used to provide information about the distribution of the four genotypes for each individual U_j. After suppressing markers from the model, we treat the distribution of U_j conditional on markers as the prior distribution of U_j in subsequent MCMC analysis.

2.4.2. The Parameters

The parameters in the analysis include population mean b, environmental error variance σ^2, the number of QTL q, the locations of the QTL $\lambda = \{\lambda_i\}_{q\times1}$, the allelic effects of founders $\mathbf{A}$, the dominance effects $\mathbf{D}$, and the epistatic effects $\mathbf{H}$. The values for U_j are considered as missing. For multiple QTL, U_j needs one more subscript i to index the QTL. Therefore, U_{ij} denotes the genotype of individual j at the ith QTL. Later, we will use $\mathbf{U}_j = \{U_{ij}\}_{q\times1}$ to denote the vector for the (unobserved) genotypic configurations for all the q QTL of individual j.

2.4.3. The Likelihood Function

Define $\boldsymbol{\theta}$ as a vector containing all the parameters detailed thus far and the missing genotypic configuration $\mathbf{U}_j$. Given $\boldsymbol{\theta}$, we can construct the likelihood function, which is proportional to the conditional probability density of the data. Let us use $p(x)$ and $p(y|x)$ as generic symbols for the density and conditional density functions, respectively; the actual forms depend on the arguments rather than the symbol p. The likelihood function is

$$p(\mathbf{y}|\theta) = \prod_{j=1}^{N} p(y_j|\theta) \propto \frac{1}{(\sigma^2)^{N/2}} \exp\left[-\frac{1}{2\sigma^2} \sum_{j=1}^{N} (y_j - b - g_j)^2\right] \qquad (11)$$

If the phenotypic value has a distribution other than Normal, we simply replace Eq. (11) by the appropriate density. For example, if the phenotype is a binary disease, y_j should be modeled as a Bernoulli variable with a probability

$$p(y_j|\theta) = [\Phi(\theta)]^{y_j}[1 - \Phi(\theta)]^{1-y_j} \qquad (12)$$

where

$$\Phi(\theta) = \int_{-\infty}^{0} \frac{1}{\sqrt{2\pi}} \exp\left[-\frac{1}{2}(x - b - g_j)^2\right]dx \qquad (13)$$

In binary data analysis, the residual variance cannot be estimated but set to $\sigma^2 = 1$.

2.4.4. Prior Probability Densities

We need to specify the prior density for the parameters and the distribution of the missing values given the parameters. For convenience, we choose the following prior:

$$p(\theta) = p(b)p(\sigma^2)p(q)p(\lambda)p(\mathbf{A}|q)p(\mathbf{D}|q)p(\mathbf{H}|q)p(\mathbf{U}|q, \lambda) \qquad (14)$$

Uniform priors are chosen for b and σ^2. A Poisson prior is used for q; that is, $p(q) = \dfrac{\mu^q e^{-\mu}}{q!}$, where μ is the Poisson prior mean for the number of QTL. The positions of QTL have a joint prior of $p(\lambda) = \displaystyle\prod_{i=1}^{q} p(\lambda_i)$, where each $p(\lambda_i)$ is uniform across the whole genome [i.e., $p(\lambda_i) \propto$ constant]. The joint prior for the allelic effects if $p(\mathbf{A}) = \displaystyle\prod_{i=1}^{q}\prod_{k=1}^{n} p(a(k, i))$, where $a(k, i) \sim N(0, \sigma^2_{A(i)}) \; \forall i$. The joint prior for the dominance effects is

$$p(\mathbf{D}) = \prod_{i=1}^{q}\prod_{k=1}^{n-1}\prod_{l=k+1}^{n} p(d(k, l, i)),$$

where $d(k, l, i) \sim N(0, \sigma^2_{D(i)}) \; \forall i$. Similiarly,

$$p(\mathbf{H}) = \prod_{i=1}^{q-1} \prod_{r=i+1}^{q} \left[\prod_{k=1}^{n} \prod_{i=1}^{n} p(h(k, l, t)) \right]$$

where $h(k, l, t) \sim N(0, \sigma^2_{H(t)})$ for $t = 1, \ldots, q(q - 1)/2$.

The hyperparameters, $\sigma^2_{A(i)}$ and $\sigma^2_{D(i)}$, are the prior variances for the allelic and dominance effects respectively for the ith QTL, and $\sigma^2_{H(t)}$ is the prior variance for the tth pairwise additive-by-additive epistatic effects.

2.4.5. The distribution for U_j

The joint distribution of the missing values is $p(\mathbf{U} \mid q, \lambda) = \prod_{j=1}^{N}$

$p(\mathbf{U}_j \mid q, \lambda)$ because the allelic inheritance configurations of different individuals are independent. The distribution $p(\mathbf{U}_j \mid q, \lambda)$ appears to be the prior distribution of $\mathbf{U}_j$; however, it represents the conditional distribution given marker information because we have suppressed markers from the model for simplicity. If the marker map is relatively dense and QTLs are sparsely distributed along the

genome, it is reasonable to assume $p(\mathbf{U}_j \mid q, \lambda) = \prod_{i=1}^{q} p(\mathbf{U}_{ij} \mid \lambda_i)$, where

$p(U_{ij}|\lambda_i)$ is the conditional probability of allelic inheritance configuration for j at the ith QTL, given information on the flanking markers, previously denoted by $p(U_j \mid M_{1j}, M_{2j}, \lambda_i)$ and given in Eq. (10).

2.4.6. The Posterior Probability Density

Given the complexity of the likelihood and the prior, the joint posterior probability density does not have a standard form. In addition, Bayesian inference should be made at the marginal level for each unobservable. Let us partition θ into $\theta = \{\theta_i, \theta_{-i}\}$ where θ_i is a single element of θ and θ_{-i} is a vector of the remaining elements. The marginal posterior distribution of θ_i is

$$p(\theta_i \mid \mathbf{y}) \propto \iint p(\mathbf{y} \mid \theta_i, \theta_{-i}) \, p(\theta_i, \theta_{-i}) \, d\theta_{-i} \tag{15}$$

Bayesian inference for θ_i should be made from the above marginal distribution. Unfortunately, this marginal distribution does not have an explicit expression. Numerical integration is often prohibited because of the high dimensionality of θ_{-i}. Therefore, we need to use the MCMC algorithm to simulate a sample from the joint posterior distribution $p(\theta|y)$. From the realized sample, we can infer the marginal distribution of θ_i by simply looking at the empirical distribution of θ_i, ignoring the variation of $\boldsymbol{\theta}_{-i}$. From this empirical distribution, we can calculate summary statistics such as the mean and variance for θ_i.

2.5. MCMC Algorithm

2.5.1. Background

Our target distribution is the joint posterior distribution $p(\boldsymbol{\theta}|\mathbf{y})$. With the MCMC algorithm, however, we do not directly generate the joint sample from $p(\boldsymbol{\theta}|\mathbf{y})$; instead, we only generate realizations from $p(\theta_i|\boldsymbol{\theta}_{-i}, \mathbf{y})$, the conditional posterior distribution for the ith parameter with all other variables fixed at their current values. This conditional posterior distribution is proportional to the joint posterior distribution $p(\theta_i, \boldsymbol{\theta}_{-i}|\mathbf{y})$ except that, in the conditional distribution, $\boldsymbol{\theta}_{-i}$ are treated as constants and θ_i as a variable. Starting from an initial value for $\boldsymbol{\theta}$, denoted by $\boldsymbol{\theta}^{(0)} = \{\theta_1^{(0)}, \theta_2^{(0)}, \ldots, \theta_r^{(0)}\}$, where r is the total number of parameters, we draw one parameter at a time from $p(\theta_i | \boldsymbol{\theta}_{-i}^{(0)}, \mathbf{y})$ with other parameters fixed at their initial values. After all the parameters have been drawn, we complete one cycle of the Markov chain; the updated values are denoted by $\boldsymbol{\theta}^{(1)} = \{\theta_1^{(1)}, \theta_2^{(1)}, \ldots, \theta_r^{(1)}\}$. The chain will grow and eventually reach a stationary distribution. Let C be the length of the chain. Because there is one realization of $\boldsymbol{\theta}$ in each cycle of the chain, we will have a realized sample of $\boldsymbol{\theta}$ with sample size C, denoted by $\{\boldsymbol{\theta}^{(1)}, \boldsymbol{\theta}^{(2)}, \ldots, \boldsymbol{\theta}^{(C)}\}$. Discarding data points of the first few thousand cycles (burn-in period) and thereafter saving one realization in every hundred cycles (approximately), we get a random sample of $\boldsymbol{\theta}$ drawn from $p(\boldsymbol{\theta}|\mathbf{y})$.

2.5.2. Sampling from the Chain

We now discuss how to draw θ_i from $p(\theta_i|\boldsymbol{\theta}_{-i}, \mathbf{y})$. This conditional posterior distribution usually has a standard form (e.g., Normal). In this case, we can directly sample θ_i from the standard distribution. The method is then called the Gibbs sampler (*31*). If $p(\theta_i|\boldsymbol{\theta}_{-i}, \mathbf{y})$ does not have a standard form, we will take a general acceptance–rejection approach, called the Metropolis–Hastings algorithm (*32,33*).

2.5.2.1. The Metropolis–Hastings Algorithm

Define $\boldsymbol{\theta}^{(t-1)}$ as the values simulated at the $t-1$ cycle. We want to draw $\theta_i^{(t)}$ from the target distribution $p(\theta_i | \boldsymbol{\theta}_{-i}^{(t-1)}, \mathbf{y})$. Instead of drawing $\theta_i^{(t)}$ directly from this target distribution, the Metropolis–Hastings algorithm draws a candidate θ_i^* from a proposal density, $q(\theta_i^*|\theta_i^{(t-1)})$, which is different from $p(\theta_j^*|\boldsymbol{\theta}_{-i}^{(t-1)}, \mathbf{y})$ but has a standard form. We then use the Metropolis–Hastings rule to decide whether to accept θ_i^* or not. If θ_i^* is accepted, $\theta_i^{(t)} = \theta_i^*$, otherwise $\theta_i^{(t)} = \theta_i^{(t-1)}$. In either case, we will move to the next element.

With the Metropolis–Hastings rule, we accept θ_i^* with probability min $\{1, \alpha\}$, where

$$\alpha = \frac{p(\theta_i^* \mid \boldsymbol{\theta}_{-i}^{(t-1)}, \mathbf{y}) \, q(\theta_i^{(t-1)} \mid \theta_i^*)}{p(\theta_i^{(t-1)} \mid \boldsymbol{\theta}_{-i}^{(t-1)}, \mathbf{y}) \, q(\theta_i^* \mid \theta_i^{(t-1)})} \tag{16}$$

Recall that

$$p(\theta_i^* \mid \boldsymbol{\theta}_{-i}^{(t-1)}, \mathbf{y}) = \text{const} \times p(\mathbf{y} \mid \theta_i^*, \boldsymbol{\theta}_{-i}^{(t-1)}) \, p(\theta_i^*, \boldsymbol{\theta}_{-i}^{(t-1)})$$

and

$$p(\theta_i^{(t-1)} \mid \boldsymbol{\theta}_{-i}^{(t-1)}, \mathbf{y}) = \text{const} \times p(\mathbf{y} \mid \theta_i^{(t-1)}, \boldsymbol{\theta}_{-i}^{(t-1)}) \, p(\theta_i^{(t-1)}, \boldsymbol{\theta}_{-i}^{(t-1)})$$

After cancellation of the constants, the acceptance probability becomes

$$\alpha = \frac{p(\mathbf{y} \mid \theta_i^*, \boldsymbol{\theta}_{-i}^{(t-1)}) \, p(\theta_i^*, \boldsymbol{\theta}_{-i}^{(t-1)}) \, q(\theta_i^{(t-1)} \mid \theta_i^*)}{p(\mathbf{y} \mid \theta_i^{(t-1)}, \boldsymbol{\theta}_{-i}^{(t-1)}) \, p(\theta_i^{(t-1)}, \boldsymbol{\theta}_{-i}^{(t-1)}) \, q(\theta_i^* \mid \theta_i^{(t-1)})} = r_1 r_2 r_3. \tag{17}$$

Therefore, the acceptance probability has been factorized into the product of the likelihood ratio (r_1), the prior ratio (r_2), and the proposal ratio (r_3).

2.5.2.2. CHOOSING THE PROPOSAL DENSITIES

Although the notation of the proposal density $q(\theta_i^* \mid \theta_i^{(t-1)})$ implies that this density is a probability density of θ_i^* conditional on the current value $\theta_i^{(t-1)}$, it does not have to depend on $\theta_i^{(t-1)}$. In fact, the proposal density can be chosen in an arbitrary fashion. It may be completely independent of $\theta_i^{(t-1)}$ or dependent of every thing else, including the data. However, the exact form of the proposal density determines the acceptance rate, and thus the efficiency, of the Metropolis–Hastings algorithm. The most efficient proposal density is the conditional posterior because it leads to a unity acceptance rate. As mentioned previously, this is the Gibbs sampler algorithm. However, if the conditional posterior density does not have a standard form, we should choose a proposal density with a standard form simply for convenience of generating random numbers. To increase the efficiency, the shape of the proposal density should be close to that of the conditional posterior.

We now discuss the proposal density for each variable. A uniform proposal density is used for the population mean b, the environmental variance σ^2, and the position of each QTL λ_i. Define $\theta_i^{(t-1)}$ as the current value for each of the above parameters. The proposal θ_i^* is drawn from $\theta_i^* \sim U(\theta_i^{(t-1)} - \frac{1}{2}\delta, \theta_i^{(t-1)} + \frac{1}{2}\delta)$ distribution, where δ is a small positive number called the tuning parameter. Therefore, the proposal density is $q(\theta_i^* \mid \theta_i^{(t-1)}) = 1/\delta$. The reverse density, $q(\theta_i^{(t-1)} \mid \theta_i^*)$, is identical to the proposal density, so they cancel out each other in the proposal ratio. This characterizes a random-walk Markov chain and is the original form of the Metropolis algorithm (*32*).

The indicator variables for the configuration of allelic transmission from parents to a child (U_{ij}) are sampled in a locus-by-locus and individual-by-individual basis. This allows the use of a Gibbs sampler. For each individual at a particular locus, there are only four possible configurations of allelic transmission. One can easily calculate the conditional posterior probability for each configuration and use it to draw a realized one. The conditional posterior probability for a QTL is

$$p(U_{ij} \mid \boldsymbol{\theta}_{-i}, \mathbf{y}) = \frac{p(y_j \mid U_{ij}, \boldsymbol{\theta}_{-i}) \, p(\mathbf{A} \mid q) \, p(\mathbf{D} \mid q) \, p(\mathbf{H} \mid q) \, p(U_{ij} \mid \lambda_i)}{\sum\limits_{U_{ij}} p(y_j \mid U_{ij}, \boldsymbol{\theta}_{-i}) \, p(\mathbf{A} \mid q) \, p(\mathbf{D} \mid q) \, p(\mathbf{H} \mid q) \, p(U_{ij} \mid \lambda_i)} \qquad (18)$$

where $\boldsymbol{\theta}_{-i}$ stands for all the parameters except U_{ij} and the summation in the denominator is over all the four possible genotypes for U_{ij}. It should be emphasized that the distribution of U_{ij} is highly dependent of the QTL position λ_i. Therefore, when a new λ_i is proposed, U_{ij} should be redrawn from the proposed position. The U_{ij} drawn from the proposed position, rather than the one from the old position, should be used to evaluate the acceptance probability for the new λ_i. The proposed λ_i and its corresponding U_{ij} should be accepted simultaneously. This is different from what has been suggested previously, where the proposed position was evaluated using U_{ij} from the old position (*15*). However, personal experience has shown that using the old position may lead to a QTL becoming trapped within an interval between two markers; hence, we suggest simultaneously updating U_{ij} and λ_i.

A Normal proposal density is applied to each of the genetic effects (including additive, dominance, and epistatic effects). Again, define $\theta_i^{(t-1)}$ as the current value for one of the genetic effects. The proposed θ_i^* is drawn from $\theta_i^* \sim N(\theta_i^{(t-1)}, \delta)$, where δ is a proposal variance (a tuning parameter). The proposal density is

$$q(\theta_i^* \mid \theta_i^{(t-1)}) = \frac{1}{\sqrt{2\pi\delta}} \exp\left\{ -\frac{1}{2\delta} (\theta_i^* - \theta_i^{(t-1)})^2 \right\} \qquad (19)$$

The reverse density $q(\theta_i^{(t-1)} \mid \theta_i^*)$ is, again, identical to the proposal density, leading to a unity proposal ratio.

2.5.2.3. UPDATING THE NUMBER OF QTL (q)

The Metropolis–Hastings algorithm described earlier can be used for updating all unobservables except q, the number of QTL. This is because q itself also defines the dimension of the model and the Metropolis–Hastings algorithm in its original form only works when the dimensionality of the model is fixed.

Green (*19*) developed a reversible-jump MCMC algorithm to accomplish the variable dimension problem. Sillanpää and Arjas (*15*) applied this method to QTL mapping for inference of the number of QTL. Instead of randomly drawing a proposed QTL number and using the Metropolis–Hastings rule to accept it, here we only consider one of two possibilities: adding a new QTL to the model (with a predetermined probability P_a) or deleting an existing QTL from the model (with probability $P_d = 1 - P_a$). Because q is also the dimension of the model, when q changes, the set of parameters will change accordingly. Let us define the set of unobservables under the current model (with q QTL) by $\theta^{(t-1)}$. If we propose adding a QTL, the new QTL number becomes $q* = q + 1$. We should propose a new position and all other variables associated with the added QTL. Define the additional unobservables after a new QTL has been added by **v.** The proposed set of parameters becomes $\theta* = \{\theta^{(t-1)}, v\}$. If **v** is drawn independently from $\theta^{(t-1)}$, the proposal is $q(\theta* \mid \theta^{(t-1)}) = p_a q(v)$, where $q(v)$ is the proposal density from which the variables associated to the new QTL are drawn. The reverse density is $q(\theta^{(t-1)} \mid \theta*) = p_d / (q + 1)$. Therefore, the acceptance probability is min $\{1, \alpha\}$, where

$$\alpha = \frac{p(y \mid \theta*)\, p(\theta*)\, p(q*)\, q(\theta^{(t-1)} \mid \theta*)}{p(y \mid \theta^{(t-1)})\, p(\theta^{(t-1)})\, p(q)\, q(\theta* \mid \theta^{(t-1)})} \tag{20}$$

where $p(q*) = \mu^{q+1}\, e^{-\mu} / (q + 1)!$ and $p(q) = \mu^q e^{-\mu}/q!$ are the prior probabilities for the new and old numbers of QTL, respectively. The prior density for the new model is $p(\theta*) = p(\theta^{(t-1)})\, p(v)$, where $p(v)$ is the prior density for **v.** Note that $p(v)$ is, in general, different from the proposal density $q(v)$. The above acceptance probability can be simplified as

$$\alpha = \frac{p(y \mid \theta*)\, p(v)\mu p_d}{p(y \mid \theta^{(t-1)})\, q(v)(q+1)^2\, P_a} \tag{21}$$

If the proposed QTL is accepted, all variables associated to it are simultaneously accepted. Deleting a QTL simply takes the reverse process. Define the current model with q QTLs by $\theta^{(t-1)}$ and the proposed model with $q* = q - 1$ QTLs by $\theta*$. Further defining the variables associated to the deleted QTL by **v,** we get $\theta^{(t-1)} = \{\theta*, v\}$. Therefore, the proposal density is $q(\theta* \mid \theta^{(t-1)}) = p_d / q$ and the reverse density is $q(\theta^{(t-1)} \mid \theta*) = p_a q(v)$. After some algebraic simplification, we have the following acceptance probability:

$$\alpha = \frac{p(y \mid \theta*)\, q(v)q^2 p_a}{p(y \mid \theta^{(t-1)})\, p(v)\, \mu p_d} \tag{22}$$

2.5.3. Overview

The MCMC algorithm starts with given values of the hyperparameters (parameters in the prior distributions) and the initial values for all the unknowns generated from their prior distributions $\boldsymbol{\theta}^{(0)}$ and proceeds with the following updating steps:

1. Update the allelic effects **A,** the dominance effects **D,** and the epistatic effects **H** of the founders.
2. Update the population mean b and the residual variance σ^2.
3. Update QTL location $\boldsymbol{\lambda}$ and the allelic inheritance configurations of QTL $\mathbf{U}_j$ simultaneously.
4. Update the QTL number q.

After the burn-in period, realizations of $\boldsymbol{\theta}$ are sampled from the chain and stored. Once enough realizations have been sampled, empirical posterior distributions for parameters in $\boldsymbol{\theta}$ can be created from the posterior sample.

3. Interpretation

Unlike maximum likelihood, Bayesian mapping does not result in a significance test; therefore, results generated from Bayesian analysis should be interpreted in a different way. The product of the MCMC algorithm is a realized sample of all unknown variables drawn from the joint posterior distribution. The posterior sample contains all of the information we need to infer the statistical properties of the parameters. Therefore, the MCMC algorithm serves as an experiment to generate data. Upon completion of the experiment, we need to summarize the results and draw conclusions. In fact, the statistical properties of parameters (means and variances) are "observed" from the data rather than inferred as in usual data analyses. This is because the sampled data points are directly made on the parameters.

3.1. Summary Statistics

The most informative summary statement from the posterior sample is the frequency table for each parameter of interest. The table may be converted into a histogram, a visual representation of the posterior density. The posterior mean, posterior variance, and credibility interval are also easily obtained from the posterior sample. The posterior mean or posterior mode of a parameter may be compared to the point estimate obtained using the maximum likelihood analysis. The 95% credibility interval is defined as

$$\Pr(a \le \theta_i \le b \mid \mathbf{y}) = \int_a^b p(\theta_i \mid \mathbf{y}) \, d\theta_i = 0.95 \tag{23}$$

where a and b are found such that $b - a$ is minimum among all other values that satisfy Eq. (23). Note that $p(\theta_i \mid \mathbf{y})$ is simply obtained from the joint posterior sample by ignoring the variation of $\boldsymbol{\theta}_{-i}$. The Bayesian credibility interval appears similar to, but has a quite different meaning from the confidence interval in significance test. The 95% credibility interval is a statement of conditional probability (i.e., conditional on observed data, the probability that θ_i lies between a and b is 0.95). The confidence interval in a significance test, however, defines an interval based on observed data. Because the interval is a function of the data, it varies from one experiment to another. The 95% confidence interval is defined in such a way that if the experiment were repeated many times, 95% of the times the intervals would cover the true parameter value. Because Bayesian inference refers to a statement of conditional probability given data in the current experiment, it never intends to make an inference about the hypothetical future experiments.

3.1.1. Locating the QTL Under a Single-QTL Model

The summary statistics of the posterior distribution are useful for QTL parameters when a single QTL is fitted to the model. The most important parameter of interest is the location of the QTL in the genome, λ. The marginal posterior distribution of QTL position can be depicted via plotting the number (frequency) of hits by the QTL in a short interval against the genome location of the interval. The regions frequently hit by the QTL are candidate locations for the QTL. The uncertainty of each candidate region is reflected by the width of the peak in the posterior density.

3.1.2. Locating QTL Under a Multiple-QTL Model

For multiple QTL, we use the reversible-jump MCMC for the change of model dimension. As the number of QTL frequently changes, most QTL have lost their identities. For instance, the first QTL in one observation may not be the first one in another observation if new QTL have been added. When the QTLs lose their identities, the posterior distributions of the corresponding QTL effects also lose their meanings. Although the posterior distributions of q, b, and σ^2 are still meaningful in the multiple-QTL model, we must seek alternative representations of the summary statistics for other QTL parameters. As mentioned in **Subheading 5.1.1,** the posterior density of the location of a QTL is estimated by the proportion of the number of hits by the QTL to a short interval surrounding that location. When a QTL loses its identity, we are unable to keep track of the hits by individual QTL; rather, we can only keep record of the total number of hits to a particular interval. Multiple hits to a short interval may be the result of different hits of the same QTL from different observations or of multiple hits by different QTL from the same observation. As a consequence, we completely ignore the origins of the hits and record the total number of hits by QTL along the whole genome. We then divide the whole genome into many equal-distant short intervals, say 1 cM, and count the number of hits to each short interval. The proportion of the hits to each interval, $P(t)$, is plotted against *t*, the genome location of the interval. In contrast to a single-QTL model, the curve is no longer called the posterior density of QTL location; rather, it is called the QTL intensity profile. Therefore, the posterior density of QTL location and QTL intensity profile are used interchangeably only under a single-QTL model.

3.1.3. Estimating the Genetic Effects Under a Multiple-QTL Model

Similarly, when the identity of a QTL is lost, the effects associated to individual QTL also lose their meanings. Corresponding to the QTL intensity profile, we calculate the average effect for each of the short intervals of the genome (sum of the QTL effects of multiple hits divided by the number of hits) and form a profile for the QTL effect, $E(t)$. For the candidate regions of QTL (regions repeatedly hit by QTL), we can visualize the average effect of QTL in those regions. It should be cautious that sometimes the profile of the QTL effect may be misleading. We have noted that regions rarely hit by QTL can sometime show a large average effect. So, the effect profile is only meaningful for regions with high QTL intensity. We propose a weighted QTL intensity, which takes the product of the QTL intensity and QTL effect, denoted by $W(t) = P(t)E(t)$. This weighted QTL intensity will eliminate the peaks in the regions rarely hit by QTL, even if the average effect in the regions may be large. There is one weighted QTL intensity profile for each QTL effect. By looking at the weighted QTL intensity profiles of all effects, we can tell the sources of variation of the detected QTL in a particular region of the genome.

3.2. Bayesian Mapping in Humans

With slight modification, the Bayesian mapping statistics developed here can be applied to QTL analysis in humans. The only difference between human pedigrees and multiple line crosses of plants that needs to be considered in modifying the method is the difference in the number of founders. Human pedigrees usually contain a much larger number of founders than plants, making the statistical inference of QTL effects more difficult. When the number of founders becomes large, information content per effect becomes small, leading to a large estimation error per effect. Furthermore, the large number of effects makes the results hard to interpret. These problems can be circumvented via the random-model approach of QTL mapping. Under the random model, QTL effects are treated as random effects and their variances become the parameters of interest.

Traditional methods used for human pedigree analysis cannot handle the complicated pedigrees with the high levels of inbreeding created by plant breeders. The method developed here does not have this limitation. The advantage of using such inbred pedigrees comes from the smaller number of founders

Table 2
An Example for the Input Data Format of a Marker Linkage Map

3						
1	3	0	15	31		
2	6	0	20	40	60	80	100
3	5	0	12	15	26	50	

Note: The first row of the data file contains a single numerical value (integer) for the total number of chromosomes (three in this example). The first values (integers) for subsequent rows store the chromosome ID numbers (chromosomes 1, 2, and 3 in this example). The second value of each subsequent row stores the number of markers for that chromosome (three markers for chromosome 1, six markers for chromosome 2, and five markers for chromosome 3 in this example). The third and subsequent values for each row are the marker positions measured in cM from the left end of the chromosome. For example, the first chromosome has three markers with positions 0, 15, and 31 cM, respectively. Numbers within the same row are separated by one or more spaces.

than that of noninbred pedigrees. With the smaller number of founders, one can estimate and test dominance and epistatic effects more accurately. Based on this argument, human pedigrees with high levels of inbreeding would provide a good resource for QTL mapping using the methodology outlined here.

4. Software

The computer program for implementing analyses as described in this chapter is called PlantModelQTL. The program is written in FORTRAN 77 and runs on a UNIX platform. The program code and a user manual are available from the author on request (xu@genetics.ucr.edu). The program analyzes both line crossing and pedigree data. The relevant file format is that shown in **Table 1.** In addition to the data file, the program requires another file storing the information of the marker linkage map (*see* **Table 2** for an example). The output file contains a posterior sample of all parameters of interest. Currently, summary statistics and graphical presentations of the posterior sample are not provided. However, we are developing a user-friendly program with a window interface that will be released in the near future.

5. Worked Example

5.1. The Simulated Data

The applicability of the proposed method is demonstrated by analyzing a set of simulated data. This experiment involves three inbred lines. The three lines were crossed in a factorial fashion to form a 3×3 half-diallel cross (*see* **Subheading 2.2.1.** for the definition of diallel cross). The mapping population contains the three crosses and their derived F_2 families. One hundred fifty individuals were sampled from each of the three F_2 families. One chromosome of length 100 cM was simulated. Eleven markers were placed on the chromosome at positions 0, 15, 20, 28, 37, 50, 58, 67, 80, 85, and 100 cM. Marker alleles of the three inbred lines were randomly sampled from a hypothetical population with six equally frequent alleles. This led to a possibility that the three lines might carry the same allele at a certain marker. Such a marker locus is actually uninformative. A quantitative trait was modeled as being controlled by two QTL residing on the simulated chromosome and a random environmental deviate distributed as $N(0, 1)$. The two simulated QTL were positioned at 25 cM and 65 cM, respectively (illustrated in **Fig. 2** with arrows). For each QTL, there were three allelic effects and six dominance effects. The true values of the genetic effects with necessary constraints are given in **Table 3.** For simplicity, epistatic effects were assumed to be absent and they were not included in the model. The overall population mean was set at $b = 0.0$. All individuals in the mapping populations were genotyped for markers, but only the terminal F_2 progeny had phenotypic records.

5.2. Initializing the Markov Chain

The MCMC algorithm started with no QTL. The starting values for the overall mean and the residual variance were 0.0 and 2.0, respectively. The truncated Poisson prior for the number of QTL had a mean of $\mu = 3$ and a maximum number of $l_{max} = 6$. The prior for the overall mean was uniform in the range of $[-4, 4]$. The residual variance took a uniform prior with a range of $[0.2]$. The priors for all QTL allelic and dominance effects were chosen to be Normal, $N(0, 1)$. Finally, the tuning parameters of proposals in the Metropolis–Hastings sampling were chosen to be 2.0 cM for QTL locations and 0.05 for all other parameters.

5.3. Running the MCMC Sampler

The proposed MCMC sampler was run for 10^6 cycles, after discarding the first 2000 cycles for the burn-in period. On a Sun Ultra 2 workstation, our analysis took about 7 h. The chains were thinned (saved 1 iteration in every 50 cycles) to reduce serial correlation in the stored samples so that the total number of samples kept in the post-Bayesian analysis was 20,000 for each parameter. The stored samples were subject to the post-Bayesian analysis.

5.4. Results from the Posterior Sample
5.4.1. The Number of QTL (q)

The number of QTL, the overall mean and the residual variance were inferred using all stored samples. The frequencies of the sampled values of the number

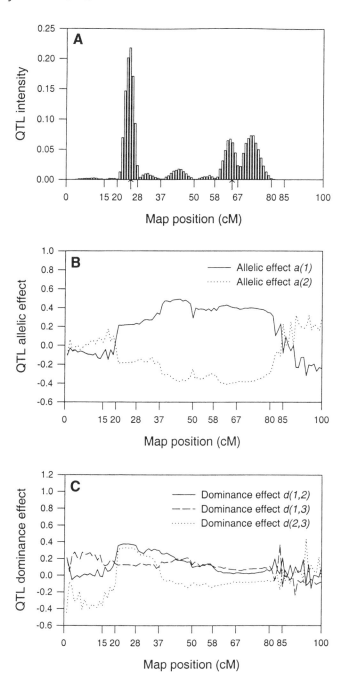

Fig. 2. (**A**) QTL intensity profile and profiles of QTL; (**B**) allelic effects; (**C**) dominance effects.

Table 3
The True Locations and Allelic and Dominance Effects for the Two
Simulated QTL

Location	Allelic effect			Dominance effect					
	$a(1)$	$a(2)$	$a(3)$	$d(1, 1)$	$d(1, 2)$	$d(1, 3)$	$d(2, 2)$	$d(2, 3)$	$d(3, 3)$
25 cM	0.3	−0.3	0.0	−0.6	0.4	0.2	−0.6	0.2	−0.4
65 cM	0.4	−0.4	0.0	0.0	0.0	0.0	0.0	0.0	0.0

Note: The allelic and dominance effects satisfy the following constraints: $a(3) = -[a(1) + a(2)]$, $d(1, 1) = -[d(1, 2) + d(1, 3)]$, $d(2, 2) + d(2, 3)]$, and $d(3, 3) = -[d(1, 3) + d(2, 3)]$.

of QTL provide an estimate of the marginal posterior distribution. The posterior mode of the number of QTL is 2, which coincides with the true QTL number. The posterior probability of $q = 2$ is $Pr(q = 2 \mid \mathbf{y}) = 0.9194$. The result strongly supports a model with two QTL in the chromosome.

5.4.2. The Locations of the QTL

Quantitative trait locus locations were inferred using the posterior QTL intensity function (*15,16*). The QTL intensity profiles are shown in **Fig. 2a.** The two major peaks of the QTL intensity fall between markers three and four (20–28 cM) and between markers seven and nine (58–80 cM), respectively.

5.4.3. Genetic Effects

For each of the QTL allelic and dominance effects, we calculated the average value within the short interval (1 cM) and then plotted the average value against the chromosomal position, forming an effect profile. For the candidate regions of QTL (regions repeatedly hit by QTL), we can visualize the size of QTL effects. The effect profiles are shown in **Figs. 2b,c.** The estimates of allelic and dominance effects, corresponding to the two major peaks on the QTL intensity profiles, are close to the true values. Note, Sillanpää and Arjas (*15*) state that the effect profile is only meaningful in the chromosomal regions where the QTL intensity is reasonably high. We used the weighted QTL intensity profiles to partition the QTL intensity profile into various components, each corresponding to one specific effect. By looking at the weighted QTL intensities, we can envisage the source of variation (additive and dominance) of the detected QTL in a particular region of the genome. The weighted QTL intensities are depicted in **Fig. 3.** From these weighted profiles, it is evident that the second QTL are completely caused by the allelic effects, rather than the dominance effects.

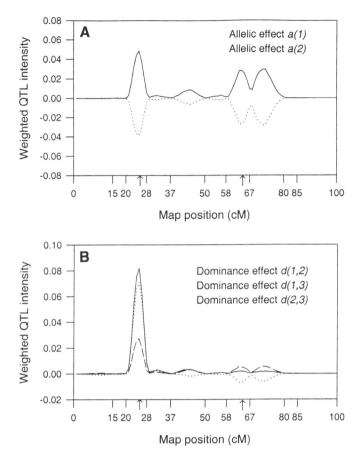

Fig. 3. Weighted QTL intensity profiles for (**A**) allelic and (**B**) dominance effects.

6. Notes

1. File preparation. It is extremely important to have individual records entered into the data sheet in chronological order. This will ensure that when generating genotypes, parents are generated before their children. If the genotype of a child is generated before its parents, the founder-allele identifiers would not necessarily be appropriately passed from the parents to the child and the method would not work.

2. Missing genotypes. For simplicity, the algorithm described in this chapter was derived under the assumptions that all markers were fully informative and there were no missing marker genotypes. However, markers that are not fully informative can be used in the computer program detailed in **Subheading 4.** In addition, the issue of missing genotypes has been reduced. For individuals with no children, missing genotypes are handled by the program. However, the problem of missing

marker genotypes in the founders and parents is difficult to handle. In real data analysis, a missing marker genotype in the founders and parents may be replaced manually by a legal genotype before the data analysis. When there are too many missing genotypes in the founders and parents, the method of the descent graph (*34*) should be adopted to sample marker genotypes.

3. Standardizing the phenotype. The Bayesian mapping statistics requires prior information and the starting values for all unknown variables. The prior distributions and starting values, however, must be chosen not too far away from the true values. The true parameter values depend on the scales and ranges of the phenotypic distribution. It is convenient to transform the phenotypic value into a standardized variable. This can be obtained using $y^* = (y - \bar{y})/s_y$, where $\bar{y}$ and s_y are the calculated average and standard deviation of y in the mapping population, respectively. When analyzing y^*, the starting values of parameters and the prior distributions can be easily chosen. For instance, given that the overall variance of y^* is approximately unity, the true residual variance must be less than 1. With the standardized phenotypic values, the computer program can use a set of intrinsic default starting values for all the unknown variables. The final results may be reported in the transformed scale or converted back into the original scale.

Acknowledgments

This research was supported by the National Institutes of Health Grant GM55321 and the USDA National Research Initiative Competitive Grants Program 00-35300-9245.

References

1. Falconer, D. S. and Mackay, T. F. C. (1996) *Introduction to Quantitative Genetics.* Longman Group, London.
2. Lynch, M. and Walsh, B. (1998) *Genetics and Analysis of Quantitative Traits.* Sinauer Associates.
3. Rebai, A. and Goffinet, B. (1993) Power of tests for QTL detection using replicated progenies derived from a diallel cross. *Theor. Appl. Genet.* **86,** 1014–1022.
4. Haley, C. S. and Knott, S. A. (1992) A simple regression method for mapping quantitative trait loci in line crosses using flanking markers. *Heredity* **69,** 315–324.
5. Martinez, O. and Curnow, R. N. (1992) Estimating the locations and the sizes of the effects of quantitative trait loci using flanking markers. *Theor. Appl. Genet.* **85,** 480–488.
6. Xu, S. (1995) A comment on the simple regression method for interval mapping. *Genetics* **141,** 1657–1659.
7. Xu, S. (1998) Further investigation on the regression method of mapping quantitative trait loci. *Heredity* **80,** 364–373.
8. Xu, S. (1998) Iteratively reweighted least squares mapping of quantitative trait loci. *Behav. Genet.* **28,** 341–355.
9. Lander, E. S. and Botstein, D. (1989) Mapping Mendelian factors underlying quantitative traits using RFLP linkage maps. *Genetics* **121,** 185–199.

10. Jansen, R. C. (1993) Interval mapping of multiple quantitative trait loci. *Genetics* **135,** 205–211.

11. Zeng, Z.-B. (1994) Precision mapping of quantitative trait loci. *Genetics* **136,** 1457–1468.

12. Hoeschele, I. and VanRaden, P. M. (1993) Bayesian analysis of linkage between genetic markers and quantitative trait loci. I. Prior knowledge. *Theor. Appl. Genet.* **85,** 953–960.

13. Hoeschele, I. and VanRaden, P. M. (1993) Bayesian analysis of linkage between genetic markers and quantitative trait loci. II. Combining prior knowledge with experimental evidence. *Theor. Appl. Genet.* **85,** 946–952.

14. Satagopan, J. M., Yandell, B. S., Newton, M. A., and Osborn, T. G. (1996) A Bayesian approach to detect quantitative trait loci using Markov chain Monte Carlo. *Genetics* **144,** 805–816.

15. Sillanpää, M. J. and Arjas, E. (1988) Bayesian mapping of multiple quantitative trait loci from incomplete inbred line cross data. *Genetics* **148,** 1373–1388.

16. Sillanpää, M. J. and Arjas, E. (1999) Bayesian mapping of multiple quantitative trait loci from incomplete outbred offspring data. *Genetics* **151,** 1605–1619.

17. Yi, N. and Xu, S. (2000) Bayesian mapping of quantitative trait loci under the IBD-based variance component model. *Genetics* **156,** 411–422.

18. Yi, N. and Xu, S. (2000) Bayesian mapping of quantitative trait loci for complex binary traits. *Genetics* **155,** 1391–1403.

19. Green, P. (1995) Reversible jump Markov chain Monte Carlo computation and Bayesian model determination. *Biometrika* **82,** 711–732.

20. Richardson, S.a.P.G. (1997) On Bayesian analysis of mixtures with an unknown number of components. *J. R. Statist. Soc. Sec. B* **59,** 731–792.

21. Steel, R.G.D. and Torrie, J. H. (1980) *Principles and Procedures of Statistics: A Biometrical Approach.* McGraw-Hill, New York.

22. Xu, S. and Atchley, W. R. (1996) Mapping quantitative trait loci for complex binary diseases using line crosses. *Genetics* **143,** 1417–1424.

23. Yi, N. and Xu, S. (1999) Mapping quantitative trait loci for complex binary traits in outbred populations. *Heredity* **82,** 668–676.

24. Yi, N. and Xu, S. (1999) A random model approach to mapping quantitative trait loci for complex binary traits in outbred populations. *Genetics* **153,** 1029–1040.

25. Kearsey, M. J. (1993) in *Plant Breeding: Principles and Prospects* (Hayward, M.D., Bosemark, N.O. and Romagosa, I., eds), Chapman & Hall, New York, pp. 163–183.

26. Lander, E. S. et al. (1987) MAPMAKER: An interactive computer package for constructing primary genetic linkage maps of experimental and natural populations. *Genomics* **1,** 174–181.

27. Stam, P. (1993) Construction of integrated genetic linkage maps by means of a new computer package: JOINMAP. *Plant J.* **3,** 739–744.

28. Cockerham, C. C. (1954) An extension of the concept of partitioning hereditary variance for analysis of covariances among relatives when epistasis is present. *Genetics* **39,** 859–882.

29. Xu, S. (1996) Computation for the full likelihood function for estimating variance at a quantitative trait locus. *Genetics* **144,** 1951–1960.

30. Haldane, J.B.S. (1919) The combination of linkage values, and the calculation of distances between the loci of linked factors. *J. Genet.* **8,** 299–309.

31. Geman S. and Geman, D. (1984) Stochastic relaxation, Gibbs distributions and the Bayesian restoration of images. *IEEE Trans. Pattern Analy. Mach. Intell.* **6,** 721–741.

32. Metropolis, N. et al. (1953) Equations of state calculations by fast computing machines. *J. Chem. Phys.* **21,** 1087–1091.

33. Hastings, W. K. (1970) Monte Carlo sampling methods using Markov chains and their applications. *Biometrika* **57,** 97–109.

34. Sobel, E. and Lange, K. (1996) Descent graphs in pedigree analysis: Applications to haplotyping, location scores, and marker-sharing statistics. *Am. J. Hum. Genet.* **58,** 1323–1337.

12

QTL Analysis in Livestock

Joao L. Rocha, Daniel Pomp, and L. Dale Van Vleck

1. Introduction

In a recent issue of *Science*, Lander and Weinberg (*1*) stated that "without doubt, the greatest achievement in biology over the past millennium has been the elucidation of the mechanism of heredity." The genetic dissection of quantitative phenotypes into Mendelian-like components, or quantitative trait loci (QTL) analysis, has provided significant insight into how complex traits are regulated and controlled. In combination with the new tools of genomics, QTL analysis promises to uncover the underlying variation in human genes that predispose to maladies such as obesity, hypertension, and diabetes and that contribute to behavioral phenotypes. This will not only yield informative diagnostics but may also lead to new therapies and potential cures in the future. In addition, we will begin to understand interactions between genes and the environment and between genes and other genes (epistasis), which, together, will play critical roles in implementing pharmacogenomic paradigms.

In food animal production, determining the identity of QTL is an important goal, but, nonetheless, accurate estimates of linkages to QTL are the necessary raw material to implement marker-assisted selection or marker-assisted management. These methodologies will utilize DNA marker information to improve the speed and accuracy of estimating breeding values in genetic selection programs or to tailor management practices (e.g., feeding, drug therapy) to better fit the genotypes of the animals.

Detection of QTL requires three essential stages: (1) collection of accurate phenotypic data within properly developed/existing pedigrees/populations; (2) collection of accurate genotypic data (DNA markers) within the pedigrees; and (3) statistical analysis correlating phenotypic and genotypic data, reflecting pedigree organization and structure. This chapter reviews the third step, particu-

From: *Methods in Molecular Biology: vol. 195: Quantitative Trait Loci: Methods and Protocols.*
Edited by: N. J. Camp and A. Cox © Humana Press, Inc., Totowa, NJ

larly with regard to methodologies and software in use (or proposed) for livestock populations. Although the reader is referred to previous reviews (*2–12*), a comprehensive assessment of state-of-the-art developments is offered, with consideration of relevant historical observations.

Methodological and statistical contributions have been significant in the last decade, and QTL analysis in livestock has reached a level of statistical soundness, as reflected by the considerable number of experiments showing replication and confirmation of findings (e.g., **refs.** *13–20*). However, integration of thought processes and terminologies of QTL researchers in different fields would be of considerable benefit. Solutions to problems of very similar genetic essence are often supported by terminologies that fail to recognize commonality, conveying the notion that methodologies and approaches are substantively different. Regardless of the species and underlying experimental paradigm, QTL analysis reflects a universal and unifying principle: the assessment of linkage disequilibrium in the segregation deriving from an event of double heterozygosity. The framework of reference is always a family or set of relatives, where the marker–QTL-allele phase relationships structuring the double heterozygosity of the common parent(s) of reference are disrupted only to the extent that there is recombination between the loci (*9*). All human and livestock QTL analysis stems from a 1938 article by Penrose (*21*), which represents the introduction and the initial quantification of the principle stated earlier. Taylor and Rocha (*9*) detailed the evolution of Penrose's contribution into modern experimental design for QTL detection in livestock.

The history of QTL analysis in livestock closely parallels that of the highly successful science of estimating genetic parameters and breeding values for quantitative traits (*22*), requiring increasingly sophisticated statistical methodologies in order to fully utilize existing complex data structures. These are often of an unbalanced nature, frequently encompassing missing data and nuisance parameters, and composed of large, complex pedigrees (*6,12,23,24*).

2. Methods

2.1. Crosses Between Outbred Lines

A common experimental design for QTL detection in livestock is the crossing of lines (e.g., breeds, or artificially selected populations; **Fig. 1**). In livestock populations, linkage equilibrium is expected. Thus, reverse marker–QTL phase relationships may occur in the two parents of a full-sib family with biallelic markers (*25*), complicating the statistical analysis and dramatically reducing its power (*25–27*). A cross between two lines determines linkage disequilibrium in the gametes forming the F_1 such that marker–QTL phase relationships will

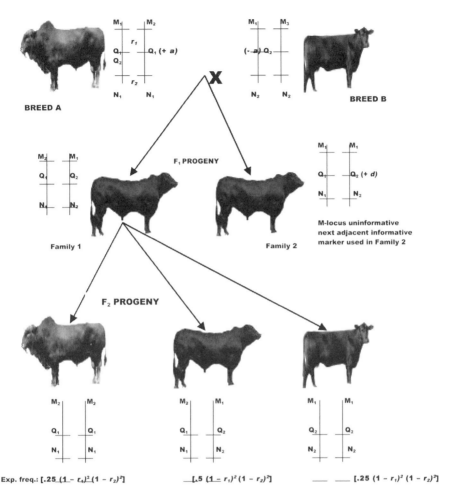

Fig. 1. A cross between outbred lines.

Recombinant classes not shown and identical genotypes assumed for both F_1 parents of this Family 1.

Ignoring double-recombinants, the expectation for the statistical contrast between the alternate double-homozygote marker-classes is (+ 2a).

Coefficients c_{ai} and c_{di} in equation (1) are computed regularly within the M-N marker-interval, conditional upon the flanking marker-information of Individual I as a function of the recombination rates r_1 and r_2.

be the same in both parents of a full-sib family (*25*). Additionally, nonrandom mating in the first generation of the cross will determine maximum parental (F_1) heterozygosity (*25*). Crossing of lines is a special case of a "full-sib" design (*see* **Subheading 2.3.**), similar to the traditional F_2 approach (*26*) used for inbred plants and animals (e.g., mice) and the power of which is considerably increased as a result of the concurrence of identical parental phases, maximal parental heterozygosity, and minimal background variation (*25,26*).

An interesting feature of this design concerns the statistical nature of QTL effects to be estimated. From a population genetics perspective, an inbred line represents an isolated, reproducible gamete, with an isolated reproducible QTL allele at each genomic location. With respect to these QTL alleles, specific statistical inferences can be made, and allelic effects are thus fixed effects in the statistical sense. In contrast, livestock populations are outbred, and individual parents of a particular experiment are only a possible sample of many from a population. The number of alleles at any given QTL is therefore unknown (*24,28,29*), and statistical inferences are usually not relative to the particular sample of alleles in the experiment, but to the overall population. Thus, with few exceptions (e.g., very large sire families in dairy or beef cattle), QTL allelic effects in livestock are random effects in the statistical sense, despite the fact that many of the analyses used to detect livestock QTL treat allelic effects as fixed effects for pragmatic reasons (*24*). Although inbred lines of livestock generally do not exist, most animals are members of a breed, sharing a higher degree of relationship than randomly chosen individuals from the species. Experimental lines having undergone long-term selection for quantitative traits will similarly have accumulated some level of inbreeding. Thus, individuals within a breed or line will simultaneously be segregating for some loci and fixed for others. Therefore, pairs of breeds/lines (especially those with large phenotypic divergence) can be treated as inbred lines from a statistical point of view for the purposes of QTL analysis. A cross between two breeds/ lines can be analyzed as an F_2 design under some assumptions, the most important of which is that the two breeds are in fixation for alternate QTL alleles while likely segregating for most marker loci with some degree of allele sharing. Inheritance of marker alleles is then traced within families, such that the breed/line of origin of each F_2 marker allele can be ascertained and the appropriate statistical contrasts evaluated (*see* **Fig. 1**).

An example of different terminologies for conceptually similar genetic designs is offered here. What is designated as "mapping by admixture linkage disequilibrium" in human populations (*30–32*) is what animal breeders designate as mapping from a cross between outbred lines. In the latter case, the admixture is complete in the first generation (fractions of 0.5 for each line), occurring in a single pulse without random mating, such that all gametic-phase disequilibrium (not resulting from linkage) vanishes in the F_2 offspring of the second generation of admixture (*32,33*).

The breed/line cross design requires F_1 marker heterozygosity, which does not always occur. Whereas Beckmann and Soller (*34*) provided the first clear theoretical indication of how to analyze such data, Haley et al. (*35*) solidly established the multimarker mapping regression approach for this particular design, as illustrated by Knott et al. (*16*). The basic statistical linear model, fitted in a least square framework and easily accommodating fixed factors and covariates, is of the type:

$$Y_i = \mu + c_{ai}a + c_{di}d + \varepsilon_i \qquad (1)$$

where Y_i is the phenotype of the *i*th F_2 individual, μ is the mean, and c_{ai} is the coefficient for the additive component for individual *i* at the assumed given location, equal to [prob(QQ) − prob(qq)] (a QTL fixed for alternative alleles Q and q is assumed in the two breeds/lines; following Falconer and Mackay (*36*), the effect of QQ is denoted "a," that of Qq is denoted as "d," and that of qq as "−a"); c_{di} is the coefficient for the dominance component for individual *i* at the given location, which is equal to prob(Qq), and ε_i are random residuals with expectation 0 and common variance (*16,35*).

The probabilities [prob(QQ) − prob(qq)] and prob(Qq) are computed at 1- to 2-cM intervals throughout the genome, conditional upon flanking marker information (*16,35;* **Fig. 1**). When the assumed location is at a fully informative marker, the probabilities depend on information from that marker only. Otherwise, the probabilities are functions of the recombination rates between the assumed location and the flanking informative markers.

A composite interval mapping approach (CIM; *37–39*) should be followed in these types of analysis. However, in outbred crosses and in livestock experimental designs in general, implementation of CIM is not straightforward because different markers will be informative in different families, and the presence of segregating QTL alleles may also be family specific (*23,29*). Knott et al. (*16*) outlined a scheme for cofactor selection in the context of an outbred cross, to adjust the analysis for unlinked QTL/polygenic effects. Based on the statistical model shown in Eq. (1), an *F*-ratio (or log odds [LOD] score) is computed at every cM to compare a model with a QTL at this location against a model without the QTL. The best estimate for QTL position is taken to be the location giving the highest *F*-ratio (*16,35*). Two-QTL models may be tested using two-dimensional searches, fitting the coefficients for two locations simultaneously (*16*). A genetic search algorithm to facilitate the implementation of multiple interacting QTL models has very recently been introduced (*40*).

Guidelines for reporting of suggestive and significant linkages (*41*) have been adopted in many livestock QTL studies. With regression approaches, suitable thresholds are often determined empirically by permutation testing (*42*). Confidence intervals for QTL location estimates may be obtained by bootstrapping (*43,44*).

The regression approach described in Eq. (1) treats the QTL effect as fixed, justifiable by the assumption of fixation of alternate alleles in the two lines. When this assumption is violated by within-line segregation of QTL alleles, there will be a random within-line variation. Perez-Enciso and Varona (*45*) recently introduced a mixed linear model procedure that provides a flexible variance component framework for QTL mapping in crosses between outbred lines and treats the average difference in allelic effects between the two breeds as a fixed effect. Additional variation within breeds is allowed through a covariance structure. They also propose partitioning the genome into a series of segments. The expected change in mean according to percentage of breed origin and the genetic variance associated with each segment are estimated using maximum likelihood [segment mapping (*45*)].

2.2. Half-Sib Designs

2.2.1. Regression Approaches

The half-sib design (*27*), sometimes designated the *daughter design* in dairy cattle, is illustrated in **Fig. 2**. This and other related approaches (**Figs. 3 and 4**) can be viewed as truncated F_2 designs, starting at the F_1 level. Given linkage equilibrium in the grandparental gametes, such that marker–QTL phase relationships may be reversed in different F_1 parents (*25*), within-family statistical analyses are required.

A multimarker mapping regression approach, deriving from **refs. 46** and **47**, has become the analytical method of choice for data from this design (e.g., **ref. 15**). Initially, the most likely haplotypes for each sire's gametes are determined (marker genotypes from dams would enhance this process, but are often too costly to justify and are seldom available). The most likely linkage phase is assumed to be the one minimizing the number of recombination events in the sire. If both phases are equally likely, one is selected at random. This process is repeated for each pair of adjacent heterozygous markers to reconstruct the two sire gametes (*15,46,47*). The QTL allele of reference for the statistical analysis is arbitrarily assigned to one of the linkage phases. The probability of inheriting the chromosomal segment of that linkage phase is calculated for every 1 or 2 cM for each sib, based on information from the closest informative markers, which will vary from sire family to sire family. Once these steps are completed, the following statistical linear model is fitted by least squares, which would easily accommodate additional fixed effects and covariates (*15,46,47*):

$$Y_{ij} = \mu + s_i + b_i X_{ij} + \varepsilon_{ij} \qquad (2)$$

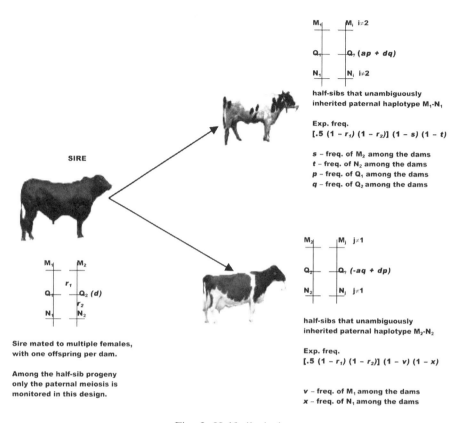

Fig. 2. Half-sib design.

Recombinant and ambiguous classes not shown. Assumes a bi-allelic QTL.

Ignoring double-recombinants, the expectation for the statistical contrast between half-sib groups above is $[a + d(q\text{-}p)]$.

The probability X_{ij} in equation (2) is computed regularly within the marker-interval M-N, conditional upon the flanking marker-information of half-sib j and as a function of the recombination rates r_1 and r_2.

where Y_{ij} is the phenotype of sib j of sire family i, s_i is the fixed effect associated with sire family i, and b_i is the average effect of the QTL allele substitution for sire i, with expectation $[a + d(q\text{-}p)]$ (**27**) if a biallelic QTL is assumed, with a and d as defined previously, and p and q are the QTL allele frequencies in the dams mated to sire i (multiple QTL alleles among the dams mated to sire i would require some reinterpretation of d, p, and q). X_{ij} is the probability of sib j of sire i inheriting the chromosomal segment for gamete one of sire i at the particular location being considered; other parameters are as defined previously. This model [Eq. (2)] allows for a maximum number of QTL alleles equal to twice the number of sires in the design (**15**). Residual sums of squares (RSS) from Eq. (2) are summed across families, and by the difference, the sum of squares explained by the QTL fitted in the model is (**15**)

$$\sum_{j=1}^{n} (Y_{ij} - \mu - s_i)^2 - \sum_{j=1}^{n} (Y_{ij} - \mu - s_i - b_i X_{ij})^2 \tag{3}$$

Larger sire-families will contribute more to overall RSS (**15**), and weighting by inverses of variances can be considered. Test statistics are then calculated at every 1 or 2 cM across the genome (**15**).

A two-stage strategy to increase experimental power has been proposed (**48**), relying on initial screening of a few progeny per sire to identify sires most likely to be heterozygous for QTL with large effects. Sires homozygous for important QTL are useless for their detection; in stage 2, only progeny of likely heterozygous sires are genotyped. A similar strategy for identification of chromosomes likely to harbor QTL was also proposed (**48**).

2.2.2. Maximum Likelihood

A maximum likelihood (ML) approach for mapping QTL in the context of a half-sib design has been proposed (**49**). The likelihood function Λ is the product of within-sire likelihoods Λ_i, which are of the following form:

$$\Lambda_i = \sum_{hsi} p(hs_i \mid M_i) \prod_{j=1}^{ni} \sum_{q=1}^{2} p(d_{ij} = q \mid hs_i, M_i) \, f(yp_{ij} \mid d_{ij} = q) \tag{4}$$

The data are assumed to be from i independent sire families, with respective dams (mates) unrelated to each other and to the sires. Sire i's mates and offspring are denoted ij (one offspring per dam). Phenotypes of progeny ij are denoted yp_{ij}, and marker genotypes of progeny, parents, and grandparents for a set of codominant loci are denoted by the prefix m (ms_i for sire i, md_{ij} for dam j mated to sire i, etc.). At each locus, the two alleles are arbitrarily denoted as ms^1_i and ms^2_i. Marker information concerning the family of sire i is pooled in vector M_i (**49**).

The L marker loci belonging to a previously known linkage group are considered simultaneously and recombination rates are assumed known from previous analyses. In (hs_i), a matrix of order L × 2, the first column, hs^1_i, corresponds to the chromosome transmitted by the grandsire to the sire, and the second column hs^2_i, corresponds to the chromosome transmitted by the grand-dam to the sire (and equivalently for hd_{ij}). At any position x within the linkage group, the hypothesis is tested that sire i is heterozygous for a QTL influencing the mean of the trait. Given the sire allele received at location x ($d_{ij} = 1$ or 2), the quantitative trait for progeny ij is assumed to be normally distributed with mean

$\mu_i^{dij} + X_{ij}\beta$ and variance σ_e^2, β being a vector of fixed effects and X_{ij} the corresponding incidence vector (for simplification, not included in Λ; *see* **ref. 49**). The penetrance function, f, is conditional on the q chromosome segment transmitted by the sire and is assumed to follow a normal distribution (*49*):

$$\left(\frac{1}{2\pi\sigma_e^2}\right)^{.5} exp\left[-0.5\left(\frac{yp_{ij} - \mu_i^q}{\sigma_e}\right)^2\right] \tag{5}$$

For computation of the remaining two components of Λ, the transmission probability $p(d_{ij} = q \mid hs_i, M_i)$ and the ordered-sire genotype probability conditional on the marker information, $p(hs_i \mid M_i)$, the reader is referred elsewhere (*49*). A number of alternative analytical strategies within the framework defined in Eq. (4) have been considered, including (1) simpler methods for handling the problem of unknown sire marker linkage phases (*50*), (2) linearization of the likelihood for relatively small QTL effects (*50*), (3) a variance components approach (*51*), (4) modeling of a biallelic QTL (*51*), and (5) heteroskedastic within-QTL variances between sire families (*51*).

Georges et al. (*14*) used ML with a mixture model similar to that defined in Eq. (4). Different sire families were analyzed independently, and likelihood ratio tests were computed by dividing the likelihood under H_a : ($\alpha_i = \mu_i^1 - \mu_i^2$ $\neq 0$; $\sigma_A^2 \neq 0$) by that under H_0 : ($\alpha_i = 0$; $\sigma_A^2 \neq 0$) (i.e., assuming no QTL segregating at the corresponding map position but still accommodating the MLE for the additive genetic variance [σ_A^2] in the likelihood). A threshold of 3 for the LOD score was chosen to indicate statistical significance based on theoretical considerations (*14*). Knott et al. (*47*) have also presented an approximate ML methodology for QTL mapping in half-sib families.

2.3. Full-Sib Designs

2.3.1. Regression Approaches

A full-sib design (*27*) is illustrated in **Fig. 3**. Least squares regression (LSR) approaches to interval mapping (*52*) with full-sib data are similar to those used in half-sib designs (*see* **ref. 53**). The basic statistical model is

$$Y_{ij} = \mu + f_i + b_{si}X_{sij} + b_{di}X_{dij} + \varepsilon_{ij} \tag{6}$$

Interpretation of statistical terms in Eq. (6) is similar to Eq. (2), but now Y_{ij} is the phenotype of sib j of full-sib family i, f_i is the fixed effect associated with full-sib family i, and because two QTL allele transmissions are traced per family (from the sire [s] and from the dam [d]), two regression terms are needed in Eq. (6). With full-sib designs, marker informativeness is particularly critical; otherwise, the capacity to ascertain allele transmission and paternal and maternal marker–QTL phase relationships may be severely hindered. Assuming fully

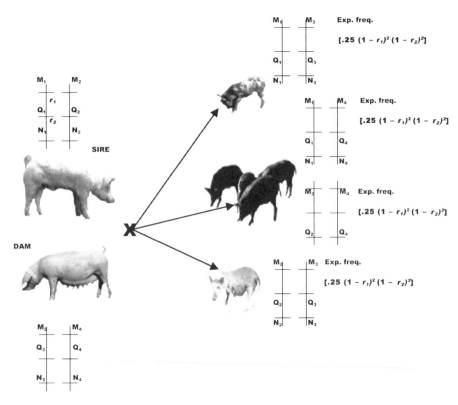

Fig. 3. Full-sib design.

Recombinant classes not shown. Assuming fully informative markers, and both parents heterozygous for the QTL, two statistical contrasts can be established among the full-sib progeny: one associated with the alternate paternal alleles inherited; the other with the alternate maternal alleles inherited. Ignoring double-recombinants, and based on the appropriate pairs of the non-recombinant classes shown above, each of these statistical contrasts has an expectation of $[a + d (q-p)]$ (see Fig. 2).

If more than two QTL alleles are involved, interpretation of a and d parameters above needs to be slightly readjusted, as they become average values across several genotypic combinations. In the context of this full-sib design, the distribution of the allele frequencies p and q in the expectation above becomes discrete as opposed to continuous in the context of the half-sib design.

informative markers (often unrealistic), the power associated with a full-sib design is roughly double that of a half-sib design (*27,54*).

2.3.2. Maximum Likelihood

Knott and Haley (*25*) introduced the following likelihood function *L* to map QTL in the context of a full-sib design, incorporating a random common-family effect:

$$L = \prod_{i=1}^{N} \oint_{-\infty}^{\infty} (2\pi\sigma_b^2)^{-0.5} \exp[-u_i^2/2\sigma_b^2] \sum_{m_s=1}^{M_s} p(m_s) \sum_{q_s=1}^{Q} \text{freq}(q_s) \sum_{m_d=1}^{M_d} p(m_d) \tag{7}$$

$$\times \sum_{q_d=1}^{Q} \text{freq}(q_d) \prod_{j=1}^{n_i} \sum_{m_j=1}^{M_j} \sum_{q_o=1}^{Q} \text{trans}(m_j, q_o \mid m_s, q_s, m_d, q_d) (2\pi\sigma_w^2)^{-0.5} \exp[-(y_{ij}-\mu-g_{q_o}-\mu_i)^2/2\sigma_w^2)]du_i$$

The first term of *L* is the random common-family effect, which is assumed to be normally distributed, with mean 0 and variance σ_b^2, and independent of the QTL and of the within-family environmental variance σ_w^2. The likelihood of the offspring phenotype given the QTL genotype (the last term of *L*) must also take account of the common-family effect (u_i). This parameter, however, is unknown and, for a given family mean, is expected to vary according to the different QTL genotypes considered for the parents. Hence, the likelihood must allow for integration over all possible values of the family effect (*25*). Apart from the common-family effect, components of *L* are analogous to those of Eq. (4), the likelihood considered in the half-sib design (*49*): *N* is the number of full-sib families, n_i is the number of full sibs in family *i*, M_j is the number of possible marker phases for offspring *j* (including whether marker haplotypes are from sire or dam); *Q* is the number of ordered genotypes at the QTL (i.e., 4), $p(m)$ is the probability of marker phase *m*, of sire *s* or dam *d*, freq(q) is the frequency of QTL genotype q, of sire *s* or dam *d*, in the parental generation, M_s and M_d are the number of possible marker phases for the sire and dam, respectively, g_{qo} is equal to *a* for Q_1Q_1, *d* for Q_1Q_2 and Q_2Q_1, and −*a* for Q_2Q_2 (*25,36*) (a bi-allelic QTL is assumed), and trans(m_j, $q_o|m_s$, q_s, m_d, q_d) is the probability of the offspring marker and QTL genotypes given the parental genotypes and phase of linkage [the probability of QTL genotypes is considered jointly with, rather than conditional on, that of observed marker genotypes (*25*)].

The QTL genotype and phase of linkage are not known for any parent and, hence, all possible genotypes and phases need to be considered (linkage equilibrium assumed in the parental generation). The *N* full-sib families are assumed unrelated with parents mated at random. A prior estimate for the recombination fraction between markers is used so that transmission probabilities can be written in terms of a single unknown parameter, the recombination fraction between one of the markers and the QTL (*25*).

A numerical approximation to the exact likelihood in Eq. (7) was proposed (*25*), replacing integration with weighted summation. To test for a QTL linked to a marker, the maximized likelihood in Eq. (7) is compared to the maximized likelihood under a model without a linked QTL. Marker data are omitted from the model under H_0, which then becomes a segregation analysis likelihood (*25*). This test is different from that implemented by Georges et al. (*14*). Knott and Haley (*25*) indicate that inflation of the test statistic may result when the test for a linked QTL is made against a model not allowing for between-family variation (including an unlinked QTL or a between-family variance component). This method [Eq. (7)] constitutes a *direct mapping approach* (*55*), with the recombination rate being a parameter over which the likelihood function is maximized, as opposed to *indirect mapping approaches* (*55*), which rely on computation of test statistics at regular genomic intervals (*15,16,35,46,47,53*).

2.4. Mixtures of Full Sibs and Half Sibs

Le Roy et al. (*56*) have proposed an ML method to map QTL with data from a mixture of large full- and half-sib families, a scenario frequently encountered in many livestock species. The methodology proposed is an extension of Eq. (4), the likelihood function introduced by Elsen et al. (*49*) for half-sib designs.

2.5. Granddaughter and Grand²-daughter Designs

The granddaughter design proposed by Weller et al. (*57*) (**Fig. 4**) represented an important innovation in experimental designs for QTL mapping, primarily in dairy cattle where pedigrees of sufficient size exist. The design is derived from the replicated progenies concept (*58,59*) and fits the structure of the progeny-testing schemes in the dairy cattle industry. In essence, the granddaughter design (*57*) amounts to a half-sib design for which the phenotype being considered and utilized for QTL mapping is a mean of grand-offspring, rather than the phenotype of the half-sib (contrast **Figs. 2** and **4**). The fact that granddaughter phenotypes are considered halves of the expectation of the marker contrasts as compared to those obtained under a half-sib design (**Figs. 2** and **4**), but the associated variances of these granddaughter contrasts will also be reduced because means are used as opposed to single measurements. This increases the power of QTL detection, requiring much less marker genotyping as opposed to more extensive phenotypic measurement (*54,57*). However, extensive phenotyping is routinely obtained in dairy bull progeny testing schemes, so little extra effort or cost is incurred.

Although the traditional granddaughter design (*57*) encompasses a half-sib structure, Van der Beek et al. (*54*) considered additional variants of the granddaughter design, such as all combinations of half- or full-sib offspring (second generation) and half- or full-sib grand-offspring (third generation).

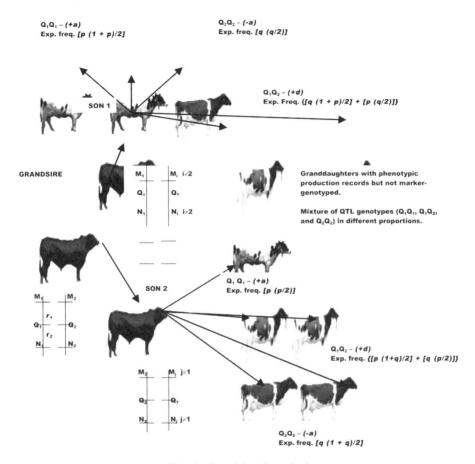

Fig. 4. Granddaughter design.

A bi-allelic QTL is assumed, recombinant marker-classes are not shown, double-recombinants are ignored, and only unambiguous paternal-haplotype transmissions are considered above (see Fig. 2).

The expectation for the statistical contrast between the two alternate mean grand offspring-values corresponding to the two alternate half-sib marker-classes above is $\frac{1}{2} [a + d (q - p)]$, which is half of the expectation for the corresponding statistical contrast in a half-sib design (see Fig. 2).

Their conclusion was that three-generation designs encompassing a full-sib-based second generation (typed for markers) and a half-sib-based third generation (with trait measurements) were most efficient in regard to genotyping for a given statistical power (**54**). They further concluded that the relative advantage decreases as heritability of the trait increases (**54**).

When means of grand-offspring are used in the analysis of a granddaughter design, each half-sib is associated with only one quantitative value (the average of his daughters' phenotypes), and, therefore, the statistical analysis becomes that for a conventional half-sib design [Eqs. (2)–(4)]. The only difference may be consideration of weighting factors (*15,60*) because some means may be based on more measurements than others (**Fig. 4**). The inverse of the variance is the weighting factor usually implemented (*15,60*).

The grand^2-daughter design proposed by Coppieters et al. (*61*) consists of a strategy for QTL confirmation, once evidence for a putative QTL emerges from a conventional granddaughter design (*57*). The method uses multimarker tracing of the segregation of the two QTL alleles from a grandsire to his maternal grandsons via nongenotyped daughters, followed by contrasting the quantitative value associated with the inheritance of these alternative homologs by the maternal grandsons. This is an effective way to rapidly confirm putative QTL in an independent sample without additional sampling or genotyping (*61*). The density of markers in the regions of interest should be increased to facilitate QTL allele tracing and compensate for missing genotypes of the dams (*61*).

2.6. Complex Pedigree Structures

2.6.1. Variance Component Approaches

Variance components (VC) approaches to interval mapping (*52*) have been developed for livestock (*24,62–64*). This is particularly relevant because prediction of *breeding values* from phenotypic records (*22*) is an integral component of genetic selection programs, having had a tremendous impact on genetic improvement in livestock species. Prediction of *breeding values* (*22*) derives from implementation of a mixed linear model incorporating fixed effects and additive genetic values of animals (the *breeding value*) as random effects with an associated variance component (*22*). A key component is the modeling of covariances among relatives with a matrix of additive genetic relationships (under no inbreeding, the fraction of genes that two individuals are, on average, expected to share identical by descent, IBD) among all members of a pedigree (*22*). Parameter estimation usually is based on restricted (or residual) maximum likelihood (REML) which maximizes the portion of the likelihood that is invariant to the fixed effects (*7,65*). Because data structures in livestock populations usually encompass large pedigrees with complex relationships, restriction to statistical methods capable of analyzing only previously described experimental designs would be a major limitation, failing to use all available information (*66,67*). Thus, incorporation of QTL interval mapping (*52*) into this VC analytical framework (*22,65*) is a significant advance that adequately models the random (statistical) nature of QTL effects in livestock populations and includes the capability to estimate the variance component associated with this random effect. The model also simultaneously accounts for residual polygenic effects while estimating QTL effects, and it adjusts predicted *breeding values* (*22*) to reflect estimated QTL effects. VC methods are robust approaches that, compared to ML methods treating QTL as fixed effects, require fewer parametric assumptions, are less sensitive to deviations from normality, and are often more tractable computationally (*24,62*).

Building on previous contributions (*68–70*), the mixed linear model introduced by Grignola et al. (*62*) is

$$Y = X\beta + Zu + ZTv + \varepsilon \tag{8}$$

where Y is an $N \times 1$ vector of phenotypes, β is a vector of fixed effects, X is a design matrix relating β to Y, u is an $n \times 1$ vector of random residual additive polygenic effects, Z is an incidence matrix relating u to y, v is a $2n \times 1$ vector of random QTL allelic effects, T is an incidence matrix relating each animal to its two QTL alleles, and ε is a vector of random residuals (*62*). The variance structures underlying Eq. (8) are

$$\text{Var}(u) = A\sigma_u^2, \text{Var}(v) = Q\sigma_v^2, \text{Var}(\varepsilon) = R\sigma_\varepsilon^2 \tag{9}$$

where A is the additive genetic relationship matrix of dimension $n \times n$, which, under no inbreeding (inbreeding can easily be accommodated), is a matrix of 1's in the diagonals and the remaining elements a_{ij} being the expected fraction of genes (alleles) that animals i and j are expected to share IBD relative to a reference base population; σ_u^2 is the residual additive polygenic variance, $Q\sigma_v^2$ is the variance–covariance matrix of the QTL allelic effects conditional on marker information, with σ_v^2 being half of the additive genetic variance explained by the QTL (also designated QTL allelic variance); R is usually an identity matrix, and σ_ε^2 is the residual variance (*62*). All of these variances are assumed to be associated with normal distributions. The expectation of $Q\sigma_v^2$ is equal to a weighted average of variance–covariance matrices conditional on all possible sets of multilocus marker genotypes given the observed marker data (*62*). Probabilities of multilocus marker genotypes are computed from the observed marker information without consideration of phenotypic information, contrary to exact mixture and Bayesian approaches (*23,29,62*).

Parameterization in Eqs. (8) and (9) circumvents the need for assumptions concerning the number of QTL alleles, often unknown in livestock populations (*24,28,29*). Effects of QTL alleles are assumed normally distributed under an *infinite alleles model* (*62*). Implementation of a REML-based VC procedure is complex, especially with a variance–covariance matrix of QTL allelic effects [Eqs. (8) and (9)] conditional on marker information, and requires estimation of a recombination parameter (*see* **refs.** *62–64* for details). Grignola et al. (*64*) expanded the model [Eqs. (8) and (9)] to include mapping of two linked QTL. The methodology appears to accommodate some degree of missing marker data (critical in complex pedigrees involving ancestors with no DNA sample), but this capability is limited (*71*). Currently, only groups of simple half- or full-sib families can be efficiently accommodated (*62–64*). Pedigree relationships among sires can be accommodated, but dams are assumed unrelated. A similar, less general REML-based VC procedure was presented by Van Arendonk et al. (*71*).

An additional consideration concerns hypothesis testing of QTL effects in the context of the model in Eqs. (8) and (9). The likelihood under the null hypothesis is evaluated at $\sigma_v^2 = 0$ (*62*). A likelihood ratio test is conducted, but the distribution is not known and empirical assessment through data permutation is computationally unfeasible (*62*). Grignola et al. (*62*) proposed the estimation of thresholds for a number of less stringent significance levels, followed by extrapolation to obtain the desired thresholds (*62,72*). Concern over robustness of likelihood ratio tests, in the framework of QTL mapping procedures using VC methods, has been raised (*73*).

A more general and flexible VC approach for QTL mapping, capable of handling considerable missing marker information and arbitrarily complex pedigree structures, is that of George et al. (*24*). The methodology is similar to the model described in Eqs. (8) and (9) and is a two-step VC approach based on interval mapping principles (*52*), which begins by utilizing available marker data and pedigree information to calculate the covariance matrices associated with a QTL at a particular position on the genome. The mixed linear model is then constructed and parameter estimates are obtained. This two-step process is repeated for each position of the genome. The approach (*24*) is highlighted by implementation of a *simulation-based algorithm* for calculating IBD probabilities (*74*) at a QTL between all pairs of individuals, given considerable missing information and pedigree complexities.

For pedigrees with incomplete marker information, direct application of *recursive* or *correlation-based algorithms* (*24*) is not possible. The matrix Q in Eq. (9) is often replaced by its expectation (*E*) conditioned on the observed marker data (M_{obs}):

$$E(Q \mid M_{obs}) = \sum_{w}^{\Omega} Q_w \, \Pr(w \mid M_{obs}) \tag{10}$$

where w is a single phase-known complete marker configuration for the pedigree from the set of all possible complete marker configurations Ω, Q_w is the covariance matrix for a putative QTL conditional on w and test position, and $\Pr(w \mid M_{obs})$ is the conditional probability of the complete marker configuration w given observed marker data M_{obs} (*24*). Each of these Q_w matrices in Eq. (10)

can be estimated via *recursive* or *correlation-based algorithms*. However, calculating the expectation of Q for pedigrees including substantial missing data presents two computational challenges. First, the number of configurations in Ω is large, and the order of summation in Eq. (10) makes the calculation infeasible (*24*). Second, exact calculation of $\Pr(w \mid M_{obs})$ is intractable (*24*). Both problems lead to utilization of simulation techniques to obtain the expectation in Eq. (10), namely Markov chain Monte Carlo (MCMC) approaches (*24*). Specifically, George et al. (*24*) implement a *multiple-site segregation sampler* that relies on the Gibbs sampler and on utilization of *segregation indicators* (*24,74*).

Variance component approaches to QTL mapping have also been developed for use in human pedigrees (*67*). Almasy and Blangero (*67*) implemented a correlation-based algorithm for the computation of IBD probabilities deriving from **ref. 75**. Once again, integration of approaches and thought processes across species would be a welcome advance in this area, where the multiplicity of related ML methodologies for complex pedigree analysis is remarkable (*24,29,62–64,66,67,71,75–86*). Although much remains to be accomplished in this respect, important steps have been initiated (*7,12,86*).

2.6.2. Maximum Likelihood

2.6.2.1. JANSEN'S MIXTURE MODEL

Assuming QTL segregate for a particular trait, the full relationship between phenotypes and possible QTL genotypes has necessarily to be a *mixture* of distributions. However, an exact *mixture analysis* can be quite demanding computationally; hence, approximate *expectation methods* have been developed that are based on normality assumptions, such as the previously described LSR approaches of Haley et al. (*35*) and Knott et al. (*46,47*) for fixed QTL effects, and the VC approaches of Grignola et al. (*62–64*) and George et al. (*24*) for random QTL effects (*29*). The ML approaches of Elsen et al. (*49*), Georges et al. (*14*), and Knott and Haley (*25*) use mixture models, but for the simplified conditions of one QTL, no relationships or dependencies among animals and no missing marker data exist.

Jansen et al. (*29*) introduced a mixture model applicable to complex population structures in which dependencies (pedigree relationships) among individuals may exist. Their methodology is based on the expectation–maximization (EM) algorithm. They proposed both a stochastic EM algorithm and a Monte Carlo EM algorithm in which a Markov chain of possible genotypic configurations is generated via the Gibbs sampler (*29*) to maximize the likelihood. They considered both single- and multiple-QTL models, with fixed random effects, and illustrated their approaches with an application to half-sib families of dairy cattle (*29*).

With θ the vector of all parameters for fixed and random model terms and for recombination and allele frequencies, the simultaneous likelihood $L(\theta)$ of all observed trait and marker data under the mixture model considered by Jansen et al. (*29*) is of the form

$$L(\theta) = f(y, h) = \sum_g P(g)f(y, h|g) \tag{11}$$

where y denotes trait values, h denotes the observed marker data, and g denotes possible genotypic configurations at all marker loci and one or more putative QTL, each with a scalar probability of occurrence $P(g)$; $f(y, h|g) = f(y|g)$ if h is consistent with g, and 0 otherwise (*29*).

Jansen et al. (*29*) evaluated models including parameters for allele frequencies of markers and QTL, for discrete or normal effects of biallelic or multiallelic QTL, and for homogeneous or heterogeneous residual variances. Compared to VC approaches previously described (*24,62–64*), their methodology (*29*) seems to offer more flexibility in handling of missing marker data and fitting of multiple QTL models. However, how their approach could parallel those of Grignola et al. and George et al. (*24,62–64*) in modeling the covariance structure among related individuals, and therefore estimation of variance components associated with random QTL effects, is not entirely clear. Consequently, the future potential of this procedure in the context of livestock QTL analysis is uncertain. The authors (*29*) describe data imputation via the Gibbs sampler that could generate "known genotypes," which would be analyzed by standard software routines for linear regression and variance components (*29*). Further developments are needed before the merits of this approach can be adequately assessed.

2.6.2.2. COMPLEX SEGREGATION AND LINKAGE ANALYSIS

Developments in ML-based complex segregation analysis have recently taken place in livestock breeding (*83,87,88*). The *finite polygenic mixed model* (*83*), an alternative to the classical mixed major-gene–polygenic model of inheritance (*76*), offers some capability for marker–QTL linkage analysis in complex pedigrees by application of the Elston–Stewart algorithm (*66*; C. Stricker, personal communication). In a sense, all QTL analysis could historically be viewed as special cases of the Elston-Stewart algorithm (*66*), which provides a general framework for quantitative trait analysis in pedigrees.

2.6.3. Bayesian Approaches

In QTL analysis, evaluation of a number of likelihood functions requires summing over the set of all possible unobserved discrete genotypes of many individuals. These likelihoods may include complex dependencies (relationships) among pedigree members, segregation of multiple QTL, occurrence of incomplete marker data in many individuals, and uncertainty with respect to a number of parameters that are not of direct relevance to the ultimate goals of the analysis [e.g., fixed effects, variance components, allele frequencies (*89*)]. The number of terms rapidly becomes too large to be calculated in an exact manner (*90*). MCMC methods and the Bayesian framework fit well for approximating these tasks numerically (*90*). Monte Carlo integration draws samples from the required distribution and MCMC samples for a long time, to construct a chain having at equilibrium a distribution equal to the distribution being approximated (*23*).

In Bayesian analysis, all model parameters and missing data ("unobservables") are treated as random variables. A full probability model is formulated considering all variables (θ) conditioned on the observed data. By applying Bayes' rule, an expression is obtained for the posterior density (*90*):

$$p\ (\theta \mid data) = [p\ (data \mid \theta)\ p\ (\theta)/p\ (data)] \tag{12}$$

where $p\ (data \mid \theta)$ is the likelihood of the data given θ, $p\ (\theta)$ is a joint prior, and $p\ (data)$ is the unconditional likelihood of the data (*90*). Nuisance parameters (not of posterior interest) are integrated out from the full posterior. MCMC methods provide feasible approximate numerical solutions to the exact evaluation of the posterior distribution, especially because the expression for the posterior density needs to be known only up to a Normalizing constant when using MCMC (*90*). Through the application of simple conditional independence assumptions, Bayesian analysis allows for a description of complex dependency structures in the joint prior $p(\theta)$. Uncertainty in one parameter is automatically incorporated into the estimation of marginal posterior distributions of other parameters (*90*). For a QTL analysis, the dimension of the parameter space (depending on the number of QTL) is treated as a random variable with an associated marginal posterior probability (*90–92*). This provides an automatic and useful feature for model selection for an analysis considering alternative multiple QTL models (*91–93*).

A frustrating aspect of current Bayesian applications in genetics is that Bayesian jargon and methodology are not well understood by many. Additionally, successful computer implementation of MCMC methods may be more an art than a scientific exercise. To obtain an MCMC realization seems to be straightforward, but to make sure that the generated sample represents the correct target distribution seems to be a different matter (*90*). To date, few analyses of real datasets have been reported, and if Bayesian approaches have real merit, a serious effort is needed to clearly elucidate the basic principles and methodologies that are involved in this implementation. For an in-depth treatment of Bayesian approaches, the reader is referred to previous reviews

(*6,12*) and recent dissertations (*23,55,90*). Understanding these works requires extensive knowledge of Bayesian principles and methodologies.

Two main Bayesian approaches have evolved for use in livestock QTL analysis. Hoeschele and VanRaden (*94,95*) defined a basic Bayesian framework for marker–QTL linkage analysis for half-sib and granddaughter designs. This included derivation of prior distributions for QTL substitution effects, QTL allele and genotype frequencies, marker–QTL recombination rates, and prior probability of linkage between a single or pair of marker loci and a QTL (*94*). Subsequently, this prior information was combined with simulated data from half-sib and granddaughter designs in a Bayesian analysis to compute the posterior probability of linkage between markers and a biallelic QTL (*95*). A prior exponential distribution of QTL effects was assumed, and if the posterior probability of linkage exceeded a limit, linkage was declared and Bayesian estimates were obtained. Estimates of QTL effects were shrunken toward the mean/mode of the exponential prior (*94,95*).

The MCMC algorithms to implement this approach (*94,95*) were developed by Thaller and Hoeschele (*96,97*). Estimators of parameters were marginal posterior means computed using a Gibbs sampler with data augmentation for marker–QTL genotypes and polygenic effects (*96,97*). MCMC versions of Bayesian tests for marker–QTL linkage (represented by an indicator variable) were also introduced (*96,97*). Uimari et al. (*98*) extended the approach to utilize information from multiple linked markers and to perform one analysis per chromosome, as opposed to analyzing each marker separately (*98*). Finally, Uimari and Hoeschele (*91*) expanded the methodology to accommodate mapping of two linked QTL. Three different MCMC schemes for testing the presence of a single or two linked QTL were compared, two of them based on the formulation of indicator variables, and the third based on model determination by *reversible-jump* MCM (*91–93*).

Hoeschele (*12*) has expanded on *genotype sampling algorithms* that are essential for implementation of MCMC Bayesian approaches and even for ML approaches such as those of Jansen et al. (*29*). Genotype sampling algorithms are necessary to obtain genotype samples for MCMC realizations and are critical for accommodating missing marker data for many individuals. Samples of genotypes derive from the joint distribution of genotypes of all pedigree members at all loci, conditional on observed marker genotypic and phenotypic data (in contrast to VC approaches that do not use phenotypic information for this purpose; *see* above; refs. *12, 23, 29,* and *62*). Hoeschele (*12*) has discussed genotype sampling algorithms based on genotypic peeling, allelic peeling, and descent graphs.

Whereas these MCMC Bayesian methodologies are focused on biallelic QTL and characterized by the utilization of reversible-jump MCMC algorithms,

Bink's Bayesian framework (in the context of granddaughter designs) is focused on normally distributed QTL effects and characterized by utilization of *simulated tempering* MCMC algorithms (*23,99–102*). First, Bink et al. (*23,99*) formulated a basic Gibbs sampling approach capable of accommodating and extracting full genetic information from ungenotyped pedigree members. A single marker linked to a QTL was considered and phenotypic information was included (*12,23,29,62*) to derive sampling distributions for augmentation of marker genotypes (*23,99*). Subsequently, the focus shifted to QTL variance component estimation through implementation of Metropolis–Hastings (M-H) algorithms, which allow for exploration of sampling spaces with nonstandard densities (*23,100*), and QTL mapping through the implementation of *simulated tempering*, a relatively new MCMC technique that improves the mixing properties of some Markov chains (*23,101*). In fact, straightforward implementation of a M-H algorithm to shuffle the QTL position within the linkage maps led to an effectively reducible Markov chain (i.e., not all possible positions were reached from a given starting position for the QTL). Bink and Van Arendonk (*102*) integrated previous developments (*99–101*) in an MCMC framework for QTL mapping and parameter estimation, facilitating augmentation of marker genotypes for ungenotyped individuals and accommodating additional dependencies (pedigree relationships) among ungenotyped dams of a granddaughter design. Although these advancements appear to create an advantage, the methods do not consider multiple QTL models in contrast to others (*91*). With both sets of methodologies [(*91,94–98*) and (*23,99–102*)], covariances among genetic effects of related individuals are taken into account via an additive genetic relationship matrix for polygenes and a gametic relationships matrix for QTL (see earlier; *refs. 24, 62–64,* and *71*).

An MCMC Bayesian framework for half-sib designs was introduced by George et al. (*55,103*). The methodology focuses on a biallelic QTL, but a monogenic model of inheritance is considered, without modeling of genetic covariances among relatives or inclusion of residual polygenic variance (*55,103*). This limitation detracts from the utility of a methodology that appears suitable primarily for estimation of QTL dominance effects (*55,103*). Reversible-jump and product-space MCMC sampler algorithms were utilized and compared (*55,103*).

Finally, Janss et al. (*104*) developed a Bayesian approach to complex segregation analysis (*55*). De Koning et al. (*105*) utilized this procedure to map QTL by obtaining posterior genotype probabilities for QTL imputed from complex segregation analyses (*104*), and subsequently conducting standard linkage analyses among these QTL genotypes, and genomewide markers. Results were not encouraging (*105*); genotypic assignments from posterior inferences were based on probability thresholds, likely yielding considerable imprecision.

3. Interpretation

For a discussion of statistical power associated with different analytical techniques and experimental designs, the reader is referred to studies addressing this important issue (*27,34,48,54,57,106–111*). Although statistical methodology for QTL analysis in livestock has reached a level of high quality, appropriate construction of 95% confidence intervals (CI) for QTL location parameters often leads to inclusion of large proportions of the target chromosomes, even when large QTL effects are detected (*16,112*) and sufficiently dense marker maps are employed. This has rendered nonselective bootstrapping (*43*) practically useless for CI construction in the context of QTL analysis (*112*). Selective bootstrapping strategies (*44*), which utilize only samples with particular properties, such as samples providing statistical evidence for the QTL or samples that support the same mode of QTL gene action and the same signs of the estimated additive and dominance effects as in the original sample, have been proposed and provide better results (*44,112*). However, even these improved strategies (*44*) lead to 95% CI that often average 20 cM in genetic distance (*112*). Assuming an average of 25 genes/cM, approximately 500 genes will be harbored within a CI spanning a particular QTL location. In addition, Visscher and Haley (*113*) and Liu and Dekkers (*114*) have established that current QTL models have limited ability to determine whether genetic variance resulting from a chromosome is contributed by a single QTL of major effect or a large number of QTL with minor effects. Thus, it is essentially impossible to extrapolate from a significant test at a particular location to identification of a list of putative candidate genes that can individually, or in combination, be responsible for the estimated effect. Obviously, increasingly sophisticated analyses, but more importantly, increasingly powerful datasets, will be necessary for refinement of estimates of QTL locations and effects. To make the leap to actual gene discovery, new tools will need to be combined with QTL analysis, including gene expression (mRNA and protein) analysis, mutational analysis, well-characterized and ordered genomic libraries, and large-scale sequencing of the expressed genomes of livestock species.

To address these issues, deriving from the study of Visscher and Haley (*113*), a number of complementary statistical tests have been proposed for a QTL analysis in the framework of a line cross (*16*). Three additional related statistical models were implemented and tested by Knott et al. (*16*) to explore biological meaning and assess the most likely genetic model underlying any statistical significance detected by the model in Eq. (1): a multiple QTL model, a single region model, and a polygenic model. With the multiple QTL model, offspring phenotypes are regressed simultaneously onto the coefficients of a and d for a number of evenly spaced marker locations along a chromosome, testing for genetic variation on the chromosome affecting the trait under consideration. Degrees of freedom for the genetic component of this model are twice the number of selected marker locations on the chromosome (*16,113*). With the single-region model, the coefficients of a and d from two selected marker locations flanking an interval are fitted. This tests for an effect associated with the flanked interval, with the analysis repeated for each interval in the chromosome. The genetic component of this model has four degrees of freedom (*16,113*). Under the polygenic model, offspring phenotypes are regressed on the proportion of each breed/line that is present along the chromosome. Some of the assumptions inherent to the fitting of this polygenic model are (1) no double recombination between selected markers, (2) means of coefficients at selected markers are weighted to account for unequal marker spacing, and (3) each equal length of a chromosome from one breed/line has the same effect in the same direction, which implies cis associations of QTL alleles in the two breeds or lines (otherwise trans effects will mask each other). If all markers in a chromosome are used, the test would be equivalent to regressing on the mean coefficients for a and d for the chromosome (*16,113*).

Comparing these tests indicates the most likely underlying genetic models for each chromosome harboring a putative QTL. If the multiple QTL model is significant, the other two models are compared with it to determine whether they provide an adequate description of the data. If one or several QTL are linked together in a small region of the chromosome, then fitting coefficients from markers flanking this region would explain most of the genetic variation associated with the chromosome and, hence, the multiple QTL model would not be a significant improvement over the single-region model. Alternatively, with many QTL linked in association in the grandparental lines, the polygenic model would provide an adequate description of the data and would not be rejected in favor of the multiple QTL model (*16,113*). Although conclusions drawn from these comparisons are somewhat limited, they may reveal clues as to the biological and genetic relevance of some of the statistically significant results detected in a QTL analysis. Similar tests could be tailored to fit experimental designs other than breed/line crosses.

Interpretation of a and d coefficients in the model in Eq. (1) was based on the assumption of alternate QTL alleles being fixed in the two crossed breeds/lines. If this assumption does not hold true, the approach may considerably lose power, and a and d become complex functions of differences between effects of QTL alleles weighted by differences in their frequency in the two lines and subject to a sampling effect as a result of parental F_1 representation in the particular experiment. Assuming that parental F_1's are a representative sample of all possible grandparental gametic combinations, a and d could then be interpreted as average additive differences and dominance deviations (at that genomic location) among all pairs of QTL alleles segregating in the two breeds/lines crossed.

4. Software

4.1. Crosses Between Outbred Lines

Software implementing methodologies described for this design (model **1**; refs. *16,* and *35*) is available for use at no cost from http://latte.cap.ed.ac.uk. This WWW site, although still in development, is user-friendly with clear instructions and detailed examples. File formats are common and easily prepared. Although the software is not available for downloading, data files may be submitted for analysis, with results provided to the user. Capabilities for data permutation (*42*) and construction of CIs by bootstrapping (*43,44*) are available.

4.2. Half-Sib Designs

Three computer programs appear to be available with capabilities to implement QTL analyses under this design (Fig. 2). **QTLMAP** (*49*) is a program written in FORTRAN 77, available upon request and at no cost from Jean-Michel Elsen (INRA; elsen@toulouse.inra.fr). The program implements ML methodology described in Eqs. (4) and (5) as well as alternative analytical strategies that were discussed under that framework (*49–51*). **HSQM** is a series of computer programs that promise to perform LSR, ML, and rank-based nonparametric (*115*) QTL analyses under half-sib designs (**Fig. 2**). Michel Georges (University of Liege; michel@stat.fmv.ulg.ac.be) has indicated that the programs are available upon request. Programs implementing LSR methodologies described in Eqs. (2) and (3) are available upon request from Chris Haley (Roslin Institute; chris.haley.@bbsrc.ac.uk).

4.3. Full-Sib Designs

From Elsen et al. (*49*), it is not clear whether **QTLMAP** will perform QTL analyses under strict full-sib designs (**Fig. 3**), but it may. **MapQTL** is a program sold from http://www.cpro.wageningen-ur.nl/cbw/mapping. This is software designed for plant-breeding applications; it implements ML-based QTL analyses for a single full-sib family, accommodating up to four QTL alleles (*116*). This limitation renders the program of little use for livestock-breeding structures.

4.4. Mixture of Full and Half Sibs

QTLMAP also implements the ML methodology introduced by Le Roy et al. (*56*), a variant of model in Eq. (4) suited to these types of family structures.

4.5. Complex Pedigree Structures

4.5.1. Variance Component Approaches

MQREMLH and **MQREMLF** are REML-based VC programs that implement methodologies introduced by Grignola et al. (*62–64*) and described in

Eqs. (8) and (9). The programs are available upon request, from Ina Hoeschele (Virginia Polytechnic Institute; inah@vt.edu). **MQREMLH** is designed for QTL mapping in half-sib and granddaughter designs (**Figs. 2** and **4**), whereas **MQREMLF** is targeted to half- and full-sib mixtures. Pedigree relationships can be accommodated only through males (**62–64,117**). These programs are written in FORTRAN 77 and run under UNIX environments. Chromosomes are analyzed singly, and two strategies are used to accommodate multiple QTL models (**117**). In strategy A, multiple QTL are mapped simultaneously with a cyclic optimization of QTL positions. In each cycle, all but one QTL are fixed at their current most likely position while the position of one of the QTLs is optimized. This procedure is performed, in turn, for each QTL until convergence is reached (**117**). Either an empty marker interval or a minimum distance between any two QTL is required to ensure estimability of both QTL positions and QTL variances (**117**). A likelihood ratio is computed for each QTL as the ratio of the likelihood with all QTL variances estimated (H_a) to the likelihood with the variance of the QTL being considered fixed at zero (H_0; **refs. 62–64** and **117**). In strategy B, for a given marker interval, one QTL at either side of the interval (flanking QTL) is fitted and the QTL within the interval is mapped while fixing the position of the flanking QTL. For each interval, a likelihood ratio test is constructed between the likelihood with variances estimated for both QTL (H_a) and the likelihood with variance fixed at zero for the QTL being mapped (H_0; **refs. 62–64** and **117**).

4.5.2. Complex Segregation and Linkage Analysis

SALP (**S**egregation **A**nd **L**inkage analysis for **P**edigrees) (**118**) is a computer program mainly designed for complex segregation analyses in complex pedigrees implementing the finite polygenic mixed-model approach of Fernando et al. (**83**) or the regressive models of Bonney et al. (**80**). Applications of the Elston-Stewart algorithm gives the program capability for two-point linkage analyses between a single biallelic QTL/major locus and a single marker with any number of alleles while accommodating a residual polygenic component (**118**). Missing marker data are not accommodated. SALP can be obtained at no cost from http://www.tz.inw.agrl.ethz.ch/~stricker/salp/.

4.5.3. Bayesian Approaches

Programs for exact Bayesian analyses for half-sib designs with relationships across families (**6**) are not currently available, but more general Bayesian programs will be available sometime in 2001 (Hoeschele, personal communication). Software developed by Sillanpaa (**90**) for Bayesian QTL analyses is aimed at plant-breeding research. Again, as with **MapQTL**, the focus is on single full-sib outbred families with up to four QTL alleles accommodated

(*90*). Sillanpaa's Bayesian software for multiple QTL mapping in outbred populations with incomplete marker data [**Multimapper/outbred** (*90*) is available at no cost from http://www.rni.helsinki.fi/~mjs/.

5. Examples in the Literature

Given the broad scope and inclusive nature of this chapter and the multitude of designs, approaches, and models used in the analysis of livestock QTL data, a single worked example is not feasible nor would it be particularly useful. Many real examples illustrating the use of most of these methodologies have been referenced in the text (*13–20,23,53,60,61,105,112,115*). Alternatively, results are available from a QTL workshop held at the 1996 biannual meeting of the International Society of Animal Genetics (*5,72*), where a systematic comparison of different QTL methodologies was conducted. Real and simulated data from a granddaughter design (*57*) comprising 20 half-sib families were analyzed by 3 different procedures: LSR, REML-VC, and Bayesian analysis (*5,72*). Bayesian analysis was performed under both a normal-effects and a biallelic QTL model. All three procedures were able to locate accurately the simulated QTL and agreed on QTL location estimates from the real dataset. However, there were important differences in estimates of QTL-associated variance, with the Bayesian analysis being sensitive to model misspecification (e.g., analyzing a simulated biallelic QTL under a normal-effects model and vice versa).

Computational advantages offered by LSR approaches were emphasized by the workshop (*72*), because they allow easy application of permutation procedures (*42*) essential for determination of significance thresholds. Although computationally demanding, Bayesian approaches were noted for their superior capabilities concerning parameter estimation under different models. REML-VC procedures were intermediate with respect to advantages and disadvantages of the other approaches (*72*). Different procedures are recommended for different stages of data analysis (*72*). A first genome scan could be conducted with LSR approaches with data permutations for threshold determination. Subsequently, genomic regions yielding evidence of suggestive or significant QTL in the first scan should then be re-evaluated with more powerful procedures for parameter estimation (*72*).

6. Notes

Several lessons and general inferences may be gleaned from this broad review of methods for QTL analysis in livestock.

1. Interval mapping. Interval mapping (*52*) approaches have become routine, with modifications of the original methodologies. Because informative markers vary from

family to family, all markers in a linkage group are simultaneously used rather than only the two flanking markers of each interval as originally considered (*52*).

2. Maximum likelihood interval mapping. Maximum likelihood interval mapping is seldom used; LSR approaches (*35,46,47*) derived from the seminal contribution of Haley and Knott in 1992 (*119*) are usually preferred. ML methods do not provide advantages in statistical power (*47,110,120*), although computationally demanding and not as robust to deviations from normality and other assumptions (*46,47*).

3. The necessity for operational simplicity. The drive to develop ever more complex statistical methodology needs to be tempered by the recognition that elements of *operational simplicity* should be retained for successful and pragmatic application of any new technology (*9*). In this respect, recent comments by Terwilliger and Goring (*121*) on roles played by the more statistically oriented in this field of research are insightful.

4. Does the method fit the data? Full utilization of, and adaptation of statistical procedures to, existing data structures are preferred to fitting data to available statistical procedures. In this regard, Bayesian approaches are appealing, although most researchers have not been exposed to those methods.

   Least squares approaches will continue to be useful as data-screening tools when large kindreds are available, especially given their ability to support data permutation necessary for statistical tests (*16,24,42,47,50,62,72*). Variance component approaches (*24,62–64*) are likely to be productive and convenient for QTL analysis in the near future and will provide a platform to tackle the complex issues of genotype × environment interaction and epistasis (*122*). Strategies for data analysis encompassing different statistical procedures at different stages of the process will likely become routine in the future (*46,72,123*).

5. The success of QTL mapping in livestock. Although a few QTL with large effects are found in nearly every study that is conducted (*13–20,60,61,112*), we have yet to find compelling evidence to dispel the wisdom of Jinks that "the number of genes found is proportional to the patience and effort which the experimenter is willing to put into their detection" (*124*). Further advances in methodology for QTL detection will likely add to the growing list of chromosomal regions of livestock harboring genes contributing to genetic variation in a variety of economically relevant complex traits.

   Quantitative trait loci analysis in livestock has successfully reached a threshold of biological and genetic relevance. However, QTL analysis has yet to reach the threshold of production relevance, enabling implementation of marker-assisted selection (*125,126*) and/or management practices. In the context of gene discovery using animal models, QTL analysis will continue to play an important role in a succession of integrated genomic applications (*127*).

Acknowledgments

We are grateful to Chris Haley (Roslin Institute, Edinburgh, UK), Ina Hoeschele (Virginia Polytechnic Institute, Blacksburg, VA, USA), Chris Stricker (Swiss Federal Institute of Technology, Zurich), Robert Elston (Case

Western Reserve University, Cleveland, OH, USA), Morris Soller (The Hebrew University of Jerusalem, Israel), Andrew George (University of Washington, Seattle, WA, USA), R. Mark Thallman (USDA-MARC, Clay Center, Nebraska), Marco Bink (DLO, Wageningen, The Netherlands), and Kari Elo (University of Nebraska–Lincoln, USA), for useful discussions and critiques of various sections of this manuscript. We thank the American Angus Association, the International Brangus Breeders Association, and the National Swine Registry for granting permission to use the photos displayed in the figures.

References

1. Lander, E. S. and Weinberg, R. A. (2000) Genomics: journey to the center of biology. *Science* **287,** 1777–1782.
2. Soller, M. (1990) Genetic mapping of the bovine genome using deoxyribonucleic acid-level markers to identify loci affecting quantitative traits of economic importance. *J. Dairy Sci.* **73,** 2628–2646.
3. Soller, M. (1991) Mapping quantitative trait loci affecting traits of economic importance in animal populations using molecular markers, in *Gene-Mapping Techniques and Applications* (Schook, L. B., Lewin, H. A., and McLaren, D. G., eds.), Marcel Dekker, New York, pp. 21–49.
4. Weller, J. I. and Ron, M. (1994) Detection and mapping quantitative trait loci in segregating populations: theory and experimental results, in Proc. 5th World Congress on Genetics Applied to Livestock Production 21, pp. 213–220.
5. Bovenhuis, H., Van Arendonk, J. A., Davis, G., Elsen, J.-M., Haley, C. S., Hill, W. G., et al. (1997) Detection and mapping of quantitative trait loci in farm animals. *Livestock Prod. Sci.* **52,** 135–144.
6. Hoeschele, I., Uimari, P., Grignola, F. E., Zhang, Q., and Gage, K. M. (1997) Advances in statistical methods to map quantitative trait loci in outbred populations. *Genetics* **147,** 1445–1457.
7. Lynch, M. and Walsh, B. (1997) *Genetics and Analysis of Quantitative Traits.* Sinauer Associates, Sunderland, MA.
8. Georges, M. (1998) Mapping genes underlying production traits in livestock, in *Animal Breeding Technology for the 21st Century* (Clark, A. J., ed.), Harwood Academic, Amsterdam, pp. 77–101.
9. Taylor, J. F. and Rocha, J. L. (1998) QTL analysis under linkage equilibrium, in *Molecular Dissection of Complex Traits* (Paterson, A. H., ed.), CRC, Boca Raton, FL, pp. 103–118.
10. Haley, C. S. (1999) Advances in quantitative trait locus mapping, in *From Jay L. Lush to Genomics: Visions for Animal Breeding and Genetics* (Dekkers, J. C., Lamont, S. J., and Rothschild, M. F., eds.), Iowa State University Press, Ames, IA, pp. 47–59.
11. Lipkin, E. and Soller, M. (2000) Quantitative trait loci in domestic animals— complex inheritance traits, in *Comparative Genomics* (Clark, M. S., ed.), Kluwer Academic, Dordrecht, pp. 123–152.

12. Hoeschele, I. (2001) Mapping quantitative trait loci in outbred pedigrees, in *Handbook of Statistical Genetics* (Balding, D. J., Bishop, M., and Cannings, C., eds.), Wiley, Chichester, in press.

13. Andersson, L., Haley, C. S., Ellegren, H., Knott, S. A., Johansson, M., Andersson, K., et al. (1994) Genetic mapping of quantitative trait loci for growth and fatness in pigs. *Science* **263**, 1771–1774.

14. Georges, M., Nielsen, D., Mackinnon, M., Mishra, A., Okimoto, R., Pasquino, A. T., et al. (1995) Mapping quantitative trait loci controlling milk production in dairy cattle by exploiting progeny testing. *Genetics* **139**, 907–920.

15. Spelman, R. J., Coppieters, W., Karim, L., Van Arendonk, J. A., and Bovenhuis, H. (1996) Quantitative trait loci for five milk production traits on chromosome six in the Dutch Holstein–Friesian population. *Genetics* **144**, 1799–1808.

16. Knott, S. A., Marklund, L., Haley, C. S., Andersson, K., Davies, W., Ellegren, H., et al. (1998) Multiple marker mapping of quantitative trait loci in a cross between outbred wild boar and Large White pigs. *Genetics* **149**, 1069–1080.

17. Walling, G. A., Archibald, A. L., Cattermole, J. A., Downing, A. C., Finlayson, H. A., Nicholson, D., et al. (1998) Mapping of quantitative trait loci on porcine chromosome 4. *Anim. Genet.* **29**, 415–424.

18. Zhang, Q., Boichard, D., Hoeschele, I., Ernst, C., Eggen, A., Murkve, B., et al. (1998) Mapping quantitative trait loci for milk production and health of dairy cattle in a large outbred pedigree. *Genetics* **149**, 1959–1973.

19. De Koning, D. J., Janss, L. L., Rattink, A. P., Van Oers, P. A., De Vries, B. J., Groenen, M. A., et al. (1999) Detection of quantitative trait loci for backfat thickness and intramuscular fat content in pigs *(Sus scrofa)*. *Genetics* **152**, 1679–1690.

20. Riquet, J., Coppieters, W., Cambisano, N., Arranz, J.-J., Berzi, P., Davis, S. K., et al. (1999) Fine-mapping of quantitative trait loci by identity by descent in outbred populations: application to milk production in dairy cattle. *Proc. Natl. Acad. Sci. USA* **96**, 9252–9257.

21. Penrose, L. S. (1938) Genetic linkage in graded human characters. *Ann. Eugen.* **8**, 233–237.

22. Henderson, C. R. (1984) *Applications of Linear Models in Animal Breeding*. University of Guelph Press, Guelph, Ontario, Canada.

23. Bink, M. C. (1998) Complex pedigree analysis to detect quantitative trait loci in dairy cattle. Ph.D. dissertation, Wageningen Agricultural University, Wageningen, The Netherlands.

24. George, A. W., Visscher, P. M., and Haley, C. S. (2000) Mapping quantitative trait loci in complex pedigrees: a two step variance component approach. *Genetics* in press.

25. Knott, S. A. and Haley, C. S. (1992) Maximum likelihood mapping of quantitative trait loci using full-sib families. *Genetics* **132**, 1211–1222.

26. Soller, M., Genizi, A., and Brody, T. (1976) On the power of experimental designs for the detection of linkage between marker loci and quantitative loci in crosses between inbred lines. *Theor. Appl. Genet.* **47**, 35–39.

27. Soller, M. and Genizi, A. (1978) The efficiency of experimental designs for the detection of linkage between a marker locus and a locus affecting a quantitative trait in segregating populations. *Biometrics* **34,** 47–55.

28. Xu, S. (1996) Computation of the full likelihood function for estimating variance at a quantitative trait locus. *Genetics* **144,** 1951–1960.

29. Jansen, R. C., Johnson, D. L., and Van Arendonk, J. A. (1998) A mixture model approach to the mapping of quantitative trait loci in complex populations with an application to multiple cattle families. *Genetics* **148,** 391–399.

30. Chakraborty, R. and Weiss, K. M. (1988) Admixture as a tool for finding linked genes and detecting that difference from allelic association between loci. *Proc. Natl. Acad. Sci. USA* **85,** 9119–9123.

31. Stephens, J. C., Briscoe, D., and O'Brien, S. J. (1994) Mapping by admixture linkage disequilibrium in human populations: limits and guidelines. *Am. J. Hum. Genet.* **55,** 809–824.

32. McKeigue, P. M. (1997) Mapping genes underlying ethnic differences in disease risk by linkage disequilibrium in recently admixed populations. *Am. J. Hum. Genet.* **60,** 188–196.

33. Baret, P. V. and Hill, W. G. (1997) Gametic disequilibrium mapping: potential application in livestock. *Anim. Breed. Abst.* **65,** 309–318.

34. Beckmann, J. S. and Soller, M. (1988) Detection of linkage between marker loci and loci affecting quantitative traits in crosses between segregating populations. *Theor. Appl. Genet.* **76,** 228–236.

35. Haley, C. S., Knott, S. A., and Elsen, J.-M. (1994) Mapping quantitative trait loci in crosses between outbred lines using least squares. *Genetics* **136,** 1195–1207.

36. Falconer, D. S. and Mackay, T. F. (1996) *Introduction to Quantitative Genetics.* Longman, Essex, UK.

37. Jansen, R. C. (1993) Interval mapping of multiple quantitative trait loci. *Genetics* **135,** 205–211.

38. Zeng, Z.-B. (1993) Theoretical basis of separation of multiple linked gene effects on mapping quantitative trait loci. *Proc. Natl. Acad. Sci. USA* **90,** 10,972–10,976.

39. Zeng, Z.-B. (1944) Precision mapping of quantitative trait loci. *Genetics* **136,** 1457–1468.

40. Carlborg, O., Andersson, L., and Kinghorn, B. P. (2000) The use of a genetic algorithm for simultaneous mapping of multiple interacting quantitative trait loci. *Genetics* **155,** 2003–2010.

41. Lander, E. S. and Kruglyak, L. (1995) Genetic dissection of complex traits: guidelines for interpreting and reporting linkage results. *Nature Genet.* **11,** 241–247.

42. Churchill, G. A. and Doerge, R. W. (1994) Empirical threshold values for quantitative trait mapping. *Genetics* **138,** 963–971.

43. Visscher, P. M., Thompson, R., and Haley, C. S. (1996) Confidence intervals in QTL mapping by bootstrapping. *Genetics* **143,** 1013–1020.

44. Lebreton, C. M. and Visscher, P. M. (1998) Empirical nonparametric bootstrap

strategies in quantitative trait loci mapping: conditioning on the genetic model. *Genetics* **148**, 525–535.

45. Perez-Enciso, M. and Varona, L. (2000) Quantitative trait loci mapping in F_2 crosses between outbred lines. *Genetics* **155**, 391–405.

46. Knott, S. A., Elsen, J.-M., and Haley, C. S. (1994) Multiple marker mapping of quantitative trait loci in half-sib populations, in Proc. 5th World Congress on Genetics Applied to Livestock Production 21, pp. 33–36.

47. Knott, S. A., Elsen, J.-M., and Haley, C. S. (1996) Methods for multiple-marker mapping of quantitative trait loci in half-sib populations. *Theor. Appl. Genet.* **93**, 71–80.

48. Du, F.-X. and Woodward, B. W. (1997) A two-stage half-sib design for mapping quantitative trait loci in food animals. *J. Dairy Sci.* **80**, 2580–2591.

49. Elsen, J.-M., Mangin, B., Goffinet, B., Boichard, D., and Le Roy, P. (1999) Alternative models for QTL detection in livestock. I. General introduction. *Genet. Sel. Evol.* **31**, 213–224.

50. Mangin, B., Goffinet, B., Le Roy, P., Boichard, D., and Elsen J.-M. (1999) Alternative models for QTL detection in livestock. II. Likelihood approximations and sire marker genotype estimations. *Genet. Sel. Evol.* **31**, 225–237.

51. Goffinet, B., Le Roy, P., Boichard, D., Elsen, J.-M., and Mangin, B. (1999) Alternative models for QTL detection in livestock. III. Heteroskedastic model and models corresponding to several distributions of the QTL effect. *Genet. Sel. Evol.* **31**, 341–350.

52. Lander, E. S. and Botstein, D. (1989) Mapping Mendelian factors underlying quantitative traits using RFLP linkage maps. *Genetics* **121**, 185–199.

53. Van Kaam, J. B., Van Arendonk, J. A., Groenen, M. A., Bovenhuis, H., Vereijken, A. L., Crooijmans, R. P., et al. (1998) Whole genome scan for quantitative trait loci affecting body weight in chickens using a three generation design. *Livestock Prod. Sci.* **54**, 133–150.

54. Van der Beek, S., Van Arendonk, J. A., and Groen, A. F. (1995) Power of two- and three-generation QTL mapping experiments in an outbred population containing full-sib or half-sib families. *Theor. Appl. Genet.* **91**, 1115–1124.

55. George, A. W. (1998) A Bayesian analysis for the mapping of a quantitative trait locus given half-sib data. Ph.D. dissertation. Centre in Statistical Science and Industrial Mathematics and the School of Mathematical Sciences, Queensland University of Technology, Brisbane, Australia.

56. Le Roy, P., Elsen, J.-M., Boichard, D., Mangin, B., Bidanel, J. P., and Goffinet, B. (1998) An algorithm for QTL detection in mixture of full and half sib families, in Proc. 6th World Congress on Genetics Applied to Livestock Production 26, pp. 257–260.

57. Weller, J. I., Kashi, Y., and Soller, M. (1990) Power of daughter and granddaughter designs for determining linkage between marker loci and quantitative trait loci in dairy cattle. *J. Dairy Sci.* **73**, 2525–2537.

58. Cowen, N. M. (1988) The use of replicated progenies in marker-based mapping of QTL's. *Theor. Appl. Genet.* **75**, 857–862.

59. Soller, M. and Beckmann, J. S. (1990) Marker-based mapping of quantitative trait loci using replicated progenies. *Theor. Appl. Genet.* **80,** 205–208.

60. Rocha, J. L., Sanders, J. O., Cherbonnier, D. M., Lawlor, T. J., and Taylor, J. F. (1998) Blood groups and milk and type traits in dairy cattle: after forty years of research. *J. Dairy Sci.* **81,** 1663–1680.

61. Coppieters, W., Riquet, J., Arranz, J.-J., Berzi, P., Cambisano, N., Grisart, B., et al. (1998) A QTL with major effect on milk yield and composition maps to bovine chromosome 14. *Mamm. Genome* **9,** 540–544.

62. Grignola, F. E., Hoeschele, I., and Tier, B. (1996) Mapping quantitative trait loci in outcross populations via residual maximum likelihood. I. Methodology. *Genet. Sel. Evol.* **28,** 479–490.

63. Grignola, F. E., Hoeschele, I., Zhang, Q., and Thaller, G. (1996) Mapping quantitative trait loci in outcross populations via residual maximum likelihood. II. A simulation study. *Genet. Sel. Evol.* **28,** 491–504.

64. Grignola, F. E., Zhang, Q., and Hoeschele, I. (1997) Mapping linked quantitative trait loci via residual maximum likelihood. *Genet. Sel. Evol.* **29,** 529–544.

65. Searle, S. R., Casella, G., and McCulloch, C. E. (1992) *Variance Components.* Wiley, New York.

66. Elston, R. C. and Stewart, J. (1971) A general model for the genetic analysis of pedigree data. *Hum. Heredity* **21,** 523–542.

67. Almasy, L. and Blangero, J. (1998) Multipoint quantitative-trait linkage analysis in general pedigrees. *Am. J. Hum. Genet.* **62,** 1198–1211.

68. Fernando, R. L. and Grossman, M. (1989) Marker-assisted selection using best linear unbiased prediction. *Genet. Sel. Evol.* **21,** 467–477.

69. Cantet, R. J. and Smith, C. (1991) Reduced animal model for marker-assisted selection using best linear unbiased prediction. *Genet. Sel. Evol.* **23,** 221–233.

70. Wang, T., Fernando, R. L., Van der Beek, S., and Grossman, M. (1995) Covariance between relatives for a marked quantitative trait locus. *Genet. Sel. Evol.* **27,** 251–274.

71. Van Arendonk, J. A., Tier, B., Bink, M. C., and Bovenhuis, H. (1998) Restricted maximum likelihood analysis of linkage between genetic markers and quantitative trait loci for a granddaughter design. *J. Dairy Sci.* **81,** 76–84.

72. Uimari, P., Zhang, Q., Grignola, F. E., Hoeschele, I., and Thaller, G. (1996) Analysis of QTL Workshop I granddaughter design data using least-squares, residual maximum likelihood and Bayesian methods. *J. Quant. Trait Loci* 2, article 7 (http://probe.nalusda.gov:8000/otherdocs/jqtl/jqtl1996-07/).

73. Allison, D. B., Neale, M. C., Zannolli, R., Schork, N. J., Amos, C. I., and Blangero, J. (1999) Testing the robustness of the likelihood-ratio test in a variance-component quantitative-trait-loci-mapping procedure. *Am. J. Hum. Genet.* **65,** 531–544.

74. Thompson, E. A. and Heath, S. C. (1999) Estimation of conditional multilocus gene identity among relatives, in *Statistics in Molecular Biology* (Seillier-Moseiwitch, F., Donnelly, P., and Waterman, M., eds.), Springer-Verlag, New York, pp. 95–113.

75. Amos, C. I. (1994) Robust variance-components approach for assessing genetic linkage in pedigrees. *Am. J. Hum. Genet.* **54,** 535–543.

76. Morton, N. E. and MacLean, C. J. (1974) Analysis of family resemblance. III. Complex segregation analysis of quantitative traits. *Am. J. Hum. Genet.* **26,** 489–503.

77. Ott, J. (1979) Maximum likelihood estimation by counting methods under polygenic and mixed models in human pedigrees. *Am. J. Hum. Genet.* **31,** 161–175.

78. Boerwinkle, E., Chakraborty, R., and Sing, C. F. (1986) The use of measured genotype information in the analysis of quantitative phenotype in man. I. Models and analytical methods. *Am. Hum. Genet.* **50,** 181–194.

79. George, V. T. and Elston, R. C. (1987) Testing the association between polymorphic genetic markers and quantitative traits in pedigrees. *Genet. Epidemiol.* **4,** 193–201.

80. Bonney, G. E., Lathrop, G. M., and Lalouel, J.-M. (1988) Combined linkage and segregation analysis using regressive models. *Am. J. Hum. Genet.* **43,** 29–37.

81. Guo, S. W. and Thompson, E. A. (1992) A Monte Carlo method for combined segregation and linkage analysis. *Am. J. Hum. Genet.* **51,** 1111–1126.

82. Hasstedt, S. J. (1993) Variance components/major locus likelihood approximation for quantitative, polychotomous, and multivariate data. *Genet. Epidemiol.* **10,** 145–158.

83. Fernando, R. L., Stricker, C., and Elston, R. C. (1994) The finite polygenic mixed model: an alternative formulation for the mixed model of inheritance. *Theor. Appl. Genet.* **88,** 573–580.

84. Xu, S. and Atchley, W. R. (1995) A random model approach to interval mapping of quantitative trait loci. *Genetics* **141,** 1189–1197.

85. Xie, C., Gessler, D. D., and Xu, S. (1998) Combining different line crosses for mapping quantitative trait loci using the identical by descent-based variance component method. *Genetics* **149,** 1139–1146.

86. Xu, S. and Gessler, D. D. (1998) Multipoint genetic mapping of quantitative trait loci using a variable number of sibs per family. *Genet. Res., Camb.* **71,** 73–83.

87. Kinghorn, B. P., Kennedy, B. W., and Smith, C. (1993) A method of screening for genes of major effect. *Genetics* **134,** 351–360.

88. Meuwissen, T. H. and Goddard, M. E. (1997) Estimation of effects of quantitative trait loci in large complex pedigrees. *Genetics* **146,** 409–416.

89. Shoemaker, J. S., Painter, I. S., and Weir, B. S. (1999) Bayesian statistics in genetics: a guide for the uninitiated. *Trends Genet.* **15,** 354–358.

90. Sillanpaa, M. J. (1999) Bayesian QTL mapping in inbred and outbred experimental designs. Ph.D. dissertation. Rolf Nevanlinna Institute Research Reports A30, University of Helsinki, Finland.

91. Uimari, P. and Hoeschele, I. (1997) Mapping-linked quantitative trait loci using Bayesian analysis and Markov chain Monte Carlo algorithms. *Genetics* **146,** 735–743.

92. Stephens, D. A. and Fisch, R. D. (1998) Bayesian analysis of quantitative trait

locus data using *reversible jump* Markov chain Monte Carlo. *Biometrics* **54,** 1334–1347.

93. Green, P. J. (1995) *Reversible jump* Markov chain Monte Carlo computation and Bayesian model determination. *Biometrika* **82,** 711–732.

94. Hoeschele, I. and VanRaden, P. M. (1993) Bayesian analysis of linkage between genetic markers and quantitative trait loci. I. Prior knowledge. *Theor. Appl. Genet.* **85,** 953–960.

95. Hoeschele, I. and VanRaden, P. M. (1993) Bayesian analysis of linkage between genetic markers and quantitative trait loci. II. Combining prior knowledge with experimental evidence. *Theor. Appl. Genet.* **85,** 946–952.

96. Thaller, G. and Hoeschele, I. (1996) A Monte Carlo method for Bayesian analysis of linkage between single markers and quantitative trait loci. I. Methodology. *Theor. Appl. Genet.* **93,** 1161–1166.

97. Thaller, G. and Hoeschele, I. (1996) A Monte Carlo method for Bayesian analysis of linkage between single markers and quantitative trait loci. II. A simulation study. *Theor. Appl. Genet.* **93,** 1167–1174.

98. Uimari, P., Thaller, G., and Hoeschele, I. (1996) The use of multiple markers in a Bayesian method for mapping quantitative trait loci. *Genetics* **143,** 1831–1842.

99. Bink, M. C., Van Arendonk, J. A., and Quaas, R. L. (1998) Breeding value estimation with incomplete marker data. *Genet. Sel. Evol.* **30,** 45–58.

100. Bink, M. C., Quaas, R. L., and Van Arendonk, J. A. (1998) Bayesian estimation of dispersion parameters with a reduced animal model including polygenic and QTL effects. *Genet. Sel. Evol.* **30,** 103–125.

101. Bink, M. C., Janss, L. L., and Quaas, R. L. (2000) Markov chain Monte Carlo for mapping a quantitative trait locus in outbred populations. *Genet. Res. Camb.* **75,** 231–241.

102. Bink, M. C. and Van Arendonk, J. A. (1999) Detection of quantitative trait loci in outbred populations with incomplete marker data. *Genetics* **151,** 409–420.

103. George, A. W., Mengersen, K. L., and Davis, G. P. (2000) Localization of a quantitative trait locus via a Bayesian approach. *Biometrics* **56,** 40–51.

104. Janss, L. L., Thompson, R., and Van Arendonk, J. A. (1995) Application of Gibbs sampling for inference in a mixed major gene-polygenic inheritance model in animal populations. *Theor. Appl. Genet.* **91,** 1137–1147.

105. De Koning, D. J., Janss, L. L., Van Arendonk, J. A., Van Oers, P. A., and Groenen, M. A. (1998) Mapping major genes affecting meat quality in Meishan crossbreds using standard linkage software, in Proc. 6th World Congress on Genetics Applied to Livestock Production 26, pp. 410–413.

106. Luo, Z. W. (1993) The power of two experimental designs for detecting linkage between a marker locus and a locus affecting a quantitative character in a segregating population. *Genet. Sel. Evol.* **25,** 249–261.

107. Le Roy, P. and Elsen, J.-M. (1995) Numerical comparison between powers of maximum likelihood and analysis of variance methods for QTL detection in progeny test designs: the case of monogenic inheritance. *Theor. Appl. Genet.* **90,** 65–72.

108. Muranty, H. (1996) Power of tests for quantitative trait loci detection using full-sib families in different schemes. *Heredity* **76**, 156–165.

109. Alfonso, L. and Haley, C. S. (1998) Power of different F_2 schemes for QTL detection in livestock. *Anim. Sci.* **66**, 1–8.

110. Baret, P. V., Knott, S. A., and Visscher, P. M. (1998) On the use of linear regression and maximum likelihood for QTL mapping in half-sib designs. *Genet. Res. Camb.* **72**, 149–158.

111. Song, J. Z., Soller, M., and Genizi, A. (1999) The full-sib intercross line (FSIL): a QTL mapping design for outcrossing species. *Genet. Res. Camb.* **73**, 61–73.

112. Kim, J.-J. (1999) Detection of Quantitative Trait Loci for Growth and Beef Carcass Quality Traits in a Cross of *Bos taurus* × *Bos indicus* Cattle. Ph.D. dissertation, Department of Animal Science, Texas A&M University, College Station, TX.

113. Visscher, P. M. and Haley, C. S. (1996) Detection of putative quantitative trait loci in line crosses under infinitesimal genetic models. *Theor. Appl. Genet.* **93**, 691–702.

114. Liu, Z. and Dekkers, J. C. (1998) Least squares interval mapping of quantitative trait loci under the infinitesimal genetic model in outbred populations. *Genetics* **148**, 495–505.

115. Coppieters, W., Kvasz, A., Farnir, F., Arranz, J.-J., Grisart, B., Mackinnon, M., et al. (1998) A rank-based nonparametric method for mapping quantitative trait loci in outbred half-sib pedigrees: application to milk production in a granddaughter design. *Genetics* **149**, 1547–1555.

116. Maliepaard, C. and Van Ooijen, J. W. (1994) QTL mapping in a full-sib family of an outcrossing species, in *Biometrics in Plant Breeding: Applications of Molecular Markers* (Van Ooijen, J. W. and Jansen, J., eds.), DLO-Centre for Plant Breeding and Reproduction Research, Wageningen, The Netherlands, pp. 140–146.

117. Zhang, Q. and Hoeschele, I. (1998) A very brief description for using the computer program MQREMLH for multiple QTL mapping via residual maximum likelihood. *Mimeo*, Department of Dairy Science, Virginia Polytechnic Institute and State University, Blacksburg, VA.

118. Stricker, C., Fernando, R. L., and Elston, R. C. (1994) *SALP—Segregation and Linkage Analysis for Pedigrees, Release 2.0.* Swiss Federal Institute of Technology ETH, Zurich.

119. Haley, C. S. and Knott, S. A. (1992) A simple regression method for mapping quantitative trait loci in line crosses using flanking markers. *Heredity* **69**, 315–324.

120. Xu, S. (1998) Further investigation on the regression method of mapping quantitative trait loci. *Heredity* **80**, 364–373.

121. Terwilliger, J. D. and Goring, H. H. (2000) Gene mapping in the 20th and 21st centuries: statistical methods, data analysis, and experimental design. *Hum. Biol.* **72**, 63–132.

122. Rocha, J. L., Taylor, J. F., Sanders, J. O., Openshaw, S. J., and Fincher, R. (1995) Genetic markers to manipulate QTL: the additive illusion, in Proc. 44th Ann. Natl. Breeders Roundtable, pp. 12–38.

123. De Koning, D. J., Visscher, P. M., Knott, S. A., and Haley, C. S. (1998) A strategy for QTL detection in half-sib populations. *Anim. Sci.* **67,** 257–268.

124. Jinks, J. L. (1977) Discussion of Dr. Eaves' paper. *J. R. Statis. Soc. Ser. A.* **140,** 352–353.

125. Haley, C. S. and Visscher, P. M. (1998) Strategies to utilize marker-quantitative trait loci associations. *J. Dairy Sci.* **81,** 85–97.

126. Soller, M. and Medjugorac, I. (1999) A *successful marriage*: making the transition from quantitative trait locus mapping to marker-assisted selection, in *From Jay L. Lush to Genomics: Visions for Animal Breeding and Genetics* (Dekkers, J. C., Lamont, S. J., and Rothschild, M. F., eds.), Iowa State University Press, Ames, IA, pp. 85–96.

127. Gelbert, L. M. and Gregg, R. E. (1997) Will genetics really revolutionize the drug discovery process? *Curr. Opin. Biotech.* **8,** 669–674.

Index

A

A/J mice, 253, 255, 256
acceptance (*see also* Markov chain
 Monte Carlo; Gibbs sampler)
 probability (Metropolis–Hastings
  algorithm), 297–299
 /rejection step (Metropolis–
  Hastings algorithm), 143–144
accuracy, 46, 66, 203–213, 229, 311
Access, 230
ACT, 69, 75, 82–98
additive
 component, 114, 131–132, 276, 315
 effect(s), 6, 65–70, 90, 123–124,
  136, 184, 209–211,
  263–269, 284–290 (*see also*
  allelic effects)
 genetic (variance), 41–45, 62–69,
  111–112, 132–136, 145,
  319, 324 (*see also* variance
  components)
admixture, 17, 106, 314
advanced intercross, 206, 212, 216, 243
allele/allelic,
 dosage, 240
 effects, 110, 293–294, 300–306,
  314–316, 324–325 (*see also*
  additive effects)
 frequencies, 6, 15–18, 23–26, 33,
  43, 62, 71–75, 101, 119,
  142–148, 154–156, 317,
  327–328

inheritance configuration, 295
interactions, 290 (*see also*
 interactions; non-allelic
 interactions)
sharing, 42, 55, 70, 93-7
alternative hypothesis, 69, 74, 80–89,
 96, 107, 114, 124, 132–134, 172
analysis of variance (ANOVA), 3–10,
 61, 109, 113, 166–169, 175–179
ascertainment, 66–68, 70–75, 82–87, 98
 double ascertainment, 82
association, 3–13, 96, 101–114,
 122–125, 131–136, 166–167,
 170, 175, 191, 196, 200, 243, 332

B

backcross, 166, 169, 170, 172, 175–179,
 187, 191, 201–205, 208–211, 215,
 226, 228, 230, 237–241, 244, 257,
 284–286
background strain, 204
BALB/c, 255–265
Bayes
 factors, 148
 rule, 328
Bayesian MCMC, 14, 40, 75, 140–147,
 167–171, 284–285, 292–295,
 300–308, 325–336
Bayesian reversible jump MCMC, 140
Bernoulli (distribution), 285, 291, 294
biased (estimates), 90, 103, 126
biometrical model, 61–64